RECENT ADVANCES IN OPHTHALMOLOGY-15

Editors

HV Nema MS
Former Professor and Head
Department of Ophthalmology
Institute of Medical Sciences
Banaras Hindu University
Varanasi, Uttar Pradesh, India

Nitin Nema MS DNB
Professor
Department of Ophthalmology
Sri Aurobindo Medical College and
Postgraduate Institute of Medical Sciences
Indore, Madhya Pradesh, India

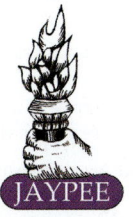

JAYPEE BROTHERS MEDICAL PUBLISHERS
The Health Sciences Publisher
New Delhi | London

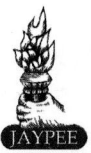
Jaypee Brothers Medical Publishers (P) Ltd

Headquarters

Jaypee Brothers Medical Publishers (P) Ltd
EMCA House, 23/23-B
Ansari Road, Daryaganj
New Delhi 110 002, India
Landline: +91-11-23272143, +91-11-23272703
+91-11-23282021, +91-11-23245672
Email: jaypee@jaypeebrothers.com

Corporate Office

Jaypee Brothers Medical Publishers (P) Ltd
4838/24, Ansari Road, Daryaganj
New Delhi 110 002, India
Phone: +91-11-43574357
Fax: +91-11-43574314
Email: jaypee@jaypeebrothers.com

Overseas Office

JP Medical Ltd
83 Victoria Street, London
SW1H 0HW (UK)
Phone: +44 20 3170 8910
Fax: +44 (0)20 3008 6180
Email: info@jpmedpub.com

Website: www.jaypeebrothers.com
Website: www.jaypeedigital.com

© 2022, Jaypee Brothers Medical Publishers

The views and opinions expressed in this book are solely those of the original contributor(s)/author(s) and do not necessarily represent those of editor(s) of the book.

All rights reserved. No part of this publication may be reproduced, stored or transmitted in any form or by any means, electronic, mechanical, photocopying, recording or otherwise, without the prior permission in writing of the publishers.

All brand names and product names used in this book are trade names, service marks, trademarks or registered trademarks of their respective owners. The publisher is not associated with any product or vendor mentioned in this book.

Medical knowledge and practice change constantly. This book is designed to provide accurate, authoritative information about the subject matter in question. However, readers are advised to check the most current information available on procedures included and check information from the manufacturer of each product to be administered, to verify the recommended dose, formula, method and duration of administration, adverse effects and contraindications. It is the responsibility of the practitioner to take all appropriate safety precautions. Neither the publisher nor the author(s)/editor(s) assume any liability for any injury and/or damage to persons or property arising from or related to use of material in this book.

This book is sold on the understanding that the publisher is not engaged in providing professional medical services. If such advice or services are required, the services of a competent medical professional should be sought.

Every effort has been made where necessary to contact holders of copyright to obtain permission to reproduce copyright material. If any have been inadvertently overlooked, the publisher will be pleased to make the necessary arrangements at the first opportunity. The **CD/DVD-ROM** (if any) provided in the sealed envelope with this book is complimentary and free of cost. **Not meant for sale**.

Inquiries for bulk sales may be solicited at: jaypee@jaypeebrothers.com

Recent Advances in Ophthalmology-15

First Edition: **2022**

ISBN: 978-93-90595-85-3

Printed at: Samrat Offset Pvt. Ltd.

Dedicated to
Our Students

Contributors

Akanksha Rai DNB
Medical Retina Fellow
Giridhar Eye Institute
Kochi, Kerala, India

Anand Rajendran FRCS DNB
Professor and Head
Retina-Vitreous Services
Aravind Eye Hospital
Chennai, Tamil Nadu, India

Asmita Mahajan MD
Senior Resident
Dr Rajendra Prasad Centre for
Ophthalmic Sciences
All India Institute of Medical Sciences
New Delhi, India

Bhanu Pangtey MS
Consultant
Retina-Vitreous Services
Aravind Eye Hospital
Madurai, Tamil Nadu, India

Chris HL Lim BSc (Med) (Hon) BMed MD MMed (Ophth)
Senior Resident
Department of Ophthalmology
National University Hospital, Singapore
Research Fellow
Singapore Eye Research Institute
Singapore

David Benet BSc MBA
Independent Researcher
Spain

Gangadhara Sundar DO FRCS (Edin) FAMS
Diplomate—The American Board of Ophthalmology
Head (Orbit and Oculofacial Surgery)
Assistant Professor
Department of Ophthalmology
National University Hospital
National University of Singapore
Singapore

Giridhar Anantharaman MS
Director and Senior Vitreoretinal Surgeon
Giridhar Eye Institute
Kochi, Kerala, India

GVN Rama Kumar MBBS MD DNB FRCS
Former Vitreoretina Fellow
Sankara Nethralaya
Consultant
Retina Surgeon and Uvea Specialist
Sankara Eye Centre
Indore, Madhya Pradesh, India

Henry Henderson MBBS DNB
MN Eye Hospitals
Chennai, Tamil Nadu, India

HV Nema MS
Former Professor and Head
Department of Ophthalmology
Institute of Medical Sciences
Banaras Hindu University
Varanasi, Uttar Pradesh, India

Ivan Seah MMed
Resident in Ophthalmology
Department of Ophthalmology
National University Hospital, Singapore
Department of Ophthalmology
Yong Loo Lin School of Medicine
National University of Singapore

Jasmine Ge MBBS
Medical Officer
Changi General Hospital, Singapore

Jorge L Alio MD PhD
Director, Professor and Chairman
Department of Ophthalmology
Universidad Miguel Hernandez, Spain

Kiran Chandran MS
Medical Retina Fellow
Giridhar Eye Institute
Kochi, Kerala, India

Lingam Gopal MS FRCS DNB MSc
Senior Consultant and Associate Professor
Department of Ophthalmology
National University Hospital, Singapore
Department of Ophthalmology
Yong Loo Lin School of Medicine
National University of Singapore
Singapore Eye Research Institute (SERI)
Singapore

Marcus Tan CJ MMed (Ophth) FRCOphth MTech (EBAC)
Associate Consultant
Division of Glaucoma and
Clinical Lecturer
Department of Ophthalmology
National University Hospital
National University of Singapore
Singapore

Mayuri Bhargava MS
Senior Resident Physician
Department of Ophthalmology
National University Hospital
Singapore

Mohana Sinnasamy MBBS DO
Consultant
Swamy Eye Clinic
Chennai, Tamil Nadu, India

Murali Ariga MS DNB FAICO (Glaucoma)
Head
Department of Ophthalmology
Sundaram Medical Foundation
Chennai, Tamil Nadu, India

Nitin Nema MS DNB
Professor
Department of Ophthalmology
Sri Aurobindo Medical College and
Postgraduate Institute of Medical Sciences
Indore, Madhya Pradesh, India

Oscar J Pellicer-Valero BSc
Intelligent Data Analysis Laboratory
Department of Electronic Engineering
ETSE (Engineering School)
Universitat de València (UV)
Valencia, Spain

Panchmi Gupta MBBS MS DNB
General Duty Medical Officer
Rajan Babu Institute of Pulmonary
Medicine and Tuberculosis
New Delhi, India

Pradeep Sharma MD FAMS
Director
Strabismus, Pediatric Ophthalmology
and Neuro-ophthalmology
Centre for Sight
New Delhi, India

Pratheeba Devi Nivean DO DNB
Director
MN Eye Hospitals
Chennai, Tamil Nadu, India

Rajiv Raman MS DNB FRCS (Ed) Hon DSc
Senior Consultant
Vitreoretinal Services
Sankara Nethralaya
Chennai, Tamil Nadu, India

Ramachandran Rajalakshmi MBBS DO MRCS (Ed) FRCS (Gl) PhD
Head (Medical Retina)
Dr Mohan's Diabetes Specialities Centre
and Madras Diabetes Research Foundation
Chennai, Tamil Nadu, India

Ramamurthy Dandapani MD MNAMS
Chairman
The Eye Foundation Group of Hospitals
Coimbatore, Tamil Nadu, India

Ray Manotosh MBBS MD (AIIMS) FRCS (Ed)
Senior Consultant
Department of Ophthalmology
National University Health System
Singapore
Associate Professor and UG Education
Director (Ophthalmology)
Yong Loo Lin School of Medicine
National University of Singapore
Singapore

Ritesh Chainani DNB
Consultant
Retina-Vitreous Services
Aravind Eye Hospital
Chennai, Tamil Nadu, India

Saba Ishrat MBBS FICO FRCS (Glasgow)
Staff Registrar
Singapore National Eye Centre (SNEC)
Singapore
Fellowship in Medical Retina and Uveitis
Moorfields Eye Hospital
London, UK

Shreesha Kumar Kodavoor
MS DNB MNAMS
Medical Superintendent
Senior Consultant
Cataract, Cornea, and Refractive Surgery
The Eye Foundation
Coimbatore, Tamil Nadu, India

Soosan Jacob MS FRCS DNB
Cornea and Lens
Dr Agarwal's Group of Eye Hospitals
Refractive and Cornea Foundation
Chennai, Tamil Nadu, India

Su Xinyi BA MBBChir (Cantab) PhD MMed
Consultant and Assistant Professor
Department of Ophthalmology
National University Hospital, Singapore
Department of Ophthalmology
Yong Loo Lin School of Medicine
National University of Singapore
Singapore Eye Research Institute (SERI)
Singapore
Institute of Molecular and Cell Biology
(IMCB), Agency for Science, Technology
and Research (A*STAR), Singapore

Sudipta Das MS
Senior Consultant
Netralayam Superspeciality Eye Hospital
and BB Eye Foundation
Kolkata, West Bengal, India

Swathi Lingam PhD
Research Fellow
Department of Ophthalmology
Yong Loo Lin School of Medicine
National University of Singapore
Institute of Molecular and Cell
Biology (IMCB), Agency for Science,
Technology and Research (A*STAR)
Singapore

Tamilarasi S MS DNB
Senior Consultant
Cataract Services
The Eye Foundation
Coimbatore, Tamil Nadu, India

Venkata Prabhakar G DNB FICO
Dr Agarwal's Group of Eye Hospitals
Chennai, Tamil Nadu, India

Vishal MY MS
Consultant
Retina-Vitreous Services
Aravind Eye Hospital
Madurai, Tamil Nadu, India

Zeng Ping liu MD
Senior Research Fellow
Department of Ophthalmology
Yong Loo Lin School of Medicine
National University of Singapore
Singapore Eye Research Institute (SERI)
Singapore
Institute of Molecular and Cell
Biology (IMCB), Agency for Science,
Technology and Research (A*STAR)
Singapore

Preface

COVID-19 originated from Wuhan, China as severe respiratory infection and became a pandemic affecting multitude of people and resulting in numerous deaths worldwide. The term COVID-19 is derived from Corona Virus Disease that was first reported in December 2019. The new strain of Corona virus (CoV-2) manifested as severe acute respiratory distress syndrome (SARS) and caused untold misery to humanity. Lingam Gopal and his colleagues have given an overview of ocular manifestations of COVID-19 infection.

In 1955, John McCarthy introduced the term artificial intelligence (AI) to describe the science of creating machines, which simulate human behavior. It is considered a branch of computer science that can perform risky or difficult task efficiently. Machine learning (ML) and deep learning (DL) recognize images in medical sciences especially in ophthalmology. Several publications have confirmed the role of AI in the diagnosis of age-related macular degeneration, diabetic retinopathy, glaucoma and retinopathy of prematurity. To train the AI system, a large number of database of retinal photographs or clinical feature data are needed. Besides problem solving, AI can help in learning, decision-making and saving time and, therefore, eases the workload. It will not be wrong to say that AI replicates human intelligence. Disadvantages of AI include high cost, addiction and unemployment.

In road of robotics in ophthalmology has shown dramatic improvement in ophthalmic surgery. Robots are performing highly complicated ophthalmic surgery with great precision. Many published reports indicate that the robotic surgery provides better results and curtails hospital stay in comparison to routine surgery. Other advantages of robotic surgery include good hand-to-eye coordination, increased dexterity, 3D view, elimination of physiological tremors, reduction in contamination, etc. Despite advantages, many hospitals have not purchased robots due to their large size necessitating a large OT and prohibitive cost.

Cell therapy is most interesting modality of treatment of degenerative diseases of the eye. Degenerated or damaged cells of retina are repaired or replaced by transplantation of stem cells. The transplanted cells have a potential to transform into new healthy cells. Some transplanted cells release growth factors, both paracrine and endocrine, to promote self-healing. The stem cell therapy is a highly effective procedure with a success rate of approximately 80%. Pluripotent cells have a capability to transform into any cell type. Gene therapy is also a type of cell therapy wherein genetic material is transported with the help of a carrier to the diseased cell.

Diabetic retinopathy and age-related macular degeneration are well-known causes of blindness in old age. Recent trends in the treatment of these diseases have been described with citation of clinical trials. In addition, optical coherence tomography angiography in posterior uveitis, serpiginous choroiditis and pachychoroid disease spectrum are included in this volume.

We hope this volume of *Recent Advances in Ophthalmology-15* will benefit postgraduate students and fellows in ophthalmology as well as practicing ophthalmologists and keep them abreast with the latest developments in ophthalmology.

HV Nema
Nitin Nema

Acknowledgments

We would like to record our grateful thanks to all authors for writing their valuable articles for *Recent Advances in Ophthalmology-15*. We are especially indebted to Dr Lingam Gopal and Dr Pradeep Sharma for submitting their articles on short notice.

Shri Jitendar P Vij (Group Chairman), Mr Ankit Vij (Managing Director) and Ms Chetna Malhotra Vohra (Associate Director—Content Strategy) of M/s Jaypee Brothers Medical Publishers (P) Ltd, New Delhi, India, deserve our sincere appreciation for their keen interest in the publication of *Recent Advances Series in Ophthalmology*.

Contents

1. **COVID-19 and the Eye** *(Critical Appraisal of Cause and Effect Relationship)* 1
   Lingam Gopal, Su Xinyi, Ivan Seah
   - The Eye as a Portal of Entry for the Virus *2*
   - Clinical Recommendations *3*
   - Ocular Manifestations in Patients with COVID-19 Systemic Infection *4*

2. **Artificial Intelligence in Ophthalmology** 16
   David Benet, Oscar J Pellicer-Valero, Jorge L Alio
   - Artificial Intelligence Algorithms in Ophthalmology *18*
   - Application of Artificial Intelligence in Ocular Diseases *24*
   - *Discussion*: Potential Advantages, Limitations, and Risks of Artificial Intelligence in the Diagnosis and Treatment of Eye Disease *30*

3. **Robotic Surgery in Ophthalmology and Orbitofacial Surgery** 36
   Marcus Tan CJ, Gangadhara Sundar
   - Principles and Concepts *37*
   - Current Applications in Ophthalmology *38*
   - Fifth Generation Wireless (5G) *43*
   - The Future *44*

4. **Advances in Corneal Crosslinking** 47
   Chris HL Lim, Ray Manotosh
   - Proposed Mechanism of Action *48*
   - Indications *49*
   - Techniques and Reported Efficacy *51*
   - Contraindications *56*
   - Risks and Complications *56*

5. **Artificial Intelligence in the Diagnosis of Glaucoma** 61
   Murali Ariga, Mohana Sinnasamy, Pratheeba Devi Nivean, Henry Henderson
   - Artificial Intelligence and its Subsets *62*
   - Optical Coherence Tomography *69*
   - Visual Field Analysis *70*
   - Current Limitations *71*

6. **Optical Coherence Tomography Angiography in Posterior Uveitis** 78
   Saba Ishrat, Panchmi Gupta, Jasmine Ge
   - Interpretation of Angio-optical Coherence Tomography *79*
   - Spectrum of Abnormal Vascular Changes in Uveitides *80*
   - Optical Coherence Tomography Angiography versus Fluorescein Angiography in Uveitis *81*
   - Optical Coherence Tomography Angiography versus Indocyanine Green Angiography in Uveitis *81*
   - Applications of Optical Coherence Tomography Angiography in Ocular Inflammation *83*
   - Optical Coherence Tomography Angiography Findings in Inflammatory Choroidal Neovascularization *94*
   - Limitations of Optical Coherence Tomography Angiography *97*

7. **Serpiginous Choroiditis** 103
   GVN Rama Kumar
   - Epidemiology *104*
   - Etiology *105*
   - Clinical Features *106*
   - Histopathology *107*
   - Diagnosis *107*
   - Complications *112*
   - Management *113*
   - Differential Diagnosis *115*

8. **Pachychoroid: The Disease Spectrum** 120
   Anand Rajendran, Ritesh Chainani, Bhanu Pangtey, MY Vishal
   Pachyvessels Morphology *121*

9. **Glued Intrascleral Haptic Fixation of Intraocular Lens** 129
   Venkata Prabhakar G, Soosan Jacob
   - Principle *130*
   - Preoperative Evaluation *130*
   - *Technique*: Step-by-Step Approach *130*
   - Nuances *132*
   - Complications *135*

10. **Advances in Phacoemulsification** 138
    Shreesha Kumar Kodavoor, Tamilarasi S, Ramamurthy Dandapani
    - Advances in Phacomachines *138*
    - Femtosecond Laser Platforms *140*
    - Advances in Microscopes *141*

- Advances in Capsulorhexis *143*
- Other Technologies for Capsulotomy *145*
- Advances in Nucleus Management in Phacoemulsification *146*
- Advances in Toric Alignment during Phacoemulsification *147*
- Image-guided Cataract Surgery *147*
- Intraoperative Wavefront Aberrometry [Optiwave Refractive Analysis (ORA) System] *149*
- Intraoperative Optical Coherence Tomography *149*

11. Recent Trends in the Management of Diabetic Retinopathy 152
Rajiv Raman, Sudipta Das, Ramachandran Rajalakshmi

- Epidemiology *153*
- Classification and Clinical Features *155*
- Investigations *160*
- Treatment *164*
- Management of Proliferative Diabetic Retinopathy *170*
- Surgical Pathoanatomy *174*
- Surgical Techniques *175*
- Complications *177*
- Outcome *178*

12. Current Trends in the Management of Neovascular Age-related Macular Degeneration 187
Giridhar Anantharaman, Kiran Chandran, Akanksha Rai

- Timeline in the Management of Wet Age-related Macular Degeneration *187*
- Treatment Regimen for Neovascular Age-related Macular Degeneration using Antivascular Endothelial Growth Factor Monotherapy *190*

13. Newer Approaches to Management of Retinal Degenerative Disorders: Gene Therapy and Cell Replacement Therapy 204
Lingam Gopal, Su Xinyi, Mayuri Bhargava, Zeng Ping Iiu, Swathi Lingam

- **Gene Therapy** *205*
  - Polymorphisms and Mutations *205*
  - Gene Therapy Approaches *208*
- **Cell Therapy for Retinal Disorders** *213*
  - Stem Cells and Regeneration *213*
  - The Eye as a Target for Cell-based Therapy *213*
  - Cells Proposed to be Replaced *215*
  - Rationale for Cell-based Therapy *216*
  - Replacement versus Rejuvenation *222*
  - Immunogenicity of Retinal Progenitor Cells Transplantation *224*

14. **Ocular Myasthenia Gravis** 229
    Asmita Mahajan, Pradeep Sharma
    - Pathophysiology *230*
    - Clinical Features *230*
    - Diagnosis *231*
    - Electrophysiologic Testing *233*
    - Imaging Studies *233*
    - Treatment *234*

Index *239*

CHAPTER 1

COVID-19 and the Eye
(Critical Appraisal of Cause and Effect Relationship)

Lingam Gopal, Su Xinyi, Ivan Seah

ABSTRACT

Severe acute respiratory syndrome coronavirus 2 (SARS-CoV-2) causes the disease coronavirus disease 2019 (COVID-19) and this has been responsible for a pandemic that is still raging across the world and causing significant morbidity and mortality. The disease is mostly spread by droplet infection and primarily causes respiratory symptoms and fever. The eye has been found to be affected in a number of patients. However, the relationship between the viral infection and the ocular manifestations has not always been clear. In most cases the evidence was circumstantial. The eye has also been mooted as a potential portal for the entry of the virus into the body. Hence, ophthalmologists have to introduce a number of measures in their practice to eliminate the risk of transmission of the virus by this route.

Keywords: COVID-19, retinal vein occlusion, conjunctivitis, central retinal artery occlusion, cranial nerve palsy.

INTRODUCTION

Severe acute respiratory syndrome coronavirus-2 (SARS-CoV-2) is a single-stranded enveloped ribonucleic acid (RNA) virus belonging to the family "Coronaviridae" and one among the seven viruses in this family to affect humans.[1] The virus causes a disease that has been termed "coronavirus disease 2019 (COVID-19)".

The eye and ophthalmology have received a fair bit of attention in the context of COVID-19. The first knowledge of the disease was made known to the medical fraternity by an ophthalmologist Dr Li Wenliang. He himself succumbed to COVID-19 which he contacted from a patient of angle closure glaucoma whom he was treating.

The present pandemic caused by SARS-CoV-2 is still active as of writing this article and several countries are grappling with the second or third wave. As of 1st May 2021, the World Health Organization COVID-19 Dashboard reports 151,110,310 confirmed cases with 3,158,792 deaths.[2] Literature on COVID-19 is abounding and rightly so. A number of articles have reflected on the role of the eye as a gateway to the virus entry as well as on the ocular manifestations in patients with COVID-19. A number of review articles have summarized the published literature on ocular manifestations from time to time.

However, the cause-and-effect relationship between the viral infection and the ocular manifestations is not established in most cases. In this review, we summarize the available information and analyze the level of evidence that connects the COVID-19 with the eye.

THE EYE AS A PORTAL OF ENTRY FOR THE VIRUS

The viral envelope has large club-shaped spikes (peplomers). The binding of the virus to host cells is mediated by the spike protein that binds to angiotensin-convertase enzyme 2 (ACE-2) receptor. Cellular entry also depends on the presence of type II transmembrane serine protease (TMPRSS2).[3] Coexpression of these two receptors is said to be important for the virus entry since TMPRSS2 cleaves the ACE-2 and the spike (S) protein thus facilitating the host-virus interaction. Coexpression of these two receptors has been demonstrated in several tissues including lung, liver, kidney, and brain. While some studies on conjunctival and corneal specimens have revealed that ACE-2 receptors are expressed in human conjunctival cells but not TMPRSS2,[4] other studies have shown expression of both ACE-2 and TMPRSS2 as well as dendritic cell-specific intracellular adhesion molecule 3-grabbing nonintegrin (DC-SIGN), DC-SIGN-related protein (DC-SIGNR) in both conjunctival and corneal cells.[5,6] Studies have also pointed out that the virus could use alternate pathways to entry such as CD26/DPP4, trypsin, cathepsin L, TMPRSS11d (as was implicated in Middle East respiratory syndrome and SARS-CoV).[7]

A recent in-vitro study highlighted the possibility of infection of ocular tissues such as the conjunctival cells. In this study by Hui et al., SARS-CoV-2 was able to infect human conjunctival explant cultures and could also undergo productive replication, resulting in higher viral titers.[8] Interestingly, in a separate study by Miner et al., SARS-CoV-2 was not capable of replicating in human corneal explants.[9] While it is tempting to infer from these results the difference in susceptibility of both tissue types to SARS-CoV-2, it should be noted that the possibility of ocular infection is affected not only by the cellular susceptibility but also dynamic factors such as mucosal immunity, tear film dynamics, and lacrimal clearance. These factors can play a part in reducing the residence time of the virus on the ocular surface, thereby limiting the chance of infection. As such, the evidence available should be interpreted with caution. Interestingly, Wei et al. also reported the development of respiratory tract infection after three rhesus macaques were inoculated with SARS-CoV-2 via the conjunctival route.[10] Further studies should seek to determine the similarities between the conjunctival tissue of these macaques and human conjunctival tissue. The dynamic factors described above should also be investigated to determine its effect on SARS-CoV-2 infection of ocular tissue.

Many respiratory viruses including adenovirus and influenza virus have ocular tropism and cause conjunctivitis frequently. With coronaviruses in general, this has been reported only rarely.[11] Hong et al. have analyzed the ocular symptoms preceding the onset of COVID-19 infection using questionnaires with the hypothesis that an altered ocular surface such as dry eye could potentially increase risk of entry of the virus through ocular surface. Their study does not show any increased incidence of dry eye symptoms before onset of COVID-19 systemically. However, 6 of the 56 patients had ocular symptoms several days before the systemic symptoms.[12]

SARS-CoV-2 in tears: Several studies have been done to try and identify the virus in the tears of COVID-19 patients with and without ocular symptoms.[13,14] In general, positive identification of virus from tears has been very low. Polymerase chain reaction (PCR) positivity was reported in 0.38% in specimens from patients who had ocular symptoms while if all PCR results were pooled irrespective of presence or absence of ocular symptoms the positivity was 0.04%.

However, a single case report by Chen et al. is illuminating in some respects.[15] 13 days after systemic symptoms the patient developed conjunctivitis. Conjunctival swab testing for PCR of the virus was positive on 14th and 17th day and became negative on 19th day. The level of virus was far less in conjunctival swab compared to nasopharyngeal swab. The trend of reduction in the virus in conjunctiva correlated with reduction in ocular symptoms.

Summary of published evidence that CoV-2 uses the ocular surface serving as portal for infection:
Evidence for:
- Angiotensin-converting enzyme 2 and TMPRSS2 receptor expression is present in the conjunctiva and cornea, permitting the virus to adhere to the cells and then gain entry.
- Small percentage of patients have ocular symptoms several days before systemic manifestation.

Evidence against:
- Polymerase chain reaction positivity from tears is very low even in established COVID systemic infection.
- Polymerase chain reaction positivity from tears is low in COVID patients despite the presence of ocular symptoms.

CLINICAL RECOMMENDATIONS

However, in the milieu of the pandemic, it is important that ophthalmologists ensure protective measures are taken while examining all patients, to minimize risk of inadvertent spread between patients and physicians, particularly as many asymptomatic patients may harbor virus in the tears.

Regardless, the risk of spread from nasopharyngeal route remains higher than via ocular routes.

Protective measures that we should comply with to avoid contamination via tears include the following:
- Avoid touching the eye directly with hands while opening the eyelids for examination. Use either gloves or cotton buds. The gloves must be removed and disposed before performing any other action including entry of data, etc.
- Sterilization of tonometer tip—this is a common practice even outside the milieu of the pandemic, but this needs re-emphasis. Usage of tonopen with disposable tips is the best option.
- Use of disposable one-time usage minims for dilation rather than usage of a common bottle for different patients.
- Ensure proper hand sanitization is performed between cases.

OCULAR MANIFESTATIONS IN PATIENTS WITH COVID-19 SYSTEMIC INFECTION

Several publications have reported various ocular manifestations in patients with COVID-19 infections. However, the cause and effect relationship is not clear for each of the reported features.

Anterior Segment Involvement

The reported anterior segment manifestations include features of viral conjunctivitis; pseudomembranous conjunctivitis, and keratoconjunctivitis. Conjunctival infection can occur due to a local spread from pre-existing infection in nasopharynx and lungs. However, conjunctivitis has also been reported to be the first symptom in some cases. **Table 1** summarizes some of the important publications related to anterior segment manifestations with comment on level of evidence as to cause and effect relationship.

The most common anterior segment structure involved is the conjunctiva. Congestion, chemosis, and epiphora are the common symptoms. Presumably these symptoms may indicate viral conjunctivitis even if conjunctival swab is negative. However, one has to keep in mind that stay in intensive care facility can also produce conjunctival hyperemia and related signs, independent of COVID-19 or any other infection.[16]

Posterior Segment Involvement

Table 2 summarizes the reported features from important publications. These include retinal hemorrhages, cotton-wool spots, branch retinal vein occlusion (BRVO) or central retinal vein occlusion (CRVO) (mostly without associated vasculitis), central artery occlusion (CRAO), paracentral acute middle maculopathy (PAMM), optical coherence tomography (OCT)

TABLE 1: Summary of anterior segment features of COVID-19.

Wu et al.[17]—Case series—Predominant conjunctival involvement

Salient features		• 38 consecutive patients with COVID-19 infection • 73.7% had nasopharyngeal swab positive while 5.2% had conjunctival swab positive (both with ocular symptoms) • 12/38 (31.6%) patients had ocular involvement • Only one patient presented with conjunctivitis as first symptom • Ocular involvement more common with greater severity of systemic manifestation • Patients with ocular involvement more likely to have higher WBC and neutrophil count; higher procalcitonin, lactate dehydrogenase, and C-reactive protein levels • Ocular manifestations include chemosis, epiphora, conjunctival hyperemia, and conjunctival discharge • No visual disturbance
Evidence for cause and effect relationship	*Level of evidence*	Moderate
	Points for	Temporal relationship; more common ocular involvement with more severe systemic disease
	Points against	Only 2/12 had conjunctival swab positive

Kumar et al.[18]—Prospective study—0.72% conjunctivitis; one with orbital cellulitis

Salient features		• Prospective study of 2,742 COVID patients • At presentation none had ocular symptoms • 0.72% developed ocular features on follow-up • Most had conjunctivitis; one had orbital cellulitis with sinusitis • No correlation with severity of systemic disease
Evidence for cause and effect relationship	*Level of evidence*	Moderate for conjunctivitis; weak for orbital cellulitis
	Points for	Temporal relationship. ACE-2 receptor expressed in paranasal sinuses. Severe systemic disease resulting in death of patient
	Points against	Known diabetic with clinical diagnosis of possible fungal sinus infection

Contd...

Contd...

Cheema et al.[19]—Case report—Keratoconjunctivitis

Salient features	• Case report • 29-year-old female with unilateral symptoms of sore eyes, discharge, conjunctival follicles, subepithelial infiltrates, pseudodendrites, and preauricular lymphadenopathy. Suspected herpetic in origin to start with • No systemic symptoms. Nasopharyngeal swab test done since she traveled recently—was positive. Conjunctival swab sent for gonorrhea and chlamydia was weakly positive for COVID	
Evidence for cause and effect relationship	Level of evidence	Weak
	Points for	Positive PCR from nasopharyngeal swab; weakly positive conjunctival swab
	Points against	• Unilateral features strongly in favor of herpetic keratouveitis • No systemic symptoms

Navel et al.[20]—Case report—Pseudomembranous conjunctivitis

Salient features	• 63-year-old male • Had pneumonia due to COVID • On day 19 had tarsal hemorrhages, mucous filaments, pseudomembranes, superficial punctate keratitis. Membranes peeled off without bleeding • Conjunctival swab negative for COVID—done twice	
Evidence for cause and effect relationship	Level of evidence	Moderate
	Points for	Pneumonia due to COVID; positive PCR from nasopharyngeal swab; bilateral conjunctivitis
	Points against	Conjunctival swab negative despite severe pseudomembranous conjunctivitis

(ACE-2: angiotensin-converting enzyme 2; COVID: coronavirus disease; PCR: polymerase chain reaction; WBC: white blood cell count)

TABLE 2: Summary of posterior segment features of COVID-19.

Marinho et al.[24]—Case series—Hyper-reflective lesions in retinal layers on OCT

Salient features		• 12 adults between 25 and 69 years with COVID-19. Nine with PCR positive and rest antibody positive • Optical coherence tomography examination (OCT) 11–33 days after COVID symptoms • 11 had anosmia. None needed ICU • OCT: All showed hyper-reflective lesions at GCL/IPL—more in papillomacular bundle. Microhemorrhages seen • All other tests including vision normal
Evidence for cause and effect relationship	Level of evidence	Weak
	Points for	Positive PCR or antibody for COVID-19
	Points against	None had severe disease; no positive scotoma reported (asymptomatic). No follow-up data. No information on status of general health except a statement that blood parameters are normal at time of eye evaluation. Possibility of misinterpretation of the OCT

Ortiz-Egea JM et al.[25]—Case report—PAMM

Salient features		• Case report • 42-year-old anesthetist presented with positive scotoma in one eye that persisted even 30 days later • Vision normal; OCT showed hyper-reflective placoid band at level of GCL/IPL—persisted 1 month later. Features similar to PAMM • High risk of COVID-19 due to profession. PCR negative, ELISA and antibody test positive. Limited ageusia (loss of taste) for several days 3 weeks before eye symptoms. No other systemic symptoms
Evidence for cause and effect relationship	Level of evidence	Moderate
	Points for	Ageusia; antibody positive; typical features of PAMM (paramacular acute middle maculopathy)—symptoms and signs. Follow-up data present
	Points against	No systemic features of COVID-19 other than ageusia. PCR negative

Contd...

Duff et al.[26]—Case report—BRVO		
Salient features	• 74-year-old female • Controlled hyperlipidemia • Branch retinal vein occlusion (BRVO) with no evidence of vasculitis diagnosed 3 months after COVID infection. But, symptoms of blurred vision occurred while symptomatic with COVID	
Evidence for cause and effect relationship	Level of evidence	Weak
	Points for	COVID-19 positive
	Points against	Unilateral BRVO in 74-year-old female with hyperlipidemia could easily occur without COVID as well; no vasculitis
Yahalomi et al.[27]—Case report—CRVO		
Salient features	• 33-year-old healthy male • Central retinal vein occlusion (CRVO) in one eye • Had cough, fatigue, and breathlessness 20 days before vision complaints • Testing for COVID, after ocular symptoms, was negative by PCR but positive by antibody testing for IgG (not IgM) • Investigations for other prothrombotic disorders negative	
Evidence for cause and effect relationship	Level of evidence	Moderate
	Points for	Evidence of previous COVID infection; young male with no other risk factors for CRVO
	Points against	No evidence of vasculitis
Sheth et al.[28]—Case report—Hemiretinal vein occlusion		
Salient features	• 52-year-old male presented with reduced vision left eye 10 days after diagnosis of COVID-19 • Diagnosed inferior hemi-vein occlusion with macular edema with signs of periphlebitis • Systemic investigations for other causes of vein occlusion were negative • Responded well to anti-VEGF drugs and steroids	
Evidence for cause and effect relationship	Level of evidence	Moderate
	Points for	Evidence of previous COVID infection; no other risk factors for CRVO, evidence of vasculitis
	Points against	No other vasculitis in body, mild systemic disease

Contd...

Contd...

Walinjkar et al.[29]—Case report—CRVO		
Salient features	• 17-year-old female with history of polycystic ovaries not on medication presents with reduced vision in right eye of 2 days duration • Had typical features of central retinal vein occlusion • Family members had COVID-19 and recovered • Investigations for other causes of vein occlusion negative • Chest CT showed features suggesting COVID-19 although swab was negative and patient is asymptomatic. IgG antibody was positive suggesting past asymptomatic infection	
Evidence for cause and effect relationship	Level of evidence	Moderate
	Points for	Evidence of previous COVID infection; no other risk factors for CRVO
	Points against	No other vasculitis in body, asymptomatic systemic disease
Gaba et al.[30]—Case report—bilateral CRVO		
Salient features	• 40-year-old male • 3 days history of fever, cough, and shortness of breath • Blurring vision • Hypertensive and morbid obesity • Diagnosed COVID-19 with deep vein thrombosis of leg and bilateral central retinal vein occlusion • Had elevated inflammatory markers	
Evidence for cause and effect relationship	Level of evidence	Strong
	Points for	Evidence of active COVID infection; deep vein thrombosis. Bilateral CRVO, elevated inflammatory markers
	Points against	None

Contd...

Contd...

Acharya S et al.[31]—Case report—CRAO		
Salient features		• 60-year-old male • History of hypertension, dyslipidemia, coronary artery disease, and chronic obstructive pulmonary disease • Needed ventilatory support for 6 days for COVID infection, 6 days after being extubated and systemically stable, developed typical CRAO
Evidence for cause and effect relationship	Level of evidence	Weak
	Points for	Severe COVID infection
	Points against	History of hypertension, dyslipidemia, coronary artery disease. CRAO occurred when patient is systemically stable
Invernizzi A et al.—SERPICO study[32]—Cross-sectional study—nonspecific retinal features		
Salient features		• 54 COVID-19 patients and 133 unexposed subjects had fundus photographs • 24.9% had severe COVID infection • 9.25% had retinal hemorrhages, 7.4% had cotton wool spots, 11.1% had drusen; 27.7% had dilated veins; and 12.9% had tortuous vessels • On computer analysis of the fundus photos (mostly not appreciated on clinical examination), mean vein diameter was larger compared to normal for all COVID patients (severe and nonsevere); and mean arterial diameter were found larger in severe COVID patients • Longer the interval between symptoms and fundus photography, less the vein diameter • None had vision threatening issues
Evidence for cause and effect relationship	Level of evidence	Moderate
	Points for	Systematically done cross-sectional study
	Points against	Significant numbers had comorbidities such as hypertension, diabetes, etc. Increased vein diameter is detected only on computer evaluation of the fundus photographs and not clinically evident

(BRVO: branch retinal vein occlusion; COVID: coronavirus disease; CRAO: central artery occlusion; CRVO: central retinal vein occlusion; ELISA: enzyme-linked immunosorbent assay; GCL: ganglion cell layer; IPL: inner plexiform layer; OCT: optical coherence tomography; PAMM: paracentral acute middle maculopathy; PCR: polymerase chain reaction; VEGF: vascular endothelial growth factor) observation of hyper-reflective lesions in the ganglion cell layer (GCL)/inner plexiform layer (IPL)-especially in the papillomacular bundle, and larger mean retinal vein diameter in COVID patients compared to normal on computer evaluation of fundus photographs. Significantly there were no cases of frank retinitis unlike Chikungunya[21] or herpetic retinitis or macular lesions such as foveolitis that were reported in "dengue" fever.[22]

Theoretically, viral involvement of retina could potentially be caused by direct viral multiplication in form of infectious retinitis or vasculitis or be the result of intravascular coagulation associated with COVID-19.[23] However, intravascular coagulation and systemic thrombotic disorders have been mostly associated with severe COVID-19 resulting in higher mortality in this group. In contrast, most cases of retinal vein occlusion were seen in patients who were asymptomatic or recovered from a mild infection. The hyper-reflective lesions noted on OCT in the GCL/IPL are difficult to interpret in terms of COVID-19. Neither they have features of active viral infection nor do they resemble PAMM. These patients were asymptomatic with no scotoma demonstrable even when the lesions were located in the papillomacular bundle. The finding of greater mean retinal vein diameter in COVID patients may not have much significance in clinical practice.

Table 3 describes the miscellaneous ocular involvements in COVID-19. In addition to the anterior and posterior segment manifestations, extraocular muscle palsies due to involvement of cranial nerves,[33] and optic neuritis with pan uveitis have been reported.[34] Kawasaki disease is a condition that affects young children and manifests as systemic vasculitis. Observations in Italy and elsewhere have shown a sudden increase in number of cases of Kawasaki disease during the COVID epidemic.[35] While the cause and effect relationship between the two has not been established, it is hypothesized that the virus could trigger the immune disease of Kawasaki although children remain asymptomatic or suffer mild symptoms due to COVID.

Ocular Complications not Directly due to COVID-19 but may be Associated with Treatment of COVID

Patients suffering from COVID-19 systemic infection can also suffer ophthalmic complications due to the drugs administered for COVID treatment or during the treatment in intensive care facility.

Intensive Care Treatment-related Ophthalmic Issues[36]

- *Exposure of cornea and its sequelae*: Patients who are severely ill may run a risk of corneal exposure that can lead to keratitis. This is a totally avoidable complication.
- *Angle-closure glaucoma*: Prone position has been recommended for patients with respiratory symptoms since it improves the ventilation. However, prolonged prone position can precipitate angle-closure glaucoma in susceptible patients.

TABLE 3: Miscellaneous ocular involvement in COVID-19.

Dinkin M et al.[33]—Case report—3rd and 6th nerve palsies		
Salient features (Case 1) (Case 2)	• 36-year-old male with mild COVID infection developed left partial 3rd nerve and bilateral 6th nerve palsy, gait ataxia, hyporeflexia and hypesthesia 4 days after fever. MRI showed enhancement of 3rd nerve. Partial improvement with immunoglobulins • 71-year-old hypertensive female developed right 6th nerve palsy many days after fever. MRI showed optic nerve sheath enhancement but not of 6th nerve • Both positive for COVID	
Evidence for cause and effect relationship	Level of evidence	Moderate
	Points for	Temporal relationship, absence of other risk factors in case 1
	Points against	Case 2 is also hypertensive. Neither patients had severe COVID
Francois et al.[34]—Case report—Optic neuritis with pan uveitis		
Salient features	• Female in late 50s with severe bilateral pneumonia due to COVID-19 • Blurred vision on day 2 in right eye with hand movement vision, evidence of RAPD, central scotoma, impaired color vision, features of mild anterior uveitis, disk edema, mild vitritis, and inferior retinal vasculitis. No other neurological deficit. MRI and CSF examination unremarkable. Blood tests for other viral infections, toxoplasma, Borrelia, syphilis, and HIV were negative • Vision remained poor despite steroid therapy and developed severe optic atrophy	
Evidence for cause and effect relationship	Level of evidence	Moderate
	Points for	Temporal relationship. No other etiology found for the optic neuritis and pan uveitis
	Points against	Can still be an independent occurrence?
Viner RM et al.[35]—Association with Kawasaki disease		
Salient features	• Observation of a monthly 30-fold increase in Kawasaki disease in Bergamo, Italy during the height of epidemic • COVID testing—Two PCR positive and rest serology positive but testing done not same time as episode • Although Kawasaki disease is a systemic vasculitis, ocular involvement is potentially possible in the form of conjunctival congestion, anterior uveitis, superficial punctate keratitis, vitreous opacities, papilledema, etc.	
Evidence for cause and effect relationship	Level of evidence	Weak
	Points for	Observation of 30-fold increase of Kawasaki disease during the COVID epidemic
	Points against	Temporal relationship between COVID and Kawasaki not established

(COVID: coronavirus disease; CSF: cerebrospinal fluid; HIV: human immunodeficiency virus; MRI: magnetic resonance imaging; PCR: polymerase chain reaction; RAPD: relative afferent pupillary defect)

- *Ischemic optic neuropathy*: Multiple factors may contribute to compromised circulation of the optic nerve and cause ischemic optic neuropathy resulting in permanent loss of vision. This includes increased venous pressure due to prone position, raised intraocular pressure and possible hypotension due to coexisting systemic issues.

- Intubation and ventilation can sometimes produce chemosis, conjunctival congestion, and subconjunctival hemorrhages. Valsalva retinopathy like picture with preretinal hemorrhages has also been described.

Ophthalmic Complications-related to Use of Pharmacological Agents during COVID Treatment
- *Steroids*: Use of steroids is life-saving in the context of cytokine storm. In some patients acute steroid therapy can precipitate central serous retinopathy. In most, however, the effect on vision is mild and the condition reverses on cessation of steroid therapy.[37]
- *Hydroxychloroquine therapy*: The role of hydroxychloroquine in the management of COVID is controversial. While there was initial enthusiasm based on some reports from China, randomized studies have shown it to be of no value. Even when used, the dosage of the drug administered for COVID is not sufficient to cause the retinal changes. These changes are typically seen with consumption of the drug for several years.[38]
- *Antiviral therapy*: Although long-term treatment with "Ritonavir" has been shown to cause retinal pigment epithelial toxicity and macular changes,[39] such toxicity is unlikely with the short-term use as is done for COVID.
- Rhino-orbital mucormycosis has assumed importance due to multiple case reports of this dreaded fungal infection occurring in severely-ill COVID-19 patients. Long-standing diabetes and use of steroids could be contributing to the causation of this superadded infection.[40]

CONCLUSION

Infection with severe acute respiratory syndrome coronavirus 2 (SARS-CoV-2) causes a disease christened as COVID-19. The disease is spread predominantly by droplet contamination. However, the conjunctival surface has also been suggested as a portal of entry of the virus. The pathogenesis of the disease is closely connected to the expression of ACE-2 and TMPRSS2 receptors in the cells and the cytokine storm that can be triggered thereafter. Ocular involvement has been described in both case series and isolated case reports. Reported associations include conjunctivitis, keratoconjunctivitis, retinal vein and artery occlusion, extraocular muscle palsies, and optic neuritis. In addition, the treatment of COVID infections with steroids, antiviral medication, etc. can potentially cause ocular side effects. Patients with severe disease requiring intensive care are also at risk of ocular complications related to prone position, exposure keratitis, etc.

REFERENCES

1. Biodefense. (2021). COVID-19|SARS-CoV-2 Coronavirus Portal. [online] Available from https://globalbiodefense.com/novel-coronavirus-covid-19-portal/ [Last accessed May, 2021].

2. World Health Organization. (2021). WHO Coronavirus (COVID-19) Dashboard. [online] Available from https://covid19.who.int [Last accessed May, 2021].
3. Hoffmann M, Kleine-Weber H, Schroeder S, Krüger N, Herrler T, Erichsen S, et al. SARS CoV-2 cell entry depends on ACE2 and TMPRSS2 and is blocked by a clinically proven protease inhibitor. Cell. 2020;181:271-80.e8.
4. Ma D, Chen CB, Jhanji V, Xu C, Yuan XL, Liang JJ, et al. Expression of SARS-CoV-2 receptor ACE2 and TMPRSS2 in human primary conjunctival and pterygium cell lines and in mouse cornea. Eye (Lond). 2020;34(7):1212-9.
5. Roehrich H, Yuan C, Hou JH. Immunohistochemical Study of SARS-CoV-2 Viral Entry Factors in the Cornea and Ocular Surface. Cornea. 2020;39(12):1556-62.
6. Collin J, Queen R, Zerti D, Dorgau B, Georgiou M, Djidrovski I, et al. Co-expression of SARS-CoV-2 entry genes in the superficial adult human conjunctival, limbal and corneal epithelium suggests an additional route of entry via the ocular surface. Ocul Surf. 2021;19:190-200.
7. Senapati S, Banerjee P, Bhagavatula S, Kushwaha PP, Kumar S. Contributions of human ACE2 and TMPRSS2 in determining host-pathogen interaction of COVID-19. J Genet. 2021;100(1):12.
8. Hui KPY, Cheung MC, Perera RAPM, Ng KC, Bui CHT, Ho JCW, et al. Tropism, replication competence, and innate immune responses of the coronavirus SARS-CoV-2 in human respiratory tract and conjunctiva: an analysis in ex-vivo and in-vitro cultures. Lancet Respir Med. 2020;8(7):687-95.
9. Miner JJ, Platt DJ, Ghaznavi CM, Chandra P, Santeford A, Menos AM, et al. HSV-1 and Zika virus but Not SARS-CoV-2 replicate in the human cornea and are restricted by corneal type III interferon. Cell Rep. 2020;33(5):108339.
10. Deng W, Bao L, Gao H, Xiang Z, Qu Y, Song Z, et al. Ocular conjunctival inoculation of SARS-CoV-2 can cause mild COVID-19 in rhesus macaques. Nat Commun. 2020;11(1):4400.
11. Belser JA, Rota PA, Tumpey TM. Ocular tropism of respiratory viruses. Microbiol Mol Biol Rev. 2013;77(1):144-56.
12. Hong N, Yu W, Xia J, Shen Y, Yap M, Han W. Evaluation of ocular symptoms and tropism of SARS-CoV-2 in patients confirmed with COVID-19. Acta Ophthalmol. 2020;10.1111/aos.14445.
13. Seah IYJ, Anderson DE, Kang AEZ, Wang L, Rao P, Young BE, et al. Assessing Viral Shedding and Infectivity of Tears in Coronavirus Disease 2019 (COVID-19) Patients. Ophthalmology. 2020;127(7):977-9.
14. La Distia Nora R, Putera I, Khalisha DF, Septiana I, Ridwan AS, Sitompul R. Are eyes the windows to COVID-19? Systematic review and meta-analysis. BMJ Open Ophthalmol. 2020;5(1):e000563.
15. Chen L, Liu M, Zhang Z, Qiao K, Huang T, Chen M, et al. Ocular manifestations of a hospitalised patient with confirmed 2019 novel coronavirus disease. Br J Ophthalmol. 2020;104(6):748-51.
16. Saritas TB, Bozkurt B, Simsek B, Cakmak Z, Ozdemir M, Yosunkaya A. Ocular surface disorders in intensive care unit patients. Sci World J. 2013;2013:182038.
17. Wu P, Duan F, Luo C, Liu Q, Qu X, Liang L, et al. Characteristics of Ocular Findings of Patients with Coronavirus Disease 2019 (COVID-19) in Hubei Province, China. JAMA Ophthalmol. 2020;138(5):575-8.
18. Kumar KK, Sampritha UC, Prakash AA, Adappa K, Chandraprabha S, Neeraja TG, et al. Ophthalmic manifestations in the COVID-19 clinical spectrum. Indian J Ophthalmol. 2021;69(3):691-4.
19. Cheema M, Aghazadeh H, Nazarali S, Ting A, Hodges J, McFarlane A, et al. Keratoconjunctivitis as the initial medical presentation of the novel coronavirus disease 2019 (COVID-19). Can J Ophthalmol. 2020.
20. Navel V, Chiambaretta F, Dutheil F. Haemorrhagic conjunctivitis with pseudomembranous related to SARS-CoV-2. Am J Ophthalmol Case Rep. 2020;19:100735.

21. Mahendradas P, Avadhani K, Shetty R. Chikungunya and the eye: a review. J Ophthalmic Inflamm Infect. 2013;3(1):35.
22. Bacsal KE, Chee SP, Cheng CL, Flores JV. Dengue-associated maculopathy. Arch Ophthalmol. 2007;125(4):501-10.
23. Tang N, Li D, Wang X, Sun Z. Abnormal coagulation parameters are associated with poor prognosis in patients with novel coronavirus pneumonia. J Thromb Haemost. 2020;18(4):844-7.
24. Marinho PM, Marcos AAA, Romano AC, Nascimento H, Belfort R Jr. Retinal findings in patients with COVID-19. Lancet. 2020;395(10237):1610.
25. Ortiz-Egea JM, Ruiz-Medrano J, Ruiz-Moreno JM. Retinal imaging study diagnoses in COVID-19: a case report. J Med Case Rep. 2021;15(1):15.
26. Duff SM, Wilde M, Khurshid G. Branch Retinal Vein Occlusion in a COVID-19 Positive Patient. Cureus. 2021;13(2):e13586.
27. Yahalomi T, Pikkel J, Arnon R, Pessach Y. Central retinal vein occlusion in a young healthy COVID-19 patient: a case report. Am J Ophthalmol Case Rep. 2020;20:100992.
28. Sheth JU, Narayanan R, Goyal J, Goyal V. Retinal vein occlusion in COVID-19: a novel entity. Indian J Ophthalmol. 2020;68(10):2291-3.
29. Walinjkar JA, Makhija SC, Sharma HR, Morekar SR, Natarajan S. Central retinal vein occlusion with COVID-19 infection as the presumptive etiology. Indian J Ophthalmol. 2020;68:2572-4.
30. Gaba WH, Ahmed D, Al Nuaimi RK, Dhanhani AA, Eatamadi H. Bilateral central retinal vein occlusion in a 40-year-old man with severe coronavirus disease 2019 (COVID-19) pneumonia. Am J Case Rep. 2020;21:927691.
31. Acharya S, Diamond M, Anwar S, Glaser A, Tyagi P. Unique case of central retinal artery occlusion secondary to COVID-19 disease. IDCases. 2020;21:e00867.
32. Invernizzi A, Torre A, Parrulli S, Zicarelli F, Schiuma M, Colombo V, et al. Retinal findings in patients with COVID-19: results from the SERPICO-19 study. EClinMed. 2020;27:100550.
33. Dinkin M, Gao V, Kahan J, Bobker S, Simonetto M, Wechsler P, et al. COVID-19 presenting with ophthalmoparesis from cranial nerve palsy. Neurology. 2020;95(5): 221-3.
34. François J, Collery AS, Hayek G, Sot M, Zaidi M, Lhuillier L, et al. Coronavirus Disease 2019-Associated Ocular Neuropathy with Panuveitis: A Case Report. JAMA Ophthalmol. 2021;139(2):247-9.
35. Viner RM, Whittaker E. Kawasaki-like disease: emerging complication during the COVID-19 pandemic. Lancet. 2020;395(10239):1741-3.
36. Bertoli F, Veritti D, Danese C, Samassa F, Sarao V, Rassu N, et al. Ocular Findings in COVID-19 Patients: a review of direct manifestations and indirect effects on the eye. J Ophthalmol. 2020;2020:4827304.
37. Bevis T, Ratnakaram R, Smith MF, Bhatti MT. Visual loss due to central serous chorioretinopathy during corticosteroid treatment for giant cell arteritis. Clin Exp Ophthalmol. 2005;33(4):437-9.
38. Marmor MF, Kellner U, Lai TY, Melles RB, Mieler WF; American Academy of Ophthalmology. Recommendations on Screening for Chloroquine and Hydroxychloroquine Retinopathy (2016 Revision). Ophthalmology. 2016;123(6): 1386-94.
39. Tu Y, Poblete RJ, Freilich BD, Zarbin MA, Bhagat N. Retinal toxicity with Ritonavir. Int J Ophthalmol. 2016;9(4):640-2.
40. Mehta S, Pandey A. Rhino-orbital mucormycosis associated with COVID-19. Cureus. 2020;30;12(9):e10726.

CHAPTER 2

Artificial Intelligence in Ophthalmology

David Benet, Oscar J Pellicer-Valero, Jorge L Alio

ABSTRACT

We are living a present, and moving toward a future which will be immersed in data. This offers a unique opportunity in health care and particularly in ophthalmology to optimize patient flow and care through each of its phases. From prevention to general population screening, from clinical diagnosis to treatment optimization, and from regimen adherence to the doctor–patient relationship: an abundance of data fills our lives, and a holistic approach to current technologies is bringing such solutions closer every day.

The integration of internet of things (IoT), big data, artificial intelligence (AI), and 5G wireless transmission technology presents itself as current and future solutions for improving the patient experience throughout the healthcare pathway as well as boosting the quality of medical care with highly efficient indicators of time, efficacy, and cost.

Artificial intelligence, in particular, is the cornerstone that experts foresee as one of the greatest opportunities in history, particularly in the field of ophthalmology. This chapter provides an overview of the current state-of-the-art of this technology within the ophthalmological field (particularly regarding diabetic retinopathy, age-related macular degeneration, glaucoma, retinopathy of prematurity, keratoconus, and cataracts), explains the basis of the underlying algorithms, and defines the guidelines and foresight that will allow us to glimpse through the explosion of a new era—the digital era, which is already disrupting the present.

Several AI-based diagnosis systems for diabetic retinopathy diagnosis from fundus images have already obtained clearance by the American Food and Drug Administration (FDA), or the European Conformity (CE) marking, hence, setting an important milestone for a generalized AI deployment in the very near future. As such, this chapter attempts to provide a global perspective on the field for ophthalmologists to be able to understand and critically reflect on this new technology.

Keywords: Artificial intelligence, machine learning, deep learning, ophthalmology, retina, optical coherence tomography, age-related macular degeneration, diabetic retinopathy, glaucoma, cataract, keratoconus.

INTRODUCTION

Artificial intelligence (AI) has undergone unprecedented growth in recent years, excelling in cognitive tasks which computers were never thought capable of performing.[1] For this reason, for some time now, AI is no longer seen as "science fiction", since it already constitutes an integral part of practically every facet of our lives.

Artificial intelligence is a combination of algorithms designed with to the aim of creating machines with the same abilities as human beings. Computer science experts Stuart Russell and Peter Norvig[2] divide AI into several subtypes:

- *Systems that think like humans*: They automate activities such as decision-making, problem-solving, and learning. One example is artificial neuronal networks.
- *Systems that act like humans*: These are computers that carry out tasks in a manner similar to people. Robots fall within this category.
- *Systems that think rationally*: They attempt to emulate the rational logical thinking of humans, that is, researchers seek to create machines that can perceive reason and take appropriate action. Expert systems fall into this group.
- *Systems that act rationally*: Ideally, these try to rationally imitate human behavior as intelligent agents.

Artificial intelligence in the health-care domain has enormous and far-reaching potential in all phases of health care involving patient flow, which ranges from visual training solutions using mobile technologies to the discovery of future drugs which fall within the remit of what can be achieved with these technologies.

In the field of ophthalmology, the type of AI that has been most developed to date and really stands out is that of systems that think like humans. Nonetheless, at the present time, there are already patient-centric pilot projects that think rationally and that range from systems such as Amazon's Alexa which communicate with people to measure health indicators, to responsive platforms like "eye early detection"[3] which give visual recommendations to patients based on their answers and refer them via GPs to the closest ophthalmology centers or hospitals or even schedule virtual consultations with selected ophthalmologists. This is an example of a system that using AI and that allows to promote the visual health of the population with the objective to facilitate the early detection of diseases and reduce the time of referral to ophthalmologists. This represents an advantage to them, since they receive naïve patients in the early stages of the disease and due to this the treatment and prognosis improve significantly.

More advanced AI systems provide diabetic retinopathy (DR) diagnosis from fundus images or calculate the volume of intraretinal fluid associated to worse visual acuity and the continuous evolution of age-related macular degeneration (AMD). In both cases, AI plays an important role helping ophthalmologists in the detection of these aggressive diseases, classifying stages of the disease and predicting the visual acuity evolution.

Advances in computing and the availability of large datasets of retinal images have spurred the development of AI systems for detecting not only DR and AMD, but also other common eye diseases such as keratoconus and glaucoma.

These AI systems could improve the speed and accuracy of large-scale screening programs as well as improve access to eye examinations in underserved areas by enabling their provision at medical centers that could not otherwise offer eye care. Nevertheless, the use of AI in the clinic will inevitably raise concerns about missed diagnoses and misdiagnosis as well as the legal and ethical issues that might arise due to its use.

ARTIFICIAL INTELLIGENCE ALGORITHMS IN OPHTHALMOLOGY

According to a recently published review on this topic,[1] AI consists in the development of systems that are able to manifest intelligent behaviors. Machine learning (ML) is a subfield of AI which attempts to build algorithms that learn from experience (e.g., just by looking at data), and it is what is actually meant when the word "AI" is employed. Finally, another common concept is deep learning (DL), which is the field inside ML dealing with the design and implementation of deep neural networks (DNNs), a class of ML algorithms characterized by having many layers, hence, being very complex and powerful at solving different tasks.

Supervised Learning

Most ML algorithms (especially in the field of ophthalmology) are supervised learning algorithms, which follow the structure exemplified in **Figure 1**. As can be seen, a supervised learning model trained on DR classification is able to take an eye fundus image as input and produce a prediction (Yes/No) as output. Furthermore, such models are able to learn the task (e.g., predicting

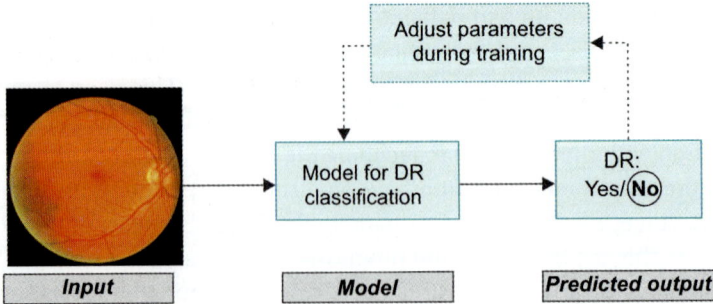

Fig. 1: Example of artificial intelligence model.
(DR: diabetic retinopathy)
Source: Image from reference 4.

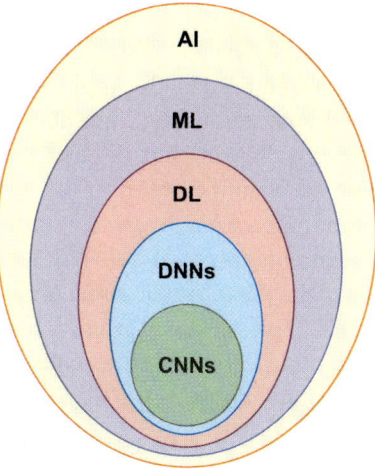

Fig. 2: Artificial intelligence (AI) hierarchy.
(CNNs: convolutional neural networks; DL: deep learning; DNNs: deep neural networks; ML: machine learning)

DR from fundus images) just by looking at hundreds of thousands of input-output pairs (e.g., a fundus image and its corresponding DR diagnostic label). During this procedure, known as training, the model automatically and progressively adjusts its parameters (which are just numbers) in order to learn the input-output relationship as accurately as possible.

Convolutional Neural Networks

Convolutional neural networks (CNNs) are a kind of supervised DL algorithm employed for dealing with images as input. In the field of ophthalmology, due to the wide availability of very informative and cost-effective imaging modalities such as fundus images and optical coherence tomography (OCT), CNNs are the most used AI algorithm. A nonexhaustive hierarchy of the field of AI can be seen in **Figure 2**.

Tasks

There are three main tasks that CNNs are usually designed to solve: (1) image classification, (2) image segmentation, and (to a lesser extent) (3) regression.

An example application of *image classification* is shown in **Figure 1**, where a fundus image is taken as input by the CNN, and a DR prediction is produced as an output. A model can be trained to predict any number of classes; for instance, in DR prediction, it is common to predict one of five possible outputs: no DR, mild, moderate, severe, and proliferative. Furthermore, unlike humans, classification models provide a probability for each class. For instance, when shown the image in **Figure 1**, a trained model might output a 95% probability of no DR, 5% probability of mild DR, and 0%

probability for the rest of classes. This allows the scientists to set the operating point of the model (which is typically set at 50% probability) to balance sensitivity and specificity as required by the application.

Image segmentation consists in the identification of some sort of anatomical structure, tissue, lesion, etc. in an image. CNNs for image segmentation take an image as input, and produce a segmentation mask as output, which is simply a map of pixel-wise classifications. An example of CNN for retinal vessel segmentation can be seen in **Figure 3**.

Finally, in *regression tasks*, the output is a real number (e.g., visual acuity, fluid volume, dosage, etc.). This has been used, for instance, for predicting visual acuity in AMD patients after being treated with antivascular endothelial growth factor (VEGF),[5] or predicting anti-VEGF requirements.[6]

Working Principles

From a high level, most CNNs for image classification have two main components: a feature extractor and a classification head, as it can be seen in **Figure 4**, where the VGG-16[7] CNN architecture has been reproduced. The feature extractor takes an image as input and transforms it into a feature vector, which is just a list of numbers (typically around 1,000) that summarizes the most important information (or features) about the image. Then, the classification head takes this feature vector as input and predicts a class probability distribution (e.g., the probability of the image belonging to each of the five DR classes) as output.

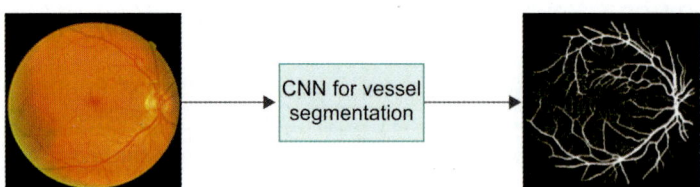

Fig. 3: Example of convolutional neural network (CNN) for vessel segmentation from fundus images.
Source: Image from reference 4.

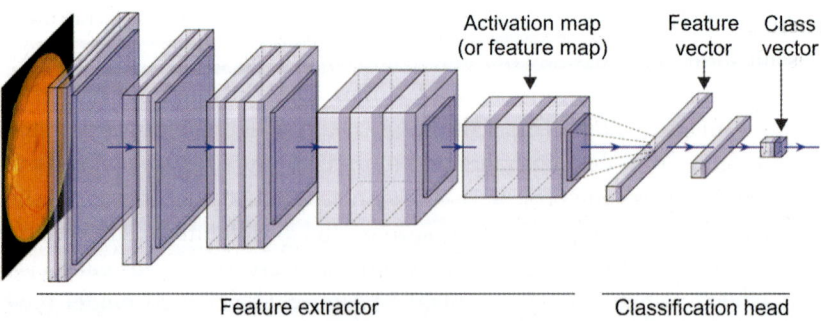

Fig. 4: VGG-16 architecture.

Internally, the feature extractor is comprised of a stack of convolutions, nonlinear activation functions, and max-pooling operations (possibly along with other operations). Convolutions are learnable filters that transform either an image into an activation map (also known as feature map), or an activation map into another activation map. A trained filter detects a specific pattern in the image (e.g., a bright spot, a change in contrast), and generates an activation map indicating where those patterns are located. Then, the next filter takes that map, and generates a further activation map, and so on. As the information travels deeper into the CNN, the detected patterns start having a more semantic meaning (e.g., hard exudates, vessel boundaries), until the final classification is performed (which is arguably the most semantic representation of the input image).

After each convolution, a nonlinear activation function is applied to each of the pixels of the resulting activation map. The most used is [ReLU(x) = max (0, x)], which simply cuts off the negative pixels of the activation map. Finally, max-pooling operations downscale the activation maps into a lower resolution (*see* **Fig. 4**). In fact, as the information travels deeper into the network, and the semantic meaning grows in importance, the spatial content of the image (e.g., where a specific pattern appears in the image) becomes more and more irrelevant (at least for the task of image classification).

Convolutional neural networks for regression share an almost identical architecture with classification of CNNs, except at the very end, where instead of predicting probabilities, a real number (or several) is predicted. CNNs for segmentation are slightly different, but share the same building blocks (convolutions, activation functions, and max-pooling).

Common Architectures and Transfer Learning

Even if sometimes the authors build a custom architecture (a precise configuration of the CNN building blocks), very often, one of several common architectures is employed instead, such as VGG16,[7] ResNet,[8] InceptionV3,[9] or InceptionV4[10] for classification (or regression) tasks, and U-net[11] for segmentation tasks. These are all known to work well for many problems, and also allow the use of a technique known as transfer learning.

Transfer learning consists in taking a CNN that has already been trained on another (typically much larger) problem, and fine-tuning it to work on another (possibly completely unrelated) problem. Usually, CNNs are pretrained on ImageNet,[12] which is a very large dataset containing >1 million images belonging to 1,000 different classes. This approach is successful because the kind of filters that CNNs learn, especially in the first few layers (e.g., a bright spot, a change in contrast), are extremely general, and can, therefore, be employed for solving many different problems, hence, a pretrained CNN provides a head start in comparison with a randomly initialized CNN.

Overfitting Assessment: Training, Validation, and Test Subsets

Convolutional neural networks are extremely powerful algorithms, which also have a high risk of overfitting. When a CNN is overfitted, it has learned the training dataset by heart, and is able to produce almost perfect predictions, but fails when exposed to images that it was not trained with. To assess this, datasets are typically split into three subsets: (1) training subset (~70% of the data), which is employed to train the CNN; (2) validation subset (~15% of the data), which is used to make design decisions (e.g., which CNN architecture to use); and (3) the test subset (~15% of the data), which contains images that have been kept secret from the CNN, and are a surrogate for what the model might find when used in clinical practice. Hence, the most interesting results are those performed on the test set. Sometimes, external validation sets are also used, which are an even harder challenge for the model, but much more representative of its real performance.

Explainability

Convolutional neural networks, as most other DL algorithms, are black boxes, which means that their internal workings cannot be easily understood by a human. However, as in most medicine applications, such an insight can be extremely helpful, or even mandatory. Even if this issue remains largely unsolved (what is an explanation anyway?), several techniques have been proposed to help visualize what parts of the image the CNN is "looking at" when a particular prediction is made. One of such techniques, known as the "integrated gradient method", is employed[13] in the task of referable DR classification, as shown in **Figure 5**. As can be seen, bright green points

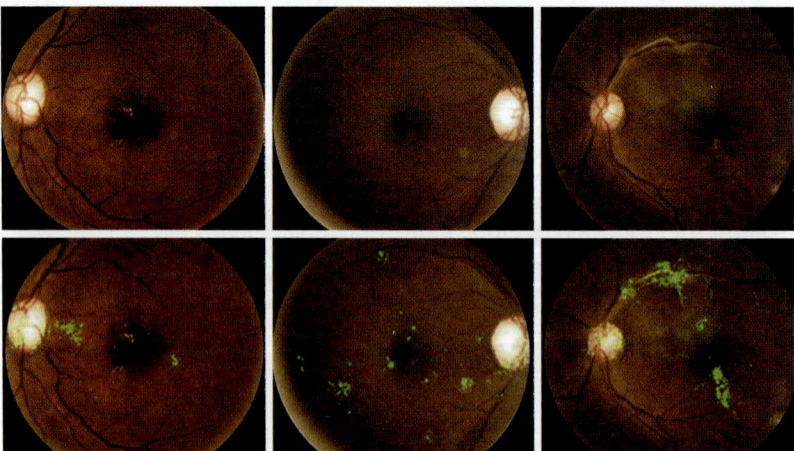

Fig. 5: Heat map visualizations using integrated gradient method in a convolutional neural network trained for referable diabetic retinopathy classification.
Source: Images from reference 13.

indicate what parts of the image are important to the CNN to perform the DR classification task.

Other Machine Learning Algorithms and Ensemble Methods

Convolutional neural networks are the state-of-the-art for dealing with images as input. However, there exist many other ML algorithms for dealing with other kinds of inputs. For numerical inputs (e.g., patient age, subretinal fluid volume, retinal thickness, visual acuity, etc.) the most employed algorithms are linear/logistic regression, feed-forward neural networks, support vector machines and decision trees. For dealing with inputs that change overtime (e.g., a patient's electronic health record), recurrent neural networks are very useful. Finally, for natural language processing (NLP) tasks, where the input is a piece of text, recurrent neural networks and transformer networks are the most popular.

Regardless of the problem or the model, ensembling is a very simple technique that generally improves the performance of the AI system. It consists in training several models on the same problem, and then taking the average (or the majority) prediction, hence, emulating the compound decision of board of experts. When applied to decision trees, the resulting algorithm is known as a random forest.

Metrics

Metrics are numbers that allow to both interpret and compare the performance of ML models. There exist several commonly employed metrics depending on the task. For classification: accuracy (fraction of correctly classified samples), sensitivity (fraction of detected positives), specificity (fraction of negatives correctly identified as such), and "area under the curve" (AUC, where the curve is obtained by varying the operating point of the model from 0 to 1). Hence, AUC is independent of the particular operating point set for the system, while the previous metrics are not. For segmentation, the above metrics can also be used (since segmentation is also a pixel-wise classification problem); however, there are specific metrics for it, such as, "Sørensen-dice similarity coefficient" (DSC, which measures the overlap between two areas or volumes, with one being a perfect overlap), or the "average boundary distance" (ABD, which measures the average error between the boundaries of two surfaces). Finally, for regression, "mean absolute error" (MAE, which represents the average error of every prediction) is a very common metric.

Developing an Artificial Intelligence System in Ophthalmology

Developing AI systems is now easier than ever, due to the very open source philosophy of the field: all frameworks and libraries (such as TensorFlow and

PyTorch) are open source, there are plenty of online resources for learning to use them, the code of the great majority of the models proposed in the literature is freely offered by the authors, etc. However, technology is not the only factor that plays a role in building a successful AI system. The following list compiles the standard procedure, as well as some recommendations:

- Find a research problem and state it in terms of inputs and outputs (e.g., the input will be a fundus image and, the output, whether it has referable DR or not). Identify the type of task to solve: image classification, segmentation, regression, etc. (e.g., DR diagnosis in fundus images is an example of image classification).
- Look for the dataset(s) that will be used for training the model (the larger the dataset, the better). If no such dataset exists, then a new one must be built: plan the recollection of the images (including authorization, patient's consent) and the labeling of the images (how many experts will label each one, how long will it take).
- Divide the dataset(s) into training, validation, and test subsets.
- Find a ML algorithm (or algorithms) that allow to model the input-output relationship defined in one, and train it (them) using the training set. Depending on the input:
  - *Images*: CNNs, either custom or common designs, such as VGG16, ResNet, etc.
  - *Numerical data*: Linear/logistic regression, feed-forward neural networks, support vector machines, and decision trees.
  - *Transient numerical data*: Recurrent neural networks.
- Decide on the final algorithm (if more than one was chosen) and the exact hyperparameters (e.g., input image resolution) by evaluating the performance on the validation set.
- Report the final metrics on the test and, if available, on the external validation sets. Also, if different experts were used to label the images, compare the performance of the model against the performance of the experts. Depending on the task, some of the most usual metrics are:
  - *Classification*: Accuracy, sensitivity, specificity, and AUC
  - *Segmentation*: Previous metrics, as well as DSC and ABD
  - *Regression*: Mean absolute error
- Generate heat map visualizations (e.g., using integrated gradient method), if possible.

APPLICATION OF ARTIFICIAL INTELLIGENCE IN OCULAR DISEASES

Diabetic Retinopathy

Diabetes and its complications are a universal health and economic concern,[14] which is only expected to worsen, especially in low- and middle-income countries (LMIC).[15] The main specific complication of the disease is DR, which affects one-third of the diabetic population, and is a sight-threatening condition caused by the damage produced to the capillaries in the retina due to high blood glucose values. Diabetic macular edema (DME) is an additional complication due to the accumulation of fluid from capillary leakage, resulting in a thickening of the retina and causing serious vision loss. This condition is typically treated with intravitreal anti-VEGF injections.

In this context, there are three main ways in which AI can be of enormous help in improving the detection and management of DR and DME:[16] (1) screening for referable DR, (2) DR stage classification, and (3) anti-VEGF outcome prediction and dose optimization.

AI-based DR screening (and stage classification) from standard eye fundus images is currently one of the most successful AI applications in medicine. Firstly, authors from many different research groups around the world have proposed systems over the last 5 years with performances equaling and sometimes even surpassing those of expert ophthalmologists and retina specialists.[13,17,18] Secondly, some of these systems have already been approved for use in several countries all around the world, such as IDx-DR,[19] the first autonomous AI to ever be approved by the USA Food and Drug Administration (FDA), or EyRIS SELENA+,[13,20] having now both Health Science Authority (HSA) certification from Singapore and CE Mark.[21] Thirdly, these systems have proven to be cost effective,[22] and may be key for healthcare systems in LMIC.

As a representative example, Krause et al.[18] train a CNN for diagnosing both DR and DME. The severity of DR is predicted using a five-point scale that follows the International Clinical Diabetic Retinopathy disease severity scale: no DR, mild, moderate, severe, and proliferative; while DME is only detected as being either referable or not. The Inception-V4 CNN model is trained with relatively large 779 × 779 fundus images as input to help in the detection of small microaneurysms and hard exudates. To train the CNN, over 1.5 million fundus images from Eye-PACS dataset were employed, and around 2,000 images from Eye-PACS-2 dataset were used for validation. Once trained, the validation results of the model were compared against three retinal specialists and three US Board-certified ophthalmologists, achieving comparable results. For instance, in the task of detecting moderate or worse DR, the median ophthalmologist achieved a sensitivity and specificity of 75.2% and 97.9% (respectively), the median retinal specialist: 74.6% and 99.3%, and the CNN model: 97.1% and 92.3%, with an AUC of 0.986. Similarly, in the task of referable DME detection, the median ophthalmologist achieved sensitivity and specificity of 91.5% and 98.7%, and the CNN model: 94.9% and 94.4%. The model, however, proved to be inferior when compared to the majority vote of either group of experts.

Anti-VEGF outcome prediction and dose optimization in DME patients is a very promising field for AI research due to the large inter-patient variability of the responses to this treatment. Although several papers have been proposed regarding treatment of AMD with anti-VEGF, very few (to the authors' knowledge) have been published in the context of DME. A custom CNN model was developed for predicting DME patient response (percentage of reduction in retinal thickness) to anti-VEGF by using a pretreatment OCT image as input.[23] Considering a reduction of 10% or more as effective, the model achieved a sensitivity and specificity of 80.1% and 85.0%.

A closely related topic is retina vessel segmentation, which can be useful in the diagnosis and screening of several diseases, including DR. In a recent review on the subject,[24] authors show that the achieved performances are at least comparable with human experts and call for the need of the assessment of cost-effectiveness of DL-based tools for retinal disease screening worldwide. As an example of such application, Arsalan et al.[4] train a custom model (which they call Vess-net, and is based on a residual U-net) for vessel segmentation from fundus images, using three different datasets, amounting to a total of around 200 images. They achieve an AUC of between 0.982 and 0.988 for every dataset, hence, surpassing state-of-the-art. It must be noted that, even if 200 images seem very few when compared to other classification problems, segmentation masks are much more informative, since they have a label for every pixel (and not just for the image as a whole) and less images are needed. Furthermore, manual segmentations are very time-consuming, so the datasets tend to be smaller.

In a recent study,[25] a very ambitious AI system was proposed for automated diagnosis of an array of eye conditions as well as general referral suggestion from OCT images, achieving AUCs above 0.99 for the majority of the conditions (and above 0.97 for all of them), therefore equaling and sometimes even surpassing, expert performance **(Fig. 6)**.

In summary, AI-based DR screening algorithms have proven effective both as a diagnostic aid,[17] and as a fully automatic system,[26] and have the potential of improving reach and effectiveness of screening programs, which is much needed in DR right now. Furthermore, anti-VEGF effectiveness prediction has a lot of potential in helping to determine the most appropriate therapy for every specific patient.

Age-related Macular Degeneration

Age-related macular degeneration (AMD) is the leading cause of vision loss in patients aged 50+ years in developed countries.[27] Although there are several risk factors associated with its onset (such as age and smoking) as well as genetic contribution, its mechanisms are yet to be fully understood. Early AMD is characterized by the appearance of yellow deposits of lipids that accumulate under the retina, called "drusen". Even if a few hard drusen can be a normal aging sign, soft large drusen can damage the macula, and are an unmistakable indication of AMD. Also, changes in the retinal pigment epithelium layer are an independent sign of late AMD.

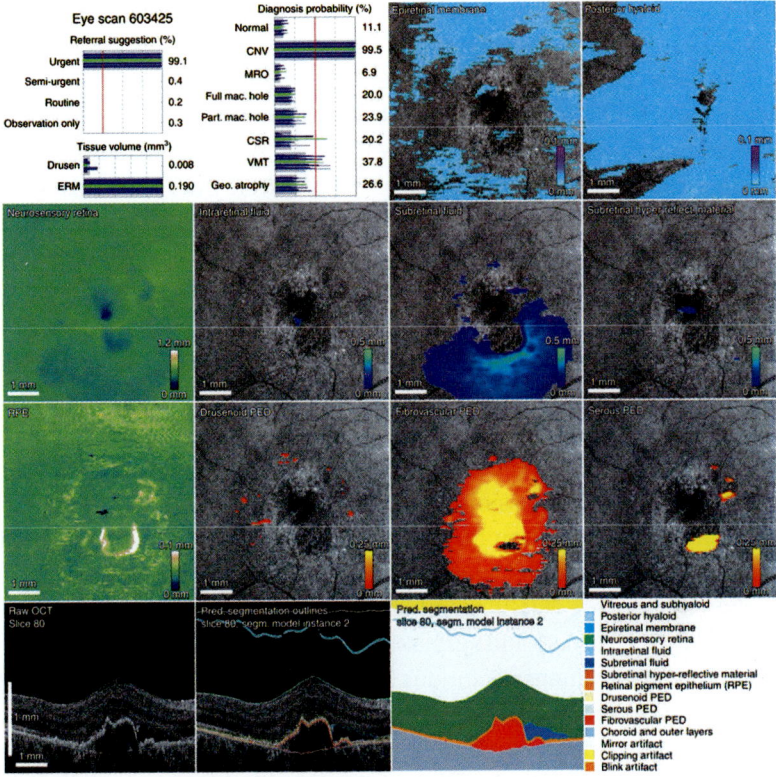

Fig. 6: Screenshot from the OCT viewer developed by De Fauw et al.[25] (CNV: choroidal neovascularization; CSR: central serous retinopathy; ERM: epiretinal membrane; MRO: maintenance, repair, and overhaul; OCT: optical coherence tomography; PED: pigment epithelial detachment; VMT: vitreomacular traction)

Currently, there is no treatment for late dry AMD, also known as "geographic atrophy" (GA), and characterized by the progressive degeneration of the retina and the photoreceptor cells, entailing a gradual and irreversible vision loss. On the contrary, for neovascular (or wet) AMD, which is characterized by the growth of new vessels in the retina, anti-VEGF drugs have been proven effective at both stopping and improving the condition of the patient. AMD stage is typically graded according to a 13-class system known as age-related eye disease study (AREDS),[28] where 1 represents normal eye, stages 2–9 indicate changes related to early or intermediate AMD, stages 10–12 represent dry, wet or both types of AMD, and stage 13 is reserved for ungradable images.[29]

Similar to DR, regarding AMD, there are two main topics in which AI systems have been proposed in the literature: AMD detection (referable/nonreferable) and staging (e.g., using AREDS system), and visual acuity (VA) prediction (typically as a result of treatment with anti-VEGF).

AI-based AMD detection and staging is a popular research question, with many papers published on the topic. For this task, there are systems using either fundus images[20,29-31] or OCTs.[32-34] For instance, Grassmann et al.[29] proposed an ensemble of six different CNNs (the predictions were combined with a random forest) for the task of performing fundus image classification according to the 13-class AREDS scale. They used the AREDS dataset for that purpose, consisting in over 120,000 images, and the Cooperative Health Research in the Region of Augsburg (KORA) dataset for external validation, consisting in over 5,000 images. They achieved an accuracy of 0.633 in the internal test dataset. However, the performance on the KORA dataset was much lower, since some of the images contained a macular reflex observed in young people, which is not present in the AREDS dataset (in which the patients all are 55+ years old). This highlights the importance of using many datasets when training a model, from as varied a population as possible, to avoid biases as much as possible. In either case, a thorough external validation is fundamental before applying any AI algorithm in clinical practice. By contrast Burlina et al.[30] used only the AREDS dataset, and trained the model on a two-class classification problem (referable/nonreferable AMD), achieving an AUC of 0.96 and surpassing human graders.

Despite the advantages of fundus imaging (such as cost and availability), OCTs are more informative for AMD detection and staging. For instance Motozawa et al.[32] trained a CNN on a dataset of around 1,500 images, and used for predicting AMD (healthy eye/nonhealthy), achieving an AUC of 0.995.

Regarding *VA prediction*, there are much fewer publications, and the topics vary slightly in nature. Aslam et al.[35] used a feed-forward neural network for predicting the VA of patient from the OCT scan, achieving a regression coefficient of 0.852 (in letters). A random forest was trained by Schmidt-Erfurth et al.[36] to predict the VA 12 months into the future, achieving a regression coefficient of 0.7 (in logMAR units) when predicting from the third month of receiving anti-VEGF treatment. Similarly, Rohm et al.[5] achieve a MAE of 0.11 logMAR when performing a similar task. Finally, Bogunovic et al.[6] developed a system to classify wet AMD patients into two anti-VEGF dose requirement groups (low and high), obtaining an AUC of 0.70 and 0.77 for each of those groups respectively.

Recently, a couple authors have studied the question of predicting the risk of a given AMD patient of progressing to late AMD.[37,38] Bhuiyan et al.[37] used the AREDS dataset and achieved a 2-year late AMD incidence prediction accuracy of 86.36% (66.88% for dry and 67.15% for wet), obtaining similar results in an external validation dataset.[37] Yim et al.[38] developed developed a system for predicting progression to wet AMD in the second eye using OCT images, and achieving a sensitivity and specificity of 80% and 55%, outperforming five out of six experts.

Age-related macular degeneration prevalence is in an upward trend and, as with DR, AI-powered systems might have the key to solving the ever-growing health and economic burden that it imposes.

Glaucoma

Glaucoma is an eye condition caused by the build-up of fluid, increasing the pressure inside the eye, and eventually damaging the optic nerve. It is a leading cause of visual impairment worldwide,[39] especially for people over the age of 60 years, with 76 million people suffering from glaucoma worldwide. Even if it can be easily treated (although it cannot be cured), its onset is typically asymptomatic, and may result in a sudden significant vision loss, hence, making screening programs paramount, an unmet need which AI can also help tackling.

There have been several publications proposing the use of AIs for referable glaucoma detection, either using fundus images as input and standard CNN for classification[20,40] or features extracted from OCTs and Radial Basis Function Network for classifications.[41] For all three papers, the authors reported AUCs between 0.931 and 0.986, which are arguably excellent results, although further validation is still needed. Apart from that, an AI was employed to obtain 16 archetypical visual field patterns for glaucoma patients.[42] The authors found that the analysis of the pattern changes in a patient as the disease progresses can be a very useful for the clinicians.

Retinopathy of Prematurity

Retinopathy of prematurity (ROP) is a vasoproliferative disorder affecting the retina of infants. In high-income countries, it only affects extremely premature infants,[43] while in middle-income countries it has a much wider reach due to the lack of appropriate screening. If treated early, a significant reduction in the percentage of unfavorable outcomes has been shown in type I ROP (8.9 vs. 15.2%), although no perfect solution exists yet.[44]

Recently, several authors have proposed AI tools for automated ROP screening from fundus images,[45-47] achieving extremely compelling results. For instance, Brown et al.[46] used a U-net CNN[11] for vessel segmentation[46] followed by an Inception-V1 CNN[48] for detection trained on over 5,000 fundus images, and achieved a sensitivity and specificity of 93% and 94% respectively detecting plus disease, and outperforming six out of eight experts. Tan et al.[47] achieved similar results in their test set: 96.6% sensitivity and 98.0% specificity with slightly worse results in an independent validation set: 93.9% sensitivity and 80.7% specificity, which highlight the importance of testing the AI models on independent validation sets.

Keratoconus

Keratoconus is characterized by a progressive thinning of the cornea resulting in corneal protrusion and scarring as well as irregular astigmatism and vision loss. Even if it can be initially managed with refractive correction, later stages of the disease require invasive procedures such as intracorneal ring segments (ICRS) implantation, corneal collagen cross-linking or even corneal transplantation.

Regarding keratoconus screening, many authors have developed AI-based systems,[49-51] achieving extremely high (above 98%) sensitivities and specificities. However, all these works incur in the limitation of using cross-validation to compute the final metrics, instead of a proper test set (or an external validation set), hence, potentially biasing the results. Regarding keratoconus management, one interesting recent publication[52] found, through clinical validation, that using an AI-guided system for ICRS implantation yielded a significant better prognosis for this intervention, hence, being the first AI in the field of keratoconus treatment.

Cataract

Cataract consists in a clouding of the lens of the eye resulting in blurry vision, faded colors, and vision loss, and representing the leading cause of blindness and visual impairment in developing countries.[39] Siddiqui et al.[53] found a recent review on the topic of AI in cataract surgery. As a summary AI has helped recently on the development of intraocular lens selection formulas, maximizing accuracy and minimizing postoperative refractive error.[54]

DISCUSSION: POTENTIAL ADVANTAGES, LIMITATIONS, AND RISKS OF ARTIFICIAL INTELLIGENCE IN THE DIAGNOSIS AND TREATMENT OF EYE DISEASE

Artificial intelligence is just one of the many tools around us, but one which has enormous potential benefits, as we saw in the previous section. The danger of AI depends completely on the use humans make of it. Obviously, the impact of the unethical use of AI can be very serious, and it is for this reason that the most powerful global organizations must define and continue to establish well-defined "rules of the game", which make the most of the advantages AI has to offer and much more may offer in the future, thus boosting its benefit to society.

In our society, AI must use transparent algorithms designed to be safe against the efforts of digital pirates. To achieve this, the use of this technology must be preceded by proper consideration and analysis of the ethical and moral implications which may arise in the short-, medium-, and long-term.

Instead of being totally dependent on AI to make important decisions in society, systems and algorithms must always be created such that their analysis is used alongside human participation, since the impact on decision-making or processes could be critical, as could the ethical risk as well as the lack of regulation for algorithm design and data privacy.

In this way, as detailed in the prior section, we can improve efficiency in healthcare management in a precise manner, making accurate diagnoses, offering personalized medicine and improving the doctor–patient relationship with a holistic use of current technologies.

Nevertheless, there are some risks associated with AI in health care and it is important to point out the three most relevant points. The first one could be the possible "errors" by AI systems that can result in patient injury or other healthcare problems, both mild and severe. Additionally, such mistakes would be especially troubling because they can impact many patients at once. The second one is related to the privacy concerns when collecting patient data, because currently there are no defined and worldwide established protocols. And the last one could be related to the nirvana fallacy. The nirvana fallacy is the informal fallacy of comparing actual things with unrealistic, idealized alternatives. In terms of AI in ophthalmology, it occurs when a new option using AI systems is compared to an ideal scenario instead of what came before it. In this case, the patient care may not be perfect after the implementation of AI and remain the same as it has always been.

At the present time, with the world engulfed in the COVID pandemic, teleophthalmology and the use of AI is emerging as a unique alternative in order to improve the detection, prediction and treatment of ocular pathologies. By way of example, the validation of the economic efficiency of AI-based telescreening for DR via teleophthalmology stands out as a model to be followed in other pathologies, ophthalmological or otherwise.

The impact of AI will be greater and will take place before we have time to prepare or anticipate, and it is very likely that it will change or disrupt almost everything we experience in our lives and in society as a whole.

This will have a positive impact in many respects, creating opportunities for individuals who are proactive and innovative in adopting new tools and following trends as changes arise, but it will also be stressful, disappointing, and bewildering for people who are unaware of the change or who are not completely prepared for it. In terms of ophthalmology, we must consider the opportunity that AI offers, both for the ophthalmologist and for the individual, for the ophthalmology department and for the hospital as an entity in its own right, while, from the patient's perspective, it will affect every stage of the patients' pathway in their pathology.

CONCLUSION

Artificial intelligence applied to ophthalmology for the purposes of detecting pathology or improving doctor–patient adherence can provide good results through the holistic use of current technologies (AI, IoT, big data, and 5G wireless technology which is currently being set up worldwide) in pathologies as severe as AMD, DR, glaucoma, keratoconus, and help in the development of precision lenses for patients with cataracts.

And following 5G, 6G will reach the market in 8 years or less with the objective of providing XR (extended reality) and high-fidelity mobile holograms, which may have many implications for remote health care. Additionally, 6G will allow for a higher security and privacy regarding personal and confidential data, which will be employed as the fuel of big data and cloud networks and the AI systems that feed on them.

Some of the challenges taken on by AI are the detection of diseases in their incipient stages, boosting access to medical care, time and costs saving and, in the field of robotics, allowing for unique health care which cannot be equaled by surgery.

Despite these challenges and risks, AI and robotics offer vast benefits which are changing all aspects of the healthcare ecosystem and improving the lives of millions of patients across the world, who have ever greater access to personalized, high-precision medicine.

Financial support: This study has been supported by the Red Temática de Investigación Cooperativa en Salud (RETICS), reference number RD16/0008/0012, Funded by Instituto de Salud Carlos III and co-funded by European Regional Development Fund (ERDF), "A way to make Europe."

REFERENCES

1. Benet-Ferrus D, Pellicer-Valero OJ. Artificial intelligence: the unstoppable revolution in ophthalmology. Surv Ophthalmol. 2021. [online] Available from: https://www.surveyophthalmol.com/article/S0039-6257(21)00076-X/fulltext [Last accessed April, 2021].
2. Russell SJ, Norvig P. Artificial Intelligence: A Modern Approach, Global Edition, 3rd edition. London, United Kingdom: Pearson; 2016. [online] Available from: https://www.pearson.ch/HigherEducation/Pearson/EAN/9781292153964/Artificial-Intelligence-A-Modern-Approach-Global-Edition. [Last accessed April, 2021].
3. EyeScreening. (2020). EyeScreening helps you perform a vision test in 5 easy steps. [online] Available from: https://www.eyescreening.eu/en/ [Last accessed April, 2021].
4. Arsalan M, Owais M, Mahmood T, Cho SW, Park KR. Aiding the diagnosis of diabetic and hypertensive retinopathy using artificial intelligence-based semantic segmentation. J Clin Med. 2019;8(9):1446.
5. Rohm M, Tresp V, Müller M, Kern C, Manakov I, Weiss M, et al. Predicting visual acuity by using machine learning in patients treated for neovascular age-related macular degeneration. Ophthalmology. 2018;125(7):1028-36.
6. Bogunovic H, Waldstein SM, Schlegl T, Langs G, Sadeghipour A, Liu X, et al. Prediction of anti-VEGF treatment requirements in neovascular AMD using a machine learning approach. Invest Ophthalmol Vis Sci. 2017;58(7):3240-8.
7. Simonyan K, Zisserman A. Very deep convolutional networks for large-scale image recognition. In: ICLR 2015—Conference Track Proceedings. 3rd International Conference on Learning Representations International Conference on Learning Representations, ICLR; 2015.
8. He K, Zhang X, Ren S, Sun J. Deep residual learning for image recognition. In: Proceedings of the IEEE Computer Society Conference on Computer Vision and Pattern Recognition. IEEE Computer Society. 2016;2016:770-8.
9. Szegedy C, Vanhoucke V, Ioffe S, Shlens J, Wojna Z. Rethinking the inception architecture for computer vision. Proc IEEE Comput Soc Conf Comput Vis Pattern Recognit. 2015;2016:2818-26.

10. Szegedy C, Ioffe S, Vanhoucke V, Alemi AA. Inception-v4, inception-ResNet and the impact of residual connections on learning. Proceedings of the Thirty-First AAAI Conference on Artificial Intelligence (AAAI-17); 2017. pp. 4278-84. [online] Available from: https://www.aaai.org/ocs/index.php/AAAI/AAAI17/paper/viewFile/14806/14311 [Last accessed April, 2021].
11. Ronneberger O, Fischer P, Brox T. U-net: Convolutional networks for biomedical image segmentation. In: Navab N, Hornegger J, Wells W, Frangi A (Eds). Medical Image Computing and Computer-Assisted Intervention—MICCAI 2015. MICCAI 2015. Lecture Notes in Computer Science, vol 9351. Springer, Cham. [online] Available from: https://doi.org/10.1007/978-3-319-24574-4_28. [Last accessed April, 2021].
12. Russakovsky O, Deng J, Su H, Krause J, Satheesh S, Ma S, et al. ImageNet large scale visual recognition challenge. Int J Comput Vis. 2015;115(3):211-52.
13. Bellemo V, Lim ZW, Lim G, Nguyen QD, Xie Y, Yip MYT, et al. Artificial intelligence using deep learning to screen for referable and vision-threatening diabetic retinopathy in Africa: a clinical validation study. Lancet Digit Health. 2019;1(1):e35-44.
14. Williams R, Karuranga S, Malanda B, Saeedi P, Basit A, Besançon S, et al. Global and regional estimates and projections of diabetes-related health expenditure: Results from the International Diabetes Federation Diabetes Atlas, 9th edition. Diabetes Res Clin Pract. 2020;162:108072.
15. Cheloni R, Gandolfi SA, Signorelli C, Odone A. Global prevalence of diabetic retinopathy: protocol for a systematic review and meta-analysis. BMJ Open. 2019;9(3):e022188.
16. Gunasekeran DV, Ting DSW, Tan GSW, Wong TY. Artificial intelligence for diabetic retinopathy screening, prediction and management. Curr Opin Ophthalmol. 2020;31(5):357-65.
17. Sayres R, Taly A, Rahimy E, Narayanaswamy A, Webster D, Devoud Coz D, et al. Using a deep learning algorithm and integrated gradients explanation to assist grading for diabetic retinopathy. Ophthalmology. 2019;126(4):552-64.
18. Krause J, Gulshan V, Rahimy E, Karth P, Widner K, Corrado GS, et al. Grader variability and the importance of reference standards for evaluating machine learning models for diabetic retinopathy. Ophthalmology. 2018;125(8):1264-72.
19. Abràmoff MD, Lavin PT, Birch M, Shah N, Folk JC. Pivotal trial of an autonomous AI-based diagnostic system for detection of diabetic retinopathy in primary care offices. Nat Digit Med. 2018;1(1):39.
20. Ting DSW, Cheung CYL, Lim G, Tan GSW, Quang ND, Gan A, et al. Development and validation of a deep learning system for diabetic retinopathy and related eye diseases using retinal images from multiethnic populations with diabetes. JAMA. 2017;318(22):2211-23.
21. EyRIS. (2021). Latest News: SELENA+ Accepted By Leading Medical Insurance Organisation In South Africa. [online] Available from: https://www.eyris.io/latest_news.cfm?id=37 [Last accessed April, 2021].
22. Xie Y, Nguyen QD, Hamzah H, Lim G, Bellemo V, Gunasekeran DV, et al. Artificial intelligence for teleophthalmology-based diabetic retinopathy screening in a national programme: an economic analysis modelling study. Lancet Digit Health. 2020;2(5):e240-9.
23. Rasti R, Allingham MJ, Mettu PS, Kavusi S, Govind K, Cousins SW, et al. Deep learning-based single-shot prediction of differential effects of anti-VEGF treatment in patients with diabetic macular edema. Biomed Opt Express. 2020;11(2):1139-52.
24. Islam MM, Poly TN, Walther BA, Yang HC, Li YC (Jack). Artificial intelligence in ophthalmology: a meta-analysis of deep learning models for retinal vessels segmentation. J Clin Med. 2020;9(4):1018.

25. De Fauw J, Ledsam JR, Romera-Paredes B, Nikolov S, Tomasev N, Blackwell S, et al. Clinically applicable deep learning for diagnosis and referral in retinal disease. Nat Med. 2018;24(9):1342-50.
26. Abràmoff MD, Lou Y, Erginay A, Clarida W, Amelon R, Folk JC, et al. Improved automated detection of diabetic retinopathy on a publicly available dataset through integration of deep learning. Invest Ophthalmol Vis Sci. 2016;57(13):5200-6.
27. Retina International. (2019). Burden: AMD—Retina International's AMD Toolkit. [online] Available from: http://amd.retinaint.org/menu/burden-of-amd-2.
28. Davis MD, Gangnon RE, Lee LY, Hubbard LD, Klein BE, Klein R, et al. The age-related eye disease study severity scale for age-related macular degeneration: AREDS Report No. 17. Arch Ophthalmol. 2005;123(11):1484-98.
29. Grassmann F, Mengelkamp J, Brandl C, Harsch S, Zimmermann ME, Linkohr B, et al. A Deep Learning Algorithm for Prediction of Age-Related Eye Disease Study Severity Scale for Age-Related Macular Degeneration from Color Fundus Photography. Ophthalmology. 2018;125(9):1410-20.
30. Burlina PM, Joshi N, Pekala M, Pacheco KD, Freund DE, Bressler NM. Automated grading of age-related macular degeneration from color fundus images using deep convolutional neural networks. JAMA Ophthalmol. 2017;135(11):1170-6.
31. Peng Y, Dharssi S, Chen Q, Keenan TD, Agrón E, Wong WT, et al. DeepSeeNet: a deep learning model for automated classification of patient-based age-related macular degeneration severity from color fundus photographs. Ophthalmology. 2019;126(4):565-75.
32. Motozawa N, An G, Takagi S, Kitahata S, Mandai M, Hirami Y, et al. Optical coherence tomography-based deep learning models for classifying normal and age-related macular degeneration and exudative and non-exudative age-related macular degeneration changes. Ophthalmol Ther. 2019;8(4):527-39.
33. Kuwayama S, Ayatsuka Y, Yanagisono D, Uta T, Usui H, Kato A, et al. Automated detection of macular diseases by optical coherence tomography and artificial intelligence machine learning of optical coherence tomography images. J Ophthalmol. 2019;2019:1-7.
34. Antony BJ, Maetschke S, Garnavi R. Automated summarisation of SDOCT volumes using deep learning: Transfer learning vs de novo trained networks PLoS One. 2019;14(5):e0203726.
35. Aslam TM, Zaki HR, Mahmood S, Ali ZC, Ahmad NA, Thorell MR, et al. Use of a Neural Net to Model: the impact of optical coherence tomography abnormalities on vision in age-related macular degeneration. Am J Ophthalmol. 2018;185:94-100.
36. Schmidt-Erfurth U, Bogunovic H, Sadeghipour A, Schlegl T, Langs G, Gerendas BS, et al. Machine learning to analyze the prognostic value of current imaging biomarkers in neovascular age-related macular degeneration. Ophthalmol Retin. 2018;2(1):24-30.
37. Bhuiyan A, Wong TY, Ting DSW, Govindaiah A, Souied EH, Smith RT. Artificial intelligence to stratify severity of age-related macular degeneration (AMD) and predict risk of progression to late AMD. Transl Vis Sci Technol. 2020;9(2):1-12.
38. Yim J, Chopra R, Spitz T, Winkens J, Obika A, Kelly C, et al. Predicting conversion to wet age-related macular degeneration using deep learning. Nat Med. 2020;26(6):892-9.
39. Flaxman SR, Bourne RRA, Resnikoff S, Ackland P, Braithwaite T, Cicinelli MV, et al. Global causes of blindness and distance vision impairment 1990–2020: a systematic review and meta-analysis. Lancet Glob Heal. 2017;5(12):e1221-34.
40. Li Z, He Y, Keel S, Meng W, Chang RT, He M. Efficacy of a Deep Learning System for Detecting Glaucomatous Optic Neuropathy Based on Color Fundus Photographs. Ophthalmology. 2018;125(8):1199-206.

41. Shigueoka LS, Vasconcellos JPC de, Schimiti RB, Reis ASC, Oliveira GO, Gomi ES, et al. Automated algorithms combining structure and function outperform general ophthalmologists in diagnosing glaucoma. PLoS One. 2018;13(12):e0207784.
42. Wang M, Shen LQ, Pasquale LR, Petrakos P, Formica S, Boland MV, et al. An artificial intelligence approach to detect visual field progression in glaucoma based on spatial pattern analysis. Invest Opthalmol Vis Sci. 2019;60(1):365-75.
43. Hartnett ME. Retinopathy of prematurity: evolving treatment with anti-vascular endothelial growth factor. Am J Ophthalmol. 2020;218:208-13.
44. Good WV, Hardy RJ, Dobson V, Palmer EA, Phelps DL, Early Treatment for Retinopathy of Prematurity Cooperative Group; et al. Final visual acuity results in the early treatment for retinopathy of prematurity study. Arch Ophthalmol. 2010;128(6):663-71.
45. Coyner AS, Swan R, Campbell JP, Ostmo S, Brown JM, Kalpathy-Cramer J, et al. Automated fundus image quality assessment in retinopathy of prematurity using deep convolutional neural networks. Ophthalmol Retin. 2019;3(5):444-50.
46. Brown JM, Campbell JP, Beers A, Chang K, Ostmo S, Chan RVP, et al. Automated diagnosis of plus disease in retinopathy of prematurity using deep convolutional neural networks. JAMA Ophthalmol. 2018;136(7):803-10.
47. Tan Z, Simkin S, Lai C, Dai S. Deep learning algorithm for automated diagnosis of retinopathy of prematurity plus disease. Transl Vis Sci Technol. 2019;8(6):23.
48. Szegedy C, Liu W, Jia Y, Sermanet P, Reed S, Anguelov D, et al. Going deeper with convolutions. 2015 IEEE Conference on Computer Vision and Pattern Recognition (CVPR). IEEE Computer Society; 2015. pp. 1-9.
49. Smadja D, Touboul D, Cohen A, Elvevåg B, Holmlund TB, Foltz PW, et al. Detection of subclinical keratoconus using an automated decision tree classification. Am J Ophthalmol. 2013;156(2):237-46.e1.
50. Souza MB, Medeiros FW, Souza DB, Garcia R, Alves MR. Evaluation of machine learning classifiers in keratoconus detection from orbscan ii examinations. Clinics (Sao Paulo). 2010;65(12):1223-8.
51. Ruiz Hidalgo I, Rodriguez P, Rozema JJ, Ní Dhubhghaill S, Zakaria N, Tassignon MJ, et al. Evaluation of a machine-learning classifier for keratoconus detection based on scheimpflug tomography. Cornea. 2016;35(6):827-32.
52. Fariselli C, Vega-Estrada A, Arnalich-Montiel F, Alio JL. Artificial neural network to guide intracorneal ring segments implantation for keratoconus treatment: a pilot study. Eye Vis (Lond). 2020;7(1):20.
53. Siddiqui AA, Ladas JG, Lee JK. Artificial intelligence in cornea, refractive, and cataract surgery. Curr Opin Ophthalmol. 2020;31(4):253-60.
54. Siddiqui AA, Ladas JG, Nutkiewicz MA, Chong JK, Marquezan MC, Hamilton D. (2018). Evaluation of New IOL Formula That Integrates Artificial Intelligence. ASCRS ASOA Annual Meeting. [online] Available from https://ascrs.confex.com/ascrs/18am/meetingapp.cgi/Paper/45603 [Last accessed April, 2021].

CHAPTER 3

Robotic Surgery in Ophthalmology and Orbitofacial Surgery

Marcus Tan CJ, Gangadhara Sundar

ABSTRACT

Robotic surgery has made great strides since its adoption from industrial use to surgical procedures in humans. Since its inception in the 1980s, there have been various attempts to apply the technology in various aspects of ophthalmic surgery. The literature reports its use on anterior segment surgery such as amniotic membrane transplantation, pterygium excision, posterior segment surgery such as epiretinal membrane peels and even orbital surgery such as endoscopic orbital decompression. We herewith share the principles of robotic surgery, highlighting the differences between the various types of robotic systems—master-slave, active and semi-active robotic systems. A futuristic insight into complementary technology including 5G networks, virtual, augmented and extended reality applications are also highlighted.

Keywords: Robotic surgery, 5G technology, augmented reality, anterior segment surgery, posterior segment surgery, orbital surgery, endoscopic surgery, orbitofacial surgery.

INTRODUCTION

Robotic surgery is an exciting field that has advanced at a dizzying pace since its introduction to modern medicine a quarter century ago. The first robot used in modern surgery, the PUMA 200 (Westinghouse Electric, Pittsburgh, PA) was a modified industrial robot deployed in 1985 that was used to position a biopsy cannula for neurosurgical stereotactic biopsies.[1] Since then, the field has grown exponentially in depth and breadth, with applications in specialties as diverse as urology, orthopedics, otolaryngology and radiosurgery, to name a few.[2] The benefits are clear: from tremor filters and motion scalers used in the NeuRobot (Shinshu University School of Medicine, Matsumoto, Japan) that pushes the limits of human dexterity in neurosurgery to the PROBOT that cuts down on repetitive cutting motions in transurethral resection of the prostate (TURP)—it is clear that robotic surgery is not only here to stay, but to flourish.[3]

This chapter provides an overview of the basic principles of robotic surgery, its relevance to the modern-day ophthalmologist and orbital surgeon, and a glimpse into the future direction that this field may take.

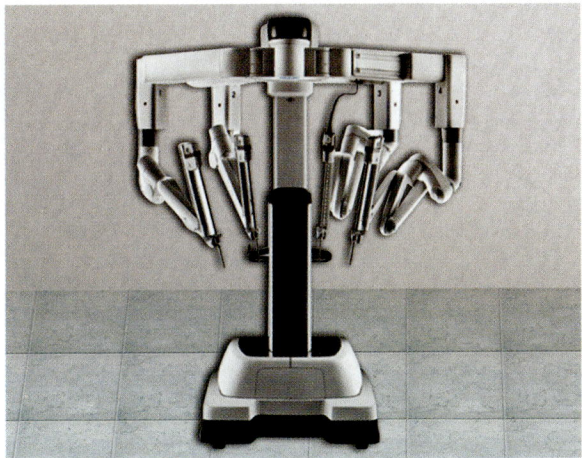

Fig. 1: Frontal view of the da Vinci Xi Surgical System.
Source: ©2021 Intuitive Surgical, Inc.

PRINCIPLES AND CONCEPTS

A surgical robot has been defined as a device that is self-powered, computer-controlled, and one that can be programmed to aid in the manipulation and positioning of surgical instruments which enables the surgeon to carry out more complex tasks.[4] Robotic systems can be broadly categorized into three types—master-slave, active, and semiactive systems.

Formal master-slave systems are often the first type of systems that one would imagine when asked about robotic surgery. These systems are fully operated by the surgeon and do not exhibit any autonomous behavior: human input is translated into movements with the appropriate filtering processes in place, such as tremor filtering or motion scaling, and this occurs in vivo. The most widely known examples of master-slave systems include the da Vinci Surgical System® (Intuitive Surgical Inc., Sunnyvale, CA) and ZEUS® (Computer Motion, Santa Barbara, CA) platforms **(Fig. 1)**.[5]

Active systems on the other hand, can be considered to be fully autonomous in their preprogrammed surgical task, with the surgeon having oversight of the task at hand. Such platforms include the PROBOT and ROBODOC described above. Although such systems are categorized as fully autonomous, this term should be interpreted within the confines of the task itself. It should be obvious that the entire surgery can be performed solely by the robot. Also, the scope of the preprogrammed task in active systems is often very narrow, meant to reduce the surgical burden of multiple repetitive movements, rather than to complete an entire surgery from start to finish.

Lastly, there are semiactive systems which bridge the gap between active and formal master-slave systems: these systems allow for some degree of surgeon input that can complement the preprogrammed element of the robot.

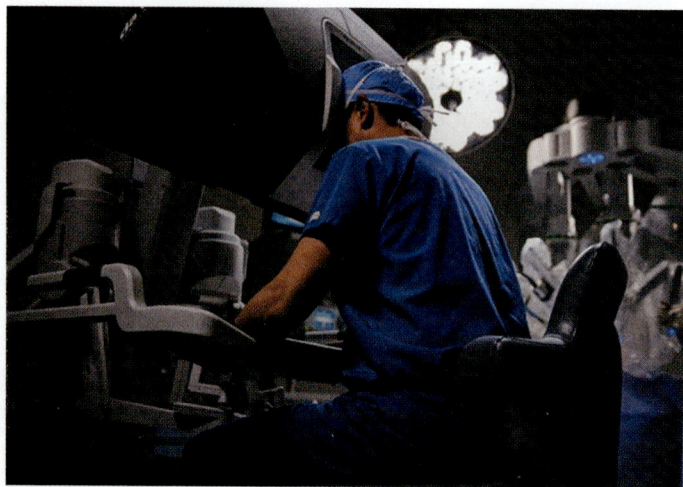

Fig. 2: Surgeon at console of the da Vinci Xi Surgical System—note the physically separate surgeon's console, allowing for the option of telesurgery.
Source: ©2021 Intuitive Surgical, Inc.

Regardless of the type of system, all surgical robots share a few common similarities. First, they allow remote control of surgeon movements and instrumentation **(Fig. 2)**. Second, there is a feedback channel whereby the surgical field can be viewed. Newer systems incorporate haptic feedback as an extra dimension. Third, they allow for modulation of the surgeon's input for more controlled, precise surgical manipulation, or to extend the physiological reach of a surgeon.[6] Many modern systems also offer telepresence or telesurgery, the ability to perform surgery from a remote location—as seen in the world's first transatlantic cholecystectomy facilitated by the ZEUS (Computer Motion, Santa Barbara, CA) system, with the operating surgeon in New York and the patient in Strasbourg, France.[7] Such systems allow surgical expertise in remote or underserved areas, and have also drawn strong interest from the defense sector due to its potential in the battlefield.

CURRENT APPLICATIONS IN OPHTHALMOLOGY

The current role of surgical robots in ophthalmology is still in its infancy. Only a handful of pioneering robotic surgeries have been performed on human eyes, notably via the da Vinci Si HD robotic Surgical System(R) (Intuitive Surgical Inc.) and the Preceyes Surgical System(R) (Preceyes BV, Eindhoven, Netherlands) as shown in **Figure 3**.

Anterior Segment Surgery

First in man robot-assisted anterior segment surgeries have been reported involving an amniotic membrane transplant (AMT) and also a pterygium excision with conjunctival autograft[8,9] **(Fig. 4)**. Following animal trials and practice with porcine eyes, both utilized the da Vinci Si HD robotic surgical

Robotic Surgery in Ophthalmology and Orbitofacial Surgery

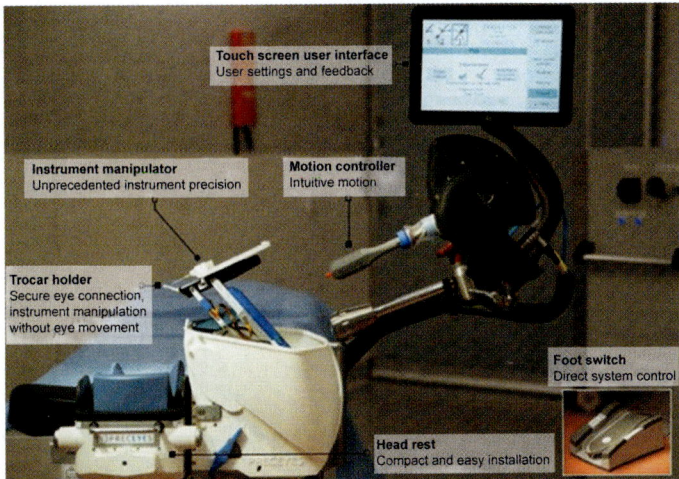

Fig. 3: The Preceyes Surgical System was used in the first successful robotic intraocular vitreoretinal surgery.

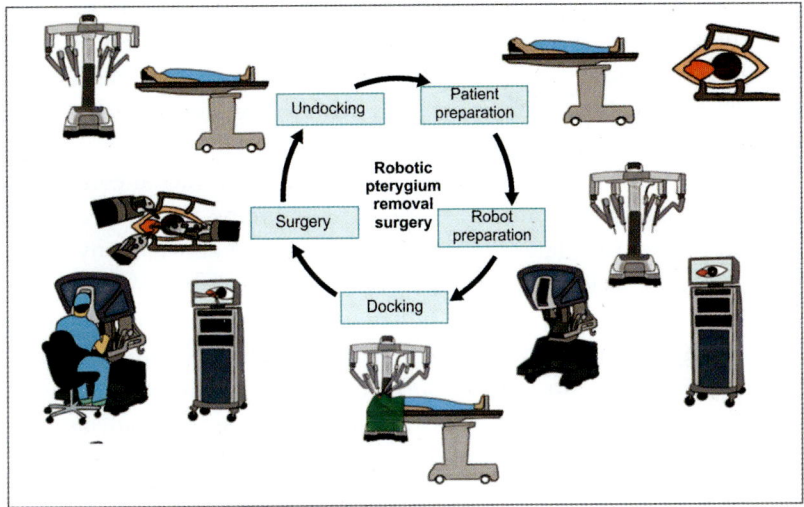

Fig. 4: Steps of robotic pterygium removal surgery. These steps are broadly used in most surgical robots currently.
Courtesy: Dr Preethi Jeyabal

system (Intuitive Surgical Inc). Three eyes were grafted with the amniotic membrane and a single patient underwent excision of a nasal and temporal pterygium with conjunctival autograft. All surgeries were uncomplicated with successful outcomes. However, the operative time was longer in both types of surgery compared to conventional methods: AMT for three eyes took a mean time of 30 min 27 sec (range 20–42 min) and the pterygium surgery took 60 min 30 sec. This was attributed to surgeon inexperience, and also the remote center of motion (pivot joint) of the robotic system being too proximal, when compared to conventional surgery. The robotic systems' remote center of motion in this case is comparable to the point of articulation of a surgeon's instrument with his fingertips. The operating team found that visualization of the operating field in terms of magnification and image quality was similar to that of a surgical microscope, and that mobility of the distally articulated arm of the robotic instrument, together with tremor filtration were advantageous especially in eyes with poor access, such as those with prominent nasal bridges or superciliary arches.

Posterior Segment Surgery

Posterior segment surgery poses a unique challenge to ophthalmologists. Three main difficulties include positioning of instruments and estimation of the force they apply, microscopic visualization, and physiological hand tremor. First, positioning of instruments within the trocar entry sites and modulation of force when doing so is important in avoiding iatrogenic injury. Second, visualization of the instrument with respect to its target site, often by utilizing the shadow it casts, is challenging for novice surgeons. Third, physiologic hand tremors have a mean amplitude of 100–150 μm, while vitreoretinal surgery requires positioning as precise as 10 μm. Together, these challenges pose a steep learning curve to most vitreoretinal surgeries that requires a high level of expertise to achieve consistently good clinical outcomes.[10]

One of the areas of vitreoretinal surgery that has attracted considerable interest for robotic assistance is epiretinal membrane (ERM) peeling—an operation that encapsulates the difficulties described above. Many types of robotic systems specific to ERM peeling have been described from as early as a decade ago, ranging from stereo vision based algorithms for motion scaling[11] to a fast sampling optical position management subsystem in the micron.[12] Most of these incorporate some form of motion attenuation or scaling and tremor filtration, as well as extended or mechanically advantageous positioning of instruments. None have been used in human eyes, with the exception of the Preceyes Surgical System (Preceyes BV, Eindhoven, Netherlands) (Preceyes).

The Preceyes was used to perform the first successful human intraocular robotic surgery, an ERM peel.[6] The system consists of a motion controller with a robotic arm that resides temporal to the patient's head, with an entry point on the globe to be aligned using an integrated electrically driven headrest. The temporal entry point allows for a reach of 130°, along with eye stabilization, tremor filtering, and motion scaling capabilities. Further developments include the capability for remote operation. A small pilot series of six patients who underwent ERM peeling with the Preceyes compared to manual surgery showed no difference in amount of retinal microtrauma, although the robotic group took longer for dissection (4 min 5 sec) compared to manual surgery (1 min 20 sec).[13]

The Preceyes was also used in a small pilot study of six patients comparing robotic assisted delivery of recombinant tissue plasminogen activator (rt-PA) via retinal vessel cannulation against manual delivery in patients with submacular hemorrhage resulting from age-related macular degeneration. Of the three patients who underwent the procedure using the Preceyes, one required completion of the injection manually. This was attributed to transient intraoperative worsening of cataract that obscured the surgical view of the cannula tip against the retina. All three eyes otherwise had the injection performed successfully.[13]

Orbital and Adnexal Surgery

Comparatively, there has been less development in robotic assisted orbital and adnexal surgery compared to posterior segment surgery. This may be due to difficult access to the surgical site for deep orbital or adnexal operations, especially for endonasal surgery, which has become an increasingly popular approach for lacrimal drainage surgery and orbital decompression.[14] There are three commercially available robotic systems for head and neck surgery—the da Vinci system, the Medrobotics Flex Robotic Systems for transoral robotic surgery (TORS), and the Medineering Robotic Endoscope Guiding System, all of which are too bulky for endoscopic orbital work.[15] Of these, only the Medineering Robotic Endoscope Guiding System has been used in endoscopic orbital surgery in a small series of eight patients undergoing endoscopic balanced orbital decompression for thyroid eye disease. The system comprises of an articulated robotic arm that holds the nasoendoscope during surgery and is positioned by a foot pedal, freeing the surgeon to use both hands.[15] No significant complications were noted and the authors found that operating time was similar to traditional endoscopic surgery, but time taken to setup the system was slightly longer (@10 minutes). This is reported to be the first use of a robotic system in orbital surgery, although the system was limited to positioning of the endoscope and did not perform the surgical procedure itself.

Strabismus Surgery

The first documented use of a surgical robotic system in strabismus surgery is limited to an experimental study on a strabismus eye model using the da Vinci Xi Surgical System (Intuitive Surgical Inc., Sunnyvale, CA).[16] The authors found that the da Vinci Xi Surgical System, a newer version of the da Vinci Surgical System, possessed the dexterity to perform almost all the steps of extraocular muscle surgery according to ICO-OSCAR (International Council of Ophthalmology's Ophthalmology Surgical Competency Assessment Rubrics) strabismus surgery guidelines, except for the forced duction tests and hooking the extraocular muscles. Similar to the case of robot-assisted orbital surgery, the authors also found that the time taken to setup the robotic system was significant, and exceeded the operative time.

As with the adoption of any new technology, cost, a longer initial setup time, and duration of surgery were common issues faced by most teams in the implementation of robotic surgery. Cost is likely to decrease with increased adoption and scale of production, much like computers and mobile phones. Setup time is expected to be reduced as bulky systems are replaced by smaller and more nimble setups. Regarding the extended duration of surgery, most authors concluded that this factor is primarily due to a learning curve, which may be reduced with practice. In summary, most of the studies looking at implementation of robotic surgery managed to show noninferiority and have concluded that it is an area brimming with potential that should be explored.

Synergistic Technologies

Robotic surgery systems, like many other modern technologies, do not exist in a vacuum. It will only achieve maximal impact when paired with other synergistic technologies. While this additional section is by no means exhaustive, it is meant to give the reader insight into the types of technologies that are likely to be paired with robotic surgical systems in the future.

Imaging

The advent of optical coherence tomography (OCT) allowed for a noncontact, in vivo imaging technique with good reproducibility and has lent itself to great clinical utility in the clinic. With spectral domain and swept source OCT, image acquisition speed and quality has improved to a point where it is now possible to utilize intraoperative OCT images to guide surgery.[17] The intraoperative OCT machine is typically mounted on the operating microscope, with newer models such as the OPMI LUMERA 700 (Carl Zeiss Meditec AG, Germany) allowing a heads up display overlaid on the operating field itself. There have already been several studies based on an intraoperative surgical robotic tool by utilizing OCT derived distance information to drive a piezoelectric micromotor, creating compensatory movements that cancels undesirable hand tremor.[18] OCT derived information in the form of a live overlay displaying anatomical layers could be used to enhance visual feedback to a surgeon who encounters difficulties in estimating depth and relevant anatomy, in the case of a hazy cornea, for example. This would be particularly useful in telerobotic surgery, where true stereopsis is currently not achievable.

Augmented and Mixed Reality

Virtual reality (VR) and its newer cousins, augmented reality (AR), and mixed reality (MR) which allow superimposition of interactive computer-generated content upon the users' surroundings have made headways in medicine and ophthalmology. Examples of such devices currently being used in the operating theater include the NGENUITY three-dimensional

(3D) visualization system (Alcon laboratories) and the TRENION 3D HD Surgical system (Carl Zeiss Meditec, Germany). The current uses for these systems are mainly for heads-up surgery, which allows for greater ergonomic comfort and the ability for shared visualization of the operating field amongst the surgical team. These would be readily incorporated into future robotic surgery systems, allowing for greater surgeon immersion and appreciation of anatomy and depth at high magnification. Visualization of the surgical field in telerobotic surgery would have to equal or surpass that of standard viewing oculars in an operating microscope before it can be widely adopted. VR, AR, and MR would be key in enabling this by presenting a faithful simulation of the actual operating field to the remote surgeon.

FIFTH GENERATION WIRELESS (5G)

One of the current bottlenecks in adoption of VR, AR, and MR is the quality and speed of wireless transmission—the large volume of data that is streamed onto such devices often exceed the limits of current wireless networks, throttling performance, which often results in a jerky, or stuttering experience. 5G, or fifth generation wireless transmission technology, promises to address this issue. The 5G features which are most relevant to healthcare include: high speed data transfer, extremely low latency [latency is defined as a delay in the data transmission-response system, and is measured in milliseconds (ms)], increased connectivity and high bandwidth, and durability within a unit area.[19] Compared to 4G long-term evolution (LTE), the current standard, 5G has a 10–100 fold improvement in transfer rate, up to 10 gigabytes per second (Gbps). It also has a network latency of <1 ms, compared with 30–50 ms for 4G LTE.

In the field of telerobotic surgery and VR/AR/MR, high transfer rates with low latencies are crucial. Many functionalities of AR/MR devices are predicated on superimposition of radiographic images onto the patient, mapping scans to the actual patient and highlighting pathology or anatomy. This is optimized only when the wireless connection is fast, responsive, and secure. With radiographic images such as computed tomography (CT) scan files commonly exceeding 0.5–1 Gigabytes, the need for 5G transfer rates is clear. The argument for low latencies is just as strong in telerobotic surgery— higher latency equals to an increased "reaction time" from the remote surgeon to the robot. Many telerobotic surgeries would simply not be possible, or too risky to perform using a high latency platform. In a 2004 study of surgeons' tolerance for latency using a porcine laparoscopic cholecystectomy model, most felt the minimum standard of latency that they felt comfortable performing surgery was 330 ms and below.[20] One would expect the standard for human surgery to be much stricter.

Though documented use of telerobotic surgery via a 5G network is limited, there has been at least one study which looked at 12 cases of telerobotic spinal surgery based on a 5G network.[21] By having a surgeon in a master control room in Beijing manipulate the telerobot remotely, the study team was able to utilize a "one to many" workflow where the leading surgeon in the master control room performed screw planning, path positioning, and image verification on up to three consecutive patients in three separate hospitals. The rest of the surgery was performed by surgeons on site. By having a senior surgeon perform the crucial task of screw placement and planning remotely, the team was able to leverage the senior surgeon's skill remotely in the other physically separate hospitals. One patient suffered a cerebrospinal fluid leak but this was attributed to nerve decompression that was performed by the surgical team on site, rather than the robotic manipulation of the screw. No other complications or network errors were encountered. The authors conclude that the 5G network was essential to overcoming the issues of transmission latency and instability in telerobotic spine surgery.

It is easy to understand why there has been much interest in 5G among proponents of robotic surgery and the growing adoption of the standard means it will only be a matter of when, not if, this would become an integral part of robotic surgery.

THE FUTURE

Having delved into the current advances and limitations of robotic surgery and its complementary technologies, we now come to the most speculative yet exciting part of this chapter—a hypothetical future that one may expect. While prediction is often an inexact science, it offers us a chance to conceptualize and work toward a better future, one that may eventually surpass our wildest ambitions.

Let us imagine a fictional patient, John—who is in his 60s and is working onboard one of many small space stations that orbit around the earth, much like the International Space Station of today. One day, while working, he accidentally hits his left eye and suffers a corneal laceration. He is quickly attended to by his crew, none of whom are ophthalmologists or trained surgeons. One of them, the crew medic, quickly puts on his headset and initiates a secure communication channel with the on-call medical team based on the earth. Using futuristic 6G technology, where the channel is free of interference and seamless, the on-call ophthalmologist, using a paired headset to see exactly what the medic sees, is able to direct the rest of the physical examination and diagnoses a full thickness laceration. He instructs that John be docked to the on-board surgical station, in preparation for the laceration repair. Required suture materials are quickly printed via the on-board 3D printer. Utilizing the telerobot in his console on the earth which provides resolution that far surpasses the human limit of 120 pixels per degree of arc, the surgeon is able to assess and repair the laceration, accurately gauging the depth and tension of his corneal suturing with the integrated surgical OCT and real time corneal topography, showing him the effects of his suture tension on astigmatism. The surgery is easily performed with the telerobot eliminating all tremor and scaling the surgeon's motions precisely. Appropriate postsurgical care is performed via the aid of MR systems, and John is able to regain good visual function. What would have been considered a sight threatening injury in years past was treated effectively, thanks to telerobotic surgery and its synergistic technologies.

While this scenario might seem unthinkable, it is a useful thought experiment where the potential challenges of future systems may be explored. It also serves to remind us that we should always strive to aim, sometimes literally, for the stars.

CONCLUSION

Robotic surgery has seen an exponential growth in the medical field across many specialties, with ophthalmology being a direct beneficiary. Being a relatively new technology, widespread adoption is limited by its cost, learning curve, risk of complications, and form factor. However, with developments in robotic engineering and the refinement of capabilities such as tremor cancelation, haptic feedback, OCT-based distance sensing, and sensor-servo functions, it will merely be a matter of time before robotic surgery is common place. Before that happens, we strongly advocate continued support and investigation into this nascent but exciting field.

ACKNOWLEDGMENTS

The authors would like to acknowledge Dr Joseph Ng and Dr Preethi Jeyabal for their kind contributions to this work.

REFERENCES

1. Kwoh YS, Hou J, Jonckheere EA, Hayati S. A robot with improved absolute positioning accuracy for CT-guided stereotactic brain surgery. IEEE Trans Biomed Eng. 1988;35(2):153-60.
2. Jeganathan VSE, Shah S. Robotic technology in ophthalmic surgery. Curr Opin Ophthalmol. 2010;21(1):75-80.
3. Harris SJ, Arambula-Cosio F, Mei Q, Hibberd RD, Davies BL, Wickham JE, et al. The Probot: an active robot for prostate resection. Proc Inst Mech Eng H. 1997;211(4):317-25.
4. Gomez G. Sabiston Textbook of Surgery, 17th edition. Emerging technology in surgery: informatics, electronics, robotics. Philadelphia. Pa: Elsevier Saunders; 2004.
5. Lane T. A short history of robotic surgery. Ann R Coll Surg Engl. 2018;100(6 Supp): 5-7.
6. de Smet MD, Naus GJL, Faridpooya K, Mura M. Robotic-assisted surgery in ophthalmology. Curr Opin Ophthalmol. 2018;29(3):248-53.
7. Gottlieb S. Surgeons perform transatlantic operation using fibreoptics. BMJ. 2001;323:713.
8. Bourcier T, Becmeur PH, Mutter D. Robotically assisted amniotic membrane transplant surgery. JAMA Ophthalmol. 2015;133(2):213-4.

9. Bourcier T, Chammas J, Becmeur PH, Danan J, Sauer A, Gaucher D, et al. Robotically assisted pterygium surgery: first human case. Cornea. 2015;34(10):1329-30.
10. Nuzzi R, Brusasco L. State-of-the-art of robotic surgery related to vision: brain and eye applications of newly available devices. Eye Brain. 2018;10:13-24.
11. Becker BC, MacLachlan RA, Lobes LA, Riviere CN. Vision-based retinal membrane peeling with a handheld robot. 2012 IEEE Int Conf Robot Autom. 2012:1075-80.
12. Adeghate J, Han Y, Routray A, Riviere C, Martel J. Membrane-peeling with a handheld tremor-cancelling robotic device for vitreoretinal surgery. Invest Ophthalmol Vis Sci. 2020;61(7):3727.
13. Edwards TL, Xue K, Meenink HCM, Beelen MJ, Naus GJL, Simunovic MP, et al. First-in-human study of the safety and viability of intraocular robotic surgery. Nat Biomed Eng. 2018;2:649-56.
14. Juniat V, Abbeel L, McGilligan JA, Curragh D, Selva D, Rajak S. Endoscopic orbital decompression by oculoplastic surgeons for proptosis in thyroid eye disease. Ophthalmic Plast Reconstr Surg. 2019;35(6):590-3.
15. Mattheis S, Schlüter A, Stähr K, Holtmann L, Höing B, Hussain T, et al. First use of a new robotic endoscope guiding system in endoscopic orbital decompression. Ear Nose Throat J. 2019:145561319885803.
16. Bourcier T, Chammas J, Gaucher D, Liverneaux P, Marescaux J, Speeg-Schatz C, et al. Robot-assisted simulated strabismus surgery. Transl Vis Sci Technol. 2019;8(3):26.
17. Leisser C, Hirnschall N, Hackl C, Döller B, Varsits R, Findl O. Diagnostic precision of a microscope-integrated intraoperative OCT device in patients with epiretinal membranes. Eur J Ophthalmol. 2018;28(3):329-32.
18. Song C, Gehlbach PL, Kang JU. Active tremor cancellation by a "smart" handheld vitreoretinal microsurgical tool using swept source optical coherence tomography. Opt Express. 2012;20(21):23414-21.
19. Li D. 5G and intelligence medicine-how the next generation of wireless technology will reconstruct healthcare? Precis Clin Med. 2019;2(4):205-8.
20. Butner SE, Ghodoussi M. Transforming a surgical robot for human telesurgery. IEEE Trans Robot Auto. 2003;19(5):818-24.
21. Tian W, Fan M, Zeng C, Liu Y, He D, Zhang Q. Telerobotic Spinal Surgery Based on 5G Network: The First 12 Cases. Neurospine. 2020;17(1):114-20.

CHAPTER 4

Advances in Corneal Crosslinking

Chris HL Lim, Ray Manotosh

ABSTRACT

Corneal crosslinking (CXL) with riboflavin and ultraviolet light (UVA) is a novel technique of strengthening corneal tissue. Riboflavin acts as a photosensitizer and its reaction with UVA facilitates formation of intra- as well as interfibrillar covalent bonds by oxidation. The primary goal of CXL is to strengthen the overall corneal biomechanics. CXL, which was initially proposed for the treatment of keratoconus, has undergone a series of modifications to overcome shortcomings of the original (Dresden) protocol. Its effectiveness has led to further adoption of this treatment modality for an increasing number of indications. These include the management of patients with infective keratitis; with a technique termed photo-activated chromophore for keratitis-corneal crosslinking (PACK-CXL), development of customized protocols (CuRV) to induce targeted stiffening, and as an adjunct to refractive laser correction surgery (LASIK Xtra and SMILE Xtra). In this chapter, we explore efforts made to improve upon the efficacy of this original technique, the growing number of indications, and safety profile of this technique.

Keywords: Collagen crosslinking, PACK-CXL, CuRV, Dresden protocol, accelerated protocol, keratoconus, infective keratitis, myopia, LASIK Xtra, SMILE Xtra.

INTRODUCTION

Corneal ectasias are a group of disorders characterized by progressive corneal steepening, thinning, and refractive changes. These include conditions such as keratoconus, pellucid marginal degeneration, keratoglobus and either postrefractive surgery or post-traumatic corneal ectasia.[1] These disorders can be progressive and debilitating, and impact upon an individual's sight and their daily functioning.

Management of patients with corneal ectasias encompasses conservative options such as spectacles and contact lenses. Surgical therapeutic options include implantation of intrastromal corneal ring segments and corneal transplantation. Although surgical management has been demonstrated to be effective, this modality of treatment is costly, labor-intensive, requires

> **BOX 1:** Indications for corneal crosslinking.
> - *Corneal ectatic disorders*:
>   – Keratoconus
>   – Pellucid marginal degeneration
>   – Terrien marginal degeneration
>   – Postrefractive surgery (such as LASIK, PRK, or radial keratotomy)
> - Bullous keratopathy
> - Microbial keratitis
> - Refractive surgery

(LASIK: laser-assisted in situ keratomileusis; PRK: photorefractive keratectomy)

highly-skilled surgical expertise and careful postoperative care to ensure good visual outcomes.[2] Corneal grafting procedures such as penetrating keratoplasties, require patients to be on life-long topical corticosteroids. There is also compromise of the globe architecture, which places patients at an increased lifetime risk of developing globe rupture.[3]

Preventive strategies to minimize progression includes advice to minimize eye rubbing, management of the itch-stimulus, and techniques to assist with structural stabilization of the cornea.[4,5] These include the use of intrastromal corneal rings, collagen crosslinking (CXL), or a combination of the above techniques.[6]

Corneal collagen crosslinking was first described by Dr Theo Seiler and his team from the University of Dresden in 1998. They demonstrated the efficacy of riboflavin 0.5% coupled with UVA irradiation in producing increased stiffness on porcine corneas.[7] Further in-vivo trials on rabbit and human eyes were performed, which led to the Food and Drug Administration (FDA) approval of corneal crosslinking in the management of patients with keratoconus and postlaser-assisted in situ keratomileusis (LASIK) ectasia in 2016.[8] Other applications of CXL have since been described **(Box 1)**.

PROPOSED MECHANISM OF ACTION

Collagen is the main structural protein in various tissues and is responsible for the integrity of various organs. Crosslinks between collagen fibrils and stromal substrates strengthens this structure. This may be driven by enzymatic, glycosylation, or oxidative pathways.

Enzymatic crosslinking occurs as part of the natural aging process. This is driven by lysyl oxidase which facilitates oxidative deamination within collagen end chains.[9] This has been suggested to account for improvements in keratometric stability of patients with keratectasias with age.

Glycosylation commonly occurs in patients with diabetes mellitus as part of the Maillard reaction and results from bonding between advanced glycosylation end products and a protein amino group.[10,11] Glycosylation products have been identified in the corneas of diabetic patients, predominantly within the epithelial, Bowman's and endothelial layers.[11]

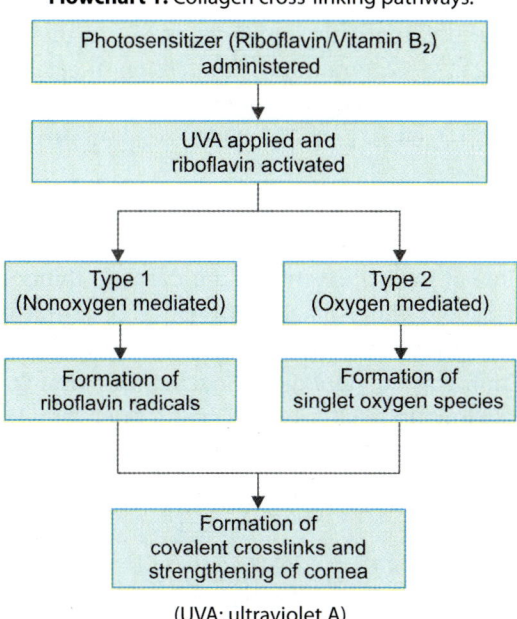

Flowchart 1: Collagen cross-linking pathways.

(UVA: ultraviolet A)

This may enhance the biomechanical strength of collagen, as reported by Kuo et al., where patients with diabetes were found to have a decreased risk of progression of keratoconus.[12]

Crosslinking, on the other hand, has been proposed to utilize both oxygen mediated and non-oxygen mediated pathways **(Flowchart 1)**.[13] Oxidative reactions form covalent bonds between collagen fibrils and stromal substrates, which occurs via chemical and structural changes initiated by the interaction between riboflavin and UV light.[13] Rapid depletion of oxygen has been observed during crosslinking procedures.[14] It has been suggested that the mechanism of action occurs through free radical formation—either singlet oxygen, excited riboflavin triplets, or changes in glycosaminoglycan synthesis.[13,15,16] Riboflavin, acting as a photoactivated chromophore, converts collagen monomers into crosslinked polymers. Riboflavin further absorbs UVA, thereby preventing injuries to deeper ocular structures.

INDICATIONS

Corneal Ectasias

CXL has been recommended to halt progression of unstable corneal ectasias. It is FDA approved and recommended for patients with keratoconus or post-refractive ectasia, although its effectiveness for other conditions such as Terrien's marginal degeneration and pellucid marginal degeneration has been reported. Parameters crucial in assessing suitability of patients include corneal tomographic or topographic changes and stability of visual acuity.

The first clinical trial of CXL for keratoconus was published in 2003.[17] 23 eyes belonging to 22 patients underwent CXL. At the last documented follow-up (mean 23.2 ± 12.9 months), progression of ectasia was ceased in 70% of patients. An average improvement in best corrected visual acuity of 1.26 lines (95% CI: −0.68 to 2.21, p = 0.026) was reported in 65% of study patients.

Pircher et al. performed a retrospective analysis of 14 eyes with a diagnosis of pellucid marginal degeneration that underwent CXL.[18] An increase in mean measurements of the cornea's thinnest point on the inferior vertical Scheimpflug image from 456 ± 74 μm at baseline to 495 ± 74 μm at 1 year of follow-up (p = 0.03) was identified. Mean K values in the central 5.0 mm zone obtained via Scheimpflug tomography remained stable at 1-year follow-up (43.37 ± 3.83 D compared with 43.72 ± 1.63 D at baseline, P = 0.78). An improvement in corrected distance visual acuity was also reported.

Microbial Keratitis

Use of CXL in the management of patients with microbial keratitis has also been described in the literature. Termed photoactivated chromophore for infectious keratitis-corneal collagen cross-linking (PACK-CXL), it has been suggested to improve healing and inhibit corneal melting.[19,20]

The effect of UVA and riboflavin has been suggested to be synergistic in this instance, with UVA directly damaging microbial deoxyribonucleic acid (DNA) and ribonucleic acid (RNA), thereby inhibiting replication.[21] Photoactivated riboflavin further releases free radicals, which damages cell membranes and nucleic acids.[22]

A systematic review investigating the combination of CXL with antimicrobial therapy found limited evidence supporting the safety and efficacy of this treatment, which was exacerbated by small sample sizes and high risks of selection and performance bias of the included randomized control trials.[23]

Bullous Keratopathy

CXL has been described in the management of patients with Fuchs' endothelial dystrophy. Use of the conventional protocol for this purpose was first reported by Ehlers et al.[24] Four out of 11 treated eyes required retreatment, while variability in visual acuity improvement was also reported. Further modifications to the conventional corneal CXL protocol include the use of intraoperative glycerol 70% or preoperative use of glucose 40% to dehydrate corneas of patients afflicted with Fuchs' endothelial dystrophy.[25,26] In both studies, reduction in central corneal thickness (CCT) and either maintenance or improvement in best corrected visual acuity (BCVA) was reported, with no further need for retreatment.

TECHNIQUES AND REPORTED EFFICACY
Dresden Protocol

The original protocol (or "Dresden" protocol) uses a UVA light source (365–370 nm) and riboflavin 0.1% (vitamin B_2) in 20% dextran (**Box 2 and Figs. 1A to D**).[17] This is typically performed under topical anesthesia with no or minimal sedation. The central 7–9 mm of corneal epithelium is debrided and riboflavin 0.1% in dextran 20% drops administered topically; first applied every 2 minutes for 30 minutes. UVA diodes are subsequently placed to provide irradiance of the central cornea of 3 mW/cm² for a treatment duration of 30 minutes and surface dose of 5.4 J/cm². Riboflavin drops are continuously administered every 5 minutes during the irradiation process.

BOX 2: Dresden protocol for collagen crosslinking.
- Eyes anesthetized with topical tetracaine 1%
- Central corneal epithelium debrided
- Riboflavin 0.1% with 20% dextran 500 instilled every 3 minutes for 30 minutes
- Ultraviolet A radiance of 3 mW/cm² irradiated continuously for 30 minutes (cumulative dose of 5.4 J/cm²)
- Cornea irrigated with balanced salt solution, topical antibiotics, and bandage contact lens applied thereafter
- Patient provided with topical corticosteroids and antibiotics for self-administration prior to discharge and tapered over a month postoperatively

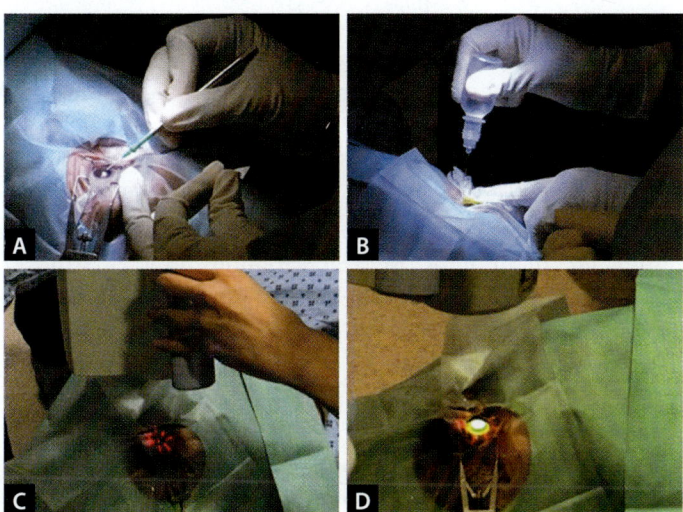

Figs. 1A to D: (A) Prepping and draping of patient followed by corneal de-epithelialization with a pterygium blade; (B) Riboflavin is applied to the corneal surface as specified in the protocol and washed off with balanced salt solution; (C) Once the corneal thickness has been determined to be of adequate thickness, precalibrated treatment parameters are counter-checked and the ultraviolet-A machine is positioned and aligned; (D) The machine is activated for the specified duration. Following which the anterior surface of the eye is irrigated with balanced salt solution and a topical antibiotic and steroid administered prior to application of a bandage contact lens.

A bandage contact lens is applied and patients are instructed to administer topical antibiotics and steroids following the procedure. Most patients are able to return to contact lenses in 1–2 weeks following treatment. A minimum corneal thickness of 400 μm following epithelial removal was recommended following safety studies establishing that cytotoxic endothelial UVA irradiance of 0.35 mW/cm² is reached at 400 μm.[27]

Criticisms of the original protocol involved the duration of this procedure and discomfort patients experienced with epithelium removal, along with associated risks. Removal of the epithelium has been associated with pain, corneal haze or scarring, development of sterile infiltrates or a diffuse lamellar keratitis type presentation, infective keratitis, and scarring which can impact upon the final visual acuity achieved.[17,28] Minimal corneal thickness for safety also precluded offering corneal CXL to patients with advanced keratoconus. Subsequent efforts at modifying this protocol to address these concerns have achieved varying degrees of success.

Accelerated Protocols

The accelerated protocol **(Box 3)** delivers a higher irradiance to the cornea to reduce the light exposure time.[29] Bunsen-Roscoe's law (BRL) of photochemical reciprocity suggests that the photochemical effect is proportional to the total energy delivered, independent of the duration of administration.[30] However, this relationship only holds over a range of exposure duration.[31] Lin et al. sought to model the relationship between exposure time and UVA intensity and have proposed a nonlinear scaling relationship.[32] Their model predicts the need for a longer exposure time for UVA intensity higher than 3 mW/cm². They have also suggested that the optimal UVA intensity ranges from 3 to 30 mW/cm².

Similar to the conventional method described above, the corneal epithelium is debrided and riboflavin 0.1% in 20% dextran is administered every minute for 10 minutes. Several variations in UVA exposure have been described in the literature to achieve a cumulative dose of 5.4 J/cm². Suggested modifications include irradiation with UVA at 30 mW/cm² for 3 minutes or 9 mW/cm² for 10 minutes.[33,34] The latter has been purported to be more effective and safer compared to higher irradiation doses.[35]

BOX 3: Accelerated protocol for collagen crosslinking.

- Eyes anesthetized with topical tetracaine 1%
- Central corneal epithelium debrided
- Riboflavin 0.1% with hydroxypropyl methylcellulose instilled every 2 minutes for 10 minutes
- Ultraviolet A radiance of 30 mW/cm² for 3 minutes 40 seconds (cumulative dose of 6.6 J/cm²)
- Cornea irrigated with balanced salt solution, topical antibiotics and bandage contact lens applied thereafter
- Patient provided with topical corticosteroids and antibiotics for self-administration prior to discharge and tapered over a month postoperatively

Transepithelial Protocols

Transepithelial protocols have been developed to obviate the need to de-epithelize the cornea and decrease discomfort associated with the procedure. This further reduces the risks of developing complications associated with denuding the epithelium, such as infective keratitis, stromal haze, and scaring and corneal melt.[36] Preservation of the epithelium increases corneal thickness and may confer further protection to the corneal endothelial cells. However, the barrier function of the epithelium limits availability of riboflavin, UVA, and oxygen within the corneal stroma—vital components to crosslinking.

This has been coupled with methods of improving riboflavin absorption including the use of topical medications [such as tetracaine, benzalkonium chloride (BAK)/ethylenediaminetetraacetic acid (EDTA), and trometamol] to loosen intraepithelial junctions, femtosecond laser facilitated intrastromal 0.1% riboflavin administration, and iontophoresis.[37-40] Hill et al. have also reported supplemental oxygen delivery as a method of optimizing the effects of corneal CXL.[41]

Caporossi et al. examined the efficacy of transepithelial crosslinking using modified riboflavin and reported evidence of corneal stability for up to 12 months. Instability at 24 months was reported with worsening of measured simulated maximum K values, increase in spherical aberration, and reduction in pachymetry readings.[42] This was particularly evident in patients aged 18 years and younger, who typically experience a more aggressive disease course. 50% of pediatric patients subsequently required retreatment with the conventional protocol due to evidence of progression.

The Boost epithelium-on protocol is a recent approach to transepithelial CXL. Several modifications have been made to overcome limitations conferred by the barrier function of the epithelium and optimize conditions for CXL. In this protocol, riboflavin concentration has been increased to 0.25%, while UVA fluence has been increased from 5.4 to 10 J/cm^2 (1 second: 1 second, pulsed).[43,44] This accounts for absorption of UVA energy by the epithelium. Identification of comparatively increased oxygen consumption of the corneal epithelium compared to the stroma has also resulted in the development and use of the Boost goggles, which creates a hyperoxic environment; with oxygen saturation >90%. This has been purported to increase oxygen diffusion by fivefold compared to normal conditions. Pulsed UVA light has also been used to increase intraoperative oxygen availability.[45]

Comparison of Conventional, Accelerated, and Epithelium-on Protocols

A comparison of the microstructural changes on imaging associated with these three methods has also been performed.[46-48] As reported by Bouheraoua et al., a demarcation line was seen in 93% of patients undergoing conventional

CXL (C-CXL), 87.5% undergoing accelerated CXL (A-CXL) and 47.7.% undergoing iontophoresis assisted CXL (I-CXL).[46] It was deepest in patients undergoing C-CXL (mean depth of 302.8 μm, SD 74.6), followed by I-CXL (212 μm, SD 36.5) and A-XCL (184.2 μm, SD 38.9). No correlation between the depth of a demarcation line seen on anterior segment optical coherence tomography (AS-OCT) and changes to visual acuity and keratometry readings has been reported.[46,48] A similar study examining the presence of a demarcation line on AS-OCT following I-CXL found demarcation lines present at a depth of between 200 and 250 μm.[49] Different iontophoresis devices were used in these studies, which may account for the variation in findings.

On confocal microscopy, the accelerated protocol was found to be associated with increased keratocyte and nerve apoptosis compared to conventional CXL.[47,46] Resolution of these differences was noted between 3 and 6 months following the procedure.[46,47]

Protocols for Thin Corneas

A minimum corneal thickness of 400 μm after epithelial removal has been suggested to minimize fallout of endothelial cell density following standard CXL.[50] The original formulation of riboflavin in the Dresden protocol contained 20% dextran T-500 which had a deturgescent effect, resulting in a reduction in corneal thickness.[51] A trial of hypoosmolar dextran-free riboflavin solution was performed by Hafezi et al. on patients with thin corneas with an average stromal thickness of 320 μm. Of 20 patients, all except one patient experienced stabilization of their corneal ectasia with no signs of endothelial damage.[52]

However, the efficacy of this approach may have its limitations, as corneal elastic modulus has been reported to be depth-dependent.[53] CXL affects predominantly the anterior stroma; as evidenced by keratocyte apoptosis and the presence of a demarcation line in the anterior stroma.[54,55] Insufficient residual anterior corneal stroma may hinder the ability to achieve a sufficient biomechanical effect conferred by CXL.[56,57]

Customized Protocols

Customized CXL utilizes targeted activation of riboflavin with customized UVA shapes to induce targeted stiffening.

Seiler et al. applied customized irradiation patterns with energy fluence of 9 mW/cm^2 (total energy levels ranging between 5.4 and 10 J/cm^2) centered over the area of maximum posterior float.[58] These results were compared against patients receiving conventional CXL. About 37% of patients receiving customized protocols (CuRV) compared to 11% of patients undergoing conventional CXL experienced flattening of two or more diopters over a 12-month follow-up period.

Al Saidi et al. performed targeted treatment of 54 adult eyes and followed these patients up over a period of 12 months.[59] Three different energy levels: 5.4, 7.2, and 10 J/cm² were applied to the area of interest with the largest energy dose focused over the central aspect of steepest posterior float. Of these, 89% of patients experienced either stability or improvement in their vision, while improvements in the uncorrected visual acuity (UCVA) demonstrated continuous improvement up till the 12-month follow-up period. 61% of patients demonstrated greater than a diopter flattening at 12 months, while none of the patients had worsening of more than a diopter. Flattening of K_{max} was also demonstrated in both groups over 6 months postoperatively with subsequent stability demonstrated. Al Ajmi reported a case series of eight eyes of four pediatric patients who underwent epithelium-off CuRV treatment with follow-up of up to 9 months.[60] Of these patients, the recorded visual acuity was either stable or demonstrated improvements following treatment.

Laser-assisted In Situ Keratomileusis Xtra and Small Incision Lenticule Extraction Xtra

Of interest would be the combination of CXL concomitantly administered to patients undergoing refractive surgery.

A study by Konstantopoulos et al. examining LASIK Xtra and small incision lenticule extraction (SMILE) Xtra protocols in LASIK rabbit ectasia models demonstrated that mean K values decreased significantly following all modalities of treatment. Mean posterior elevation following post-LASIK Xtra was reduced compared to conventional LASIK.[61] LASIK Xtra has also been reported to confer greater refractive stability with a smaller refractive shift in manifest refraction spherical equivalent at the 2-year follow-up period.[62] In a study by Tan et al. examining the efficacy of LASIK Xtra in high myopes (−8.00 to −19.00 D), 98% of patients (n = 70) undergoing LASIK Xtra achieved an uncorrected distance visual acuity of 20/25 or better at 3 months follow-up postoperatively, compared to 61% (n = 64) of patients in a retrospective consecutive control group undergoing LASIK.[63] 88% of those in the LASIK Xtra group were also within 0.50 of their intended correction, compared to 65% of patients in the LASIK-only group.

Combination Protocols

The Athens Protocol, which combines same-day topography-guided partial PRK with cornea CXL, has been further recommended for patients with ectatic conditions.[64] Patients first undergo phototherapeutic keratectomy to the central 6.5 mm to remove 50 μm of epithelium. Thereafter, topography-guided partial PRK is performed with treatment targeted toward the area of steepening to normalize the corneal surface. Mitomycin C 0.02% of 20 seconds duration is applied to the treated area before proceeding with CXL.[64] A comparison of patients with keratoconus undergoing this protocol versus those who had CXL followed by delayed topography-guided surface ablation favored combination of these procedures.[64] This included a greater improvement across measured parameters, including mean logMAR UCVA, BCVA, along with a greater mean reduction in the manifest refraction spherical equivalent and keratometry values. Patients who underwent concurrent treatment also experienced less corneal haze compared to those who were sequentially treated. Reduction in CCT and changes in endothelial cell density were similar in both groups.[65] Further concurrent treatment combinations, such as the use of CXL with phototherapeutic keratectomy and intrastromal ring segment implantation for the management of keratoconus, have also been reported and found to be effective.[66]

CONTRAINDICATIONS

Several exclusion criteria for this modality of treatment have been suggested. These include patients who are either pregnant or lactating, those with prior herpetic infections, active ophthalmic inflammation, severe central or paracentral corneal scars, severe ocular surface disease, autoimmune disorders, and a history of poor epithelial wound healing. Corneal thickness of <400 μm is a relative contraindication, which can be circumvented by modification of the composition of riboflavin solutions used.[52]

RISKS AND COMPLICATIONS

While the current long-term risk of malignancies is not well-established, UVA light is cytotoxic and possesses risks of inciting development of ocular surface neoplasia.[67] Further risks associated with CXL varies depending on the protocol used. In addition to the risks of developing a persistent epithelial defect, infective keratitis, stromal haze, scaring and corneal melt, other risks include inciting corneal endothelial decompensation and damage to the lens or the retina.[17] Development of herpetic keratouveitis and late onset of peripheral ulcerative keratitis (PUK) following CXL has also been reported.[68,69]

CONCLUSION

CXL has been widely accepted as an efficacious and safe treatment of patients with keratectasias. Significant interest has driven research to modify and augment the original Dresden protocol, and extend the application of this modality of treatment beyond the scope of patients with keratoconus and postrefractive corneal ectasia. These evolving advancements demonstrate that this form of treatment has yet to reach its full potential and further modifications may provide greater efficacy, safety, and a larger degree of customization.

ACKNOWLEDGMENTS

The authors would like to acknowledge Dr Charmaine Chai and Dr Blanche Lim for contributing the images included in this book chapter.

REFERENCES

1. Hafezi F, Kanellopoulos J, Wiltfang R, Seiler T. Corneal collagen crosslinking with riboflavin and ultraviolet A to treat induced keratectasia after laser in situ keratomileusis. J Cataract Refract Surg. 2007;33:2035-40.
2. Roussy JPF, Aubin MJ, Brunette I, Lachaine J. Cost of corneal transplantation for the Quebec healthcare system. Canadian J Ophthalmol. 2009;44:36-41.
3. Ross AH, Jones MN, Nguyen DQ, Jaycock PD, Armitage WJ, Cook SD, et al. Long-term topical steroid treatment after penetrating keratoplasty in patients with pseudophakic bullous keratopathy. Ophthalmology. 2009;116:2369-72.
4. Balasubramanian SA, Pye DC, Willcox MD. Effects of eye rubbing on the levels of protease, protease activity and cytokines in tears: relevance in keratoconus. Clin Exp Optom. 2013;96:214-8.
5. Jafri B, Lichter H, Stulting RD. Asymmetric keratoconus attributed to eye rubbing. Cornea. 2004;23:560-4.
6. Torquetti L, Berbel RF, Ferrara P. Long-term follow-up of intrastromal corneal ring segments in keratoconus. J Cataract Refract Surg. 2009;35:1768-73.
7. Spoerl E, Huhle M, Seiler T. Induction of crosslinks in corneal tissue. Exp Eye Res. 1998;66:97-103.
8. Lowes R. FDA Approves Photrexa for Corneal Crosslinking in Keratoconus. Medscape Medical News 2016. [online] Available from: https://www.medscape.com/viewarticle/862122. [Last accessed May, 2021].
9. Takaoka A, Babar N, Hogan J, Kim M, Price MO, Price FW, et al. An evaluation of lysyl oxidase-derived crosslinking in keratoconus by liquid chromatography/mass spectrometry. Invest Ophthalmol Vis Sci. 2016;57:126-36.
10. Sady C, Khosrof S, Nagaraj R. Advanced Maillard reaction and crosslinking of corneal collagen in diabetes. Biochem Biophys Res Commun. 1995;214:793-7.
11. Dawczynski J, Franke S, Blum M, Kasper M, Stein G, Strobel J. Advanced glycation end-products in corneas of patients with keratoconus. Graefe's Arch Clin Exp Ophthalmol. 2002;240:296-301.
12. Kuo IC, Broman A, Pirouzmanesh A, Melia M. Is there an association between diabetes and keratoconus? Ophthalmology. 2006;113:184-90.
13. Kamaev P, Friedman MD, Sherr E, Muller D. Photochemical kinetics of corneal cross-linking with riboflavin. Invest Ophthalmol Vis Sci. 2012;53:2360-7.
14. Richoz O, Hammer A, Tabibian D, Gatzioufas Z, Hafezi F. The biomechanical effect of corneal collagen crosslinking (CXL) with riboflavin and UV-A is oxygen dependent. Transl Vis Sci Technol. 2013;2(7):6.
15. Diniz C, Gadelha F, Michelacci Y, Campos M. Effects of riboflavin and UV upon glycosaminoglycan synthesis in human keratoconic corneas. Invest Ophthalmol Vis Sci. 2009;50:5461.
16. Ryu A, Naru E, Arakane K, Masunaga T, Shinmoto K, Nagano T, et al. Cross-linking of collagen by singlet oxygen generated with UV-A. Chem Pharmaceut Bulletin. 1997;45:1243-7.
17. Wollensak G, Spoerl E, Seiler T. Riboflavin/ultraviolet-A-induced collagen crosslinking for the treatment of keratoconus. Am J Ophthalmol. 2003;135:620-7.
18. Pircher N, Lammer J, Holzer S, Gschließer A, Schmidinger G. Corneal crosslinking for pellucid marginal degeneration. J Cataract Refract Surg. 2019;45:1163-7.

19. Iseli HP, Thiel MA, Hafezi F, Kampmeier J, Seiler T. Ultraviolet A/riboflavin corneal cross-linking for infectious keratitis associated with corneal melts. Cornea. 2008;27:590-4.
20. Makdoumi K, Mortensen J, Sorkhabi O, Malmvall BE, Crafoord S. UVA-riboflavin photochemical therapy of bacterial keratitis: a pilot study. Graefe's Arch Clin Exp Ophthalmol. 2012;250:95-102.
21. Russell AD, Hugo WB, Ayliffe GAJ. Radiation sterilization. In: Russell AD, Hugo WB, Ayliffe GAJ (Eds). Principles and Practice of Disinfection, Preservation and Sterilization. Oxford: Blackwell Scientific Ltd.; 1999. pp. 675-702.
22. Vazirani J, Vaddavalli PK. Cross-linking for microbial keratitis. Indian J Ophthalmol. 2013;61:441.
23. Davis SA, Bovelle R, Han G, Kwagyan J. Corneal collagen crosslinking for bacterial infectious keratitis. Cochrane Database Syst Rev. 2020.
24. Ehlers N, Hjortdal J. Riboflavin-ultraviolet light induced cross-linking in endothelial decompensation. Acta Ophthalmologica. 2008;86:549-51.
25. Hafezi F, Dejica P, Majo F. Modified corneal collagen crosslinking reduces corneal oedema and diurnal visual fluctuations in Fuchs dystrophy. Br J Ophthalmol. 2010;94:660-1.
26. Wollensak G, Aurich H, Wirbelauer C, Pham DT. Potential use of riboflavin/UVA crosslinking in bullous keratopathy. Ophthalmic Res. 2009;41:114-7.
27. Kolozsvári L, Nógrádi A, Hopp Bl, Bor Z. UV absorbance of the human cornea in the 240- to 400-nm range. Invest Ophthalmol Vis Sci. 2002;43:2165-8.
28. Evangelista CB, Hatch KM. Corneal collagen cross-linking complications. Semin Ophthalmol. 2018;33:29-35.
29. Rocha KM, Qian Y, Ramos-Esteban JC, Krueger RR, Herekar S. Comparative study of riboflavin-UVA cross-linking and "flash-linking" using surface wave elastometry. J Refract Surg. 2008;24:S748-51.
30. Schindl A, Rosado-Schlosser B, Trautinger F. Reciprocity regulation in photobiology: an overview. Der Hautarzt; Zeitschrift fur Dermatologie, Venerologie, und Verwandte Gebiete. 2001;52:779-85.
31. Wernli J, Schumacher S, Spoerl E, Mrochen M. The efficacy of corneal cross-linking shows a sudden decrease with very high intensity UV light and short treatment time. Invest Ophthalmol Vis Sci. 2013;54:1176-80.
32. Lin JT, Cheng DC. Modeling the efficacy profiles of UV-light activated corneal collagen crosslinking. PLoS One. 2017;12:e0175002.
33. Çınar Y, Cingü AK, Türkcü FM, Çınar T, Yüksel H, Özkurt ZG, et al. Comparison of accelerated and conventional corneal collagen cross-linking for progressive keratoconus. Cutan Ocul Toxicol. 2014;33:218-22.
34. Tomita M, Mita M, Huseynova T. Accelerated versus conventional corneal collagen crosslinking. J Cataract Refract Surg. 2014;40:1013-20.
35. Subasinghe SK, Ogbuehi KC, Dias GJ. Current perspectives on corneal collagen crosslinking (CXL). Graefe's Arch Clin Exp Ophthalmol. 2018;256:1363-84.
36. Stojanovic A, Chen X, Jin N, Zhang T, Stojanovic F, Raeder S, et al. Safety and efficacy of epithelium-on corneal collagen cross-linking using a multifactorial approach to achieve proper stromal riboflavin saturation. J Ophthalmol. 2012;2012:498435.
37. Bottós KM, Schor P, Dreyfuss JL, Nader HB, Chamon W. Effect of corneal epithelium on ultraviolet-A and riboflavin absorption. Arquivos Brasileiros de Oftalmologia. 2011;74:348-51.
38. Kissner A, Spoerl E, Jung R, Spekl K, Pillunat LE, Raiskup F. Pharmacological modification of the epithelial permeability by benzalkonium chloride in UVA/Riboflavin corneal collagen cross-linking. Curr Eye Res. 2010;35:715-21.
39. Krueger RR, Ramos-Esteban JC, Kanellopoulos AJ. Staged intrastromal delivery of riboflavin with UVA cross-linking in advanced bullous keratopathy: laboratory investigation and first clinical case. J Refract Surg. 2008;24:S730-6.

40. Majumdar S, Hippalgaonkar K, Repka MA. Effect of chitosan, benzalkonium chloride and ethylenediaminetetraacetic acid on permeation of acyclovir across isolated rabbit cornea. Int J Pharma. 2008;348:175-8.
41. Hill J, Liu C, Deardorff P, Tavakol B, Eddington W, Thompson V, et al. Optimization of oxygen dynamics, UV-A delivery, and drug formulation for accelerated Epi-on corneal crosslinking. Curr Eye Res. 2020;45:450-8.
42. Caporossi A, Mazzotta C, Paradiso AL, Baiocchi S, Marigliani D, Caporossi T. Transepithelial corneal collagen crosslinking for progressive keratoconus: 24-month clinical results. J Cataract Refract Surg. 2013;39:1157-63.
43. Liu C, Deardorff P, Adler DC, Thompson V, Gore D. Stromal oxygen dynamics during high-irradiance epi-on corneal crosslinking. Invest Ophthalmol Vis Sci. 2019; 60:325.
44. Bandara A. Epi-on Crosslinking for Keratoconus Patients in Oman: 9-months Results. World Ophthalmol Congress. 2020.
45. Cimberle M. (2019). Advances in epi-on techniques may establish new gold standard in corneal cross-linking. [online] Available from: https://www.healio.com/news/ophthalmology/20191203/advances-in-epion-techniques-may-establish-new-gold-standard-in-corneal-crosslinking. [Last accessed May, 2021].
46. Bouheraoua N, Jouve L, El Sanharawi M, Sandali O, Temstet C, Loriaut P, et al. Optical coherence tomography and confocal microscopy following three different protocols of corneal collagen-crosslinking in keratoconus. Invest Ophthalmol Vis Sci. 2014;55:7601-9.
47. Touboul D, Efron N, Smadja D, Praud D, Malet F, Colin J. Corneal confocal microscopy following conventional, transepithelial, and accelerated corneal collagen cross-linking procedures for keratoconus. J Refract Surg. 2012;28:769-75.
48. Yam JC, Chan CW, Cheng AC. Corneal collagen cross-linking demarcation line depth assessed by Visante OCT after CXL for keratoconus and corneal ectasia. J Refract Surg. 2012;28:475-81.
49. Bikbova G, Bikbov M. Transepithelial corneal collagen cross-linking by iontophoresis of riboflavin. Acta Ophthalmologica. 2014;92:e30-4.
50. Kymionis GD, Portaliou DM, Diakonis VF, Kounis GA, Panagopoulou SI, Grentzelos MA. Corneal collagen cross-linking with riboflavin and ultraviolet-A irradiation in patients with thin corneas. Am J Ophthalmol. 2012;153:24-8.
51. Holopainen JM, Krootila K. Transient corneal thinning in eyes undergoing corneal cross-linking. Am J Ophthalmol. 2011;152:533-6.
52. Hafezi F. Limitation of collagen cross-linking with hypoosmolar riboflavin solution: failure in an extremely thin cornea. Cornea. 2011;30:917-9.
53. Scarcelli G, Pineda R, Yun SH. Brillouin optical microscopy for corneal biomechanics. Invest Ophthalmol Vis Sci. 2012;53:185-90.
54. Seiler T, Hafezi F. Corneal cross-linking-induced stromal demarcation line. Cornea. 2006;25:1057-9.
55. Wollensak G, Spoerl E, Wilsch M, Seiler T. Keratocyte apoptosis after corneal collagen cross-linking using riboflavin/UVA treatment. Cornea. 2004;23:43-9.
56. Kohlhaas M, Spoerl E, Schilde T, Unger G, Wittig C, Pillunat LE. Biomechanical evidence of the distribution of cross-links in corneas treated with riboflavin and ultraviolet A light. J Cataract Refract Surg. 2006;32:279-83.
57. Steinberg J, Ahmadiyar M, Rost A, Frings A, Filev F, Katz T, et al. Anterior and posterior corneal changes after crosslinking for keratoconus. Optometr Vis Sci. 2014;91:178-86.
58. Seiler TG, Fischinger I, Koller T, Zapp D, Frueh BE, Seiler T. Customized corneal cross-linking: one-year results. Am J Ophthalmol. 2016;166:14-21.
59. Al-Saidi R. Outcome of Customised Corneal Collagen Crosslinking (CuRV) for Keratoconus Patients in Oman: 12-months results. World Ophthalmol Congress. 2020;2020.

60. Al-Ajmi M. Outcome of Customised Corneal CXL (CuRV) in Pediatric Age Group. World Ophthalmol Congress. 2020;2020.
61. Konstantopoulos A, Liu YC, Teo EP, Nyein CL, Yam GH, Mehta JS. Corneal stability of LASIK and SMILE when combined with collagen cross-linking. Transl Vis Sci Technol. 2019;8:21.
62. Kanellopoulos AJ, Asimellis G. Combined laser in situ keratomileusis and prophylactic high-fluence corneal collagen crosslinking for high myopia: two-year safety and efficacy. J Cataract Refract Surg. 2015;41:1426-33.
63. Tan J, Lytle GE, Marshall J. Consecutive laser in situ keratomileusis and accelerated corneal crosslinking in highly myopic patients: preliminary results. Eur J Ophthalmol. 2015;25:101-7.
64. Kanellopoulos AJ, Binder PS. Management of corneal ectasia after LASIK with combined, same-day, topography-guided partial transepithelial PRK and collagen cross-linking: the Athens protocol. J Refract Surg. 2011;27:323-31.
65. Kanellopoulos AJ. Comparison of sequential vs same-day simultaneous collagen cross-linking and topography-guided PRK for treatment of keratoconus. J Refract Surg. 2009;25:S812-8.
66. Elbaz U, Shen C, Lichtinger A, Zauberman NA, Goldich Y, Ziai S, et al. Accelerated versus standard corneal collagen crosslinking combined with same day phototherapeutic keratectomy and single intrastromal ring segment implantation for keratoconus. Br J Ophthalmol. 2015;99:155-9.
67. Moore JE, Atkinson SD, Azar DT, Worthington J, Downes CS, Courtney DG, et al. Protection of corneal epithelial stem cells prevents ultraviolet A damage during corneal collagen cross-linking treatment for keratoconus. Br J Ophthalmol. 2014;98:270-4.
68. Chanbour W, Mokdad I, Mouhajer A, Jarade E. Late-onset sterile peripheral ulcerative keratitis post-corneal collagen crosslinking. Cornea. 2019;38:338-43.
69. Kymionis GD, Portaliou DM, Bouzoukis DI, Suh LH, Pallikaris AI, Markomanolakis M, et al. Herpetic keratitis with iritis after corneal crosslinking with riboflavin and ultraviolet A for keratoconus. J Cataract Refract Surg. 2007;33:1982-4.

Artificial Intelligence in the Diagnosis of Glaucoma

CHAPTER 5

Murali Ariga, Mohana Sinnasamy,
Pratheeba Devi Nivean, Henry Henderson

ABSTRACT

Artificial intelligence (AI) has kindled great interest in recent times across multiple industries. Its applications have found its way in everyday activities such as face recognition, voice recognition, virtual assistance, personalized online search results, etc. In medicine, the immense potential of image recognition by AI is being tapped in diagnosis, disease classification, and grading of severity. Deep learning (DL) is applied to detect diabetic retinopathy, retinopathy of prematurity, age-related macular degeneration (ARMD), macular edema, glaucoma, etc. from fundus images, optical coherence tomography (OCT) images, and visual fields. DL algorithm has shown results comparable to human graders in many studies increasing the likelihood of AI in future health care settings. Nonetheless, it has challenges in implementation that needs to be addressed. This chapter aims to discuss the basics of AI, potential role in diagnosis of glaucoma, its ability to predict the progression of glaucoma along with benefits, and issues of AI in healthcare.

Keywords: Artificial intelligence, glaucoma, machine learning, deep learning, convoluted neural networks, artificial neural network

INTRODUCTION

The concept of artificial intelligence (AI), i.e., creating machines with human intelligence[1] has been incubating since 1956 when John McCarthy coined the term. Although AI has been under lens over half a century, the recent surgeoncy in its popularity can be attributed to the availability of large volume of data and development of hardware that can handle great volume of data. In this age of fourth industrial revolution which includes AI, autonomous vehicles, robotics, internet of things, and three-dimensional (3D) printing.[2] It has already become an integral part in our day-to-day affairs like voice recognition, face recognition, virtual assistants, smart homes, and predicting personal choices in online searches among the myriad of other applications.

Medicine involves large volume of image recognition and analysis and makes it ideal field for study by AI. Among the branches of medicine—ophthalmology, dermatology, pathology, and radiology are likely to see immense contribution from AI since these specialties involve more image analysis. The fundus images provide an opportunity to study the blood vessels noninvasively. Application of AI on this image serves as a treasure trove providing valuable insights on the health status of the individual under study and has enabled to predict the cardiovascular risk factors including age, gender, hemoglobin A1C (HbA1C), blood pressure (BP), body mass index (BMI), and major adverse cardiovascular events (MACE).[3]

Tech Giant, Google partnered with Aravind Eye Care System and Sankara Nethralaya in the development of its AI system to detect diabetic retinopathy (DR) from fundus images. They used data from EyePACS-1 and MESSIDOR-2 data set to train their AI system and showed a sensitivity of 97.5% and 96.1% in each sets.[4] The specificity of each data sets was 98.1% and 98.5%, respectively. This announcement marked the beginning of new era in medicine. It will not be long before AI will be actively aiding ophthalmologists in their day-to-day clinical decisions. Hence, learning the basic concepts of AI, machine learning (ML), and deep learning (DL) is important. This chapter strives to introduce these basic concepts and presents an overview of the recent developments in AI pertaining to glaucoma and its role in the future.

ARTIFICIAL INTELLIGENCE AND ITS SUBSETS

Artificial intelligence simply means to create intelligence like human beings artificially, i.e., algorithms are created to enable machines to process information like human brain in comparison to the current software which give step-by-step instructions in processing the input.[1]

Machine learning, a term coined by Arthur Samuel in 1959 is a subset of AI. **Figure 1** shows the relationship of AI, ML, and DL. ML is the ability to learn from data by repeated practise. As more practise gives more expertise in human beings, similarly greater the volume of data analyzed more precise output is achieved with ML **(Flowchart 1)**. The learning can be supervised or unsupervised. In supervised learning the machine is fed with details to be identified in the data. The algorithm detects the presence of features pertaining to disease conditions from test data. This system is useful to classify or grade disease conditions. Unsupervised learning involves training the algorithm with no prior labeling. The system learns by itself to

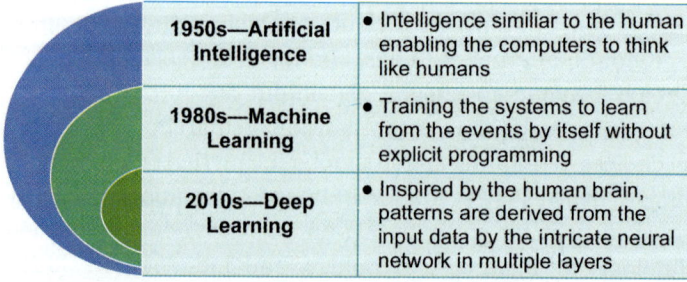

Fig. 1: Artificial intelligence and its subsets.

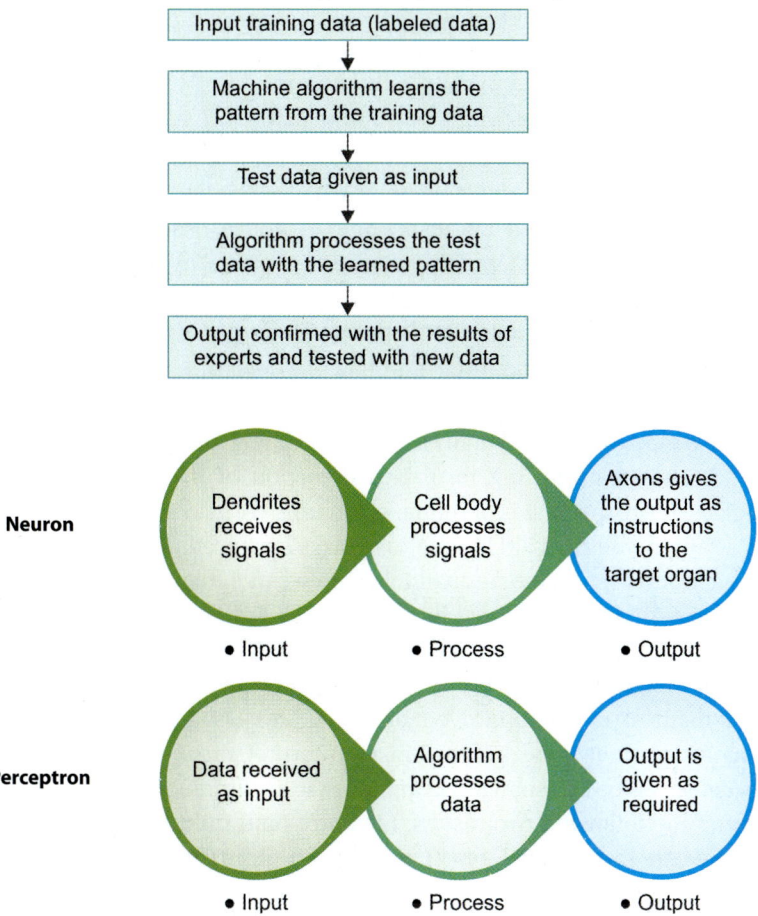

Flowchart 1: Machine learning—the steps in processing the data.

Fig. 2: *Perceptron and neuron*: Flow of processing information.

give output. This system is useful to identify associations between different factors and disease conditions.[5]

In ML, the system learns by repeated practise which can be made more efficient if multiple layers of analysis are incorporated in place of single level of learning. This is aided by DL which involves multiple layers of Convolutional Neural Networks (CNNs). These CNNs are algorithms that are commonly used to analyze visual data. CNNs are based on biological brain in that the connections and processing of perceptron (artificial neurons) mimic that of the neurons in visual cortex as shown in **Figure 2**.

In this subset of ML, each layer analyzes different aspects of input and sends the processed information to next layer for further analysis. One layer may analyze the outline of a figure, another layer the colors, another the curves, slants, and so on. The artificial neural networks (ANN) learn independently by repeating and correcting process. This is done by feeding the system a set of labeled data which ANN studies to learn the pattern as given in **Figure 3**. Later they are fed with test data which is analyzed multiple times till it achieves results equivalent to a human expert which is ready to interpret unread images.

Deep learning algorithms can be of two types: lesion-based detection systems or image-based detection system.[6] The features of the disease like microaneurysm, dot, and blot hemorrhages for DR are used to train the system in lesion-based DL algorithm. In image based algorithm, the DL identifies the pathology by studying the image pixel by pixel.[4]

Application of Artificial Intelligence in Ophthalmology

Ophthalmology is a field that handles large volume of images like fundus images, optical coherence tomography (OCT), X-rays, visual field images, corneal topography, and many more. ML is highly suitable for image analysis. It has shown promising results in detection of disease conditions from images in subspecialties of retina, glaucoma, cornea, cataract, oncology, etc. In addition, they can aid in repetitive tasks for the clinicians and detect early signs in a symptom free individual as they can detect very early signs of the disease from the images that human eyes may miss.[7]

The most promising results of AI in medicine is from the analysis of retinal images. The DL system IDx-DR developed by Abramoff et al. is the first medical device approved by Food and Drug Administration (FDA) which does not need a clinician to interpret the image.[8,9] It is designed to detect early DR changes in patients from fundus images and provides one of the following two results: (1) more than mild DR detected—refer to an eye care professional, or (2) negative for more than mild DR; rescreen in 12 months.[10]

With the help of AI, it has been possible to perform the DR screening from a smart phone-based setup. Medios AI (Remidio) an offline, smartphone-based, automated system of fundus image analysis to identify DR with

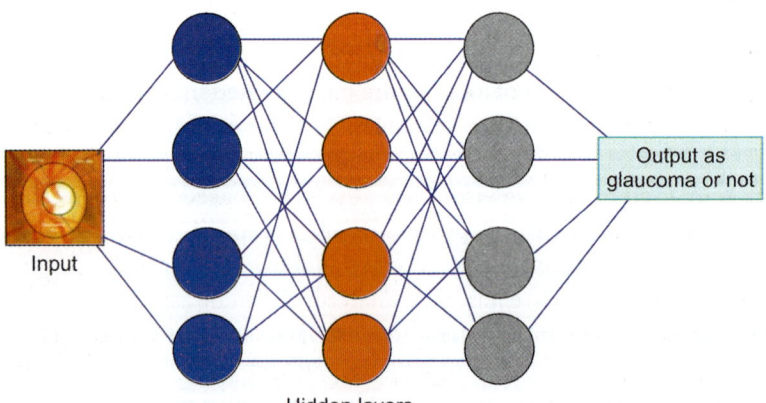

Fig. 3: Graphical representation of artificial neural network (ANN) (the fundus image is input which is analyzed by the hidden layers and the output is given).

Remedio's fundus on phone, nonmydriatic fundus camera showed 100% sensitivity and 88.4% specificity in identifying patients with DR changes that needs reference [referable DR (RDR)]. This system has the potential to revolutionize telemedicine especially screening for DR.[11]

Other studies of interest in various subspecialties of ophthalmology such as age-related macular degeneration (ARMD),[12] retinopathy of prematurity (ROP),[13] corneal ectasia,[14] keratoconus,[15] retinal detachments from fundus images,[16] pigment epithelial detachment in polypoidal choroidal vasculopathy,[17] pediatric cataract,[18] detection of refractive error from the fundus images,[19] planning for strabismus surgery,[20] and demarcate the extend of ocular surface squamous neoplasia in biopsy specimens.[21]

In addition to diagnostics, AI is being studied for intraocular lens (IOL) power calculations.[22] Online calculations using AI, Hill-RBF (radial basis function) formula is one of the best online calculators available now. Few notable studies that worked on AI applications in ophthalmology are given in the **Table 1**.

Currently, the potential of AI is being tapped extensively to detect DR. The ease of detection from fundus images, single modality to study, need for massive screening, clear guidelines for defining, and classifying the disease has made DR an ideal disease condition to study with AI.

TABLE 1: Studies on applications of AI in ophthalmology.

Area of interest	Nature of study	Sensitivity (in %)	Specificity (in %)	Developed by
DR	Idx-DR: detect referable DR	96.8	87	Abramoff et al.[9]
DR	Detecting DR (MESSIDOR data set)	87	98.1	Gulshan et al.[4]
DR	Remidio/eye ART	99.3	66.8	Rajalakshmi et al.[23]
DR	Smartphone-based AI Medios AI	100	88.4	Natarajan et al.[24]
DR	Smartphone-based AI Medios AI	98.8	86.7	Soosale B et al.[11]
Multiethnic study with DR images	Singapore National Diabetic Retinopathy Screening Program	90.5	91.6	Ting et al.[25]
Multiethnic study with AMD images		93.2	88.7	Ting et al.[25]
AMD	Identify dry AMD	83.99	99.34	Hwang et al.[26]
ROP	Detection of ROP from fundus images	82.5	98.3	Worrall et al.[27]
Glaucoma	Detection of glaucoma progression with RNFL thickness	80	73	Yousefi et al.[28]

(AI: artificial intelligence; AMD: age-related macular degeneration; DR: diabetic retinopathy; RNFL: retinal nerve fiber layer; ROP: retinopathy of prematurity)

Although glaucoma needs multiple investigations and lacks clear guidelines on definition of the disease, it can still reap the benefits of AI. It can be particularly used to derive meaningful information from multiple diagnostics. This can further aid ophthalmologists in unearthing new associations, early detection, better prediction of progression, and deciding on management plan on case-by-case basis.

Application of Artificial Intelligence in Glaucoma Diagnosis and Management

Glaucoma is a condition of chronic optic neuropathy that leads to progressive visual field defects with intraocular pressure as the only modifiable risk factor. This silent thief of sight usually presents with advanced optic disk cupping.

The diagnosis of glaucoma involves multiple procedures such as intraocular pressure (IOP) measurement, measurement of central corneal thickness, gonioscopy, examination of optic disk for disk damage, retinal nerve fiber layer (RNFL) defects, perimetry, and involves imaging techniques including anterior segment-OCT (AS-OCT), OCT, etc. In addition, the other factors such as refractive error, history of intraocular surgery, trauma, and other relevant systemic condition needs to be considered in the diagnosis of glaucoma.

Analyzing all these factors and assessing the disease severity can be daunting for the treating ophthalmologist. AI may have the potential to analyze and evaluate the data from different diagnostics and examinations to classify the stage of disease and predict its prognosis. This will be possible with an exclusively designed comprehensive algorithm which must prove its efficiency on par with experts in unlabeled data and can analyze IOP, disk changes, field defects, and other factors. Such an algorithm is still not available.[29] Nevertheless, it can be designed to integrate all the information in a meaningful manner from multiple diagnostic modalities and predict the progression of the disease which can be used to tailor individualized management plan for the patients.

Artificial intelligence helps in detection of glaucoma by:
- Detection of glaucomatous disk from fundus images
- Analyzing the RNFL thickness from OCT images
- Studying the angle structures in (AS-OCT)
- Studying the visual field images for detection and estimating the progression of glaucoma
- Automate IOP estimation by Goldmann applanation tonometry (GAT)

Optic Disk Images

Detection of glaucomatous changes in the fundus images by different DL algorithms is being studied for their accuracy and predictive potential. A list of various studies is given in the **Table 2**. In these studies, the algorithm

TABLE 2: List of studies that analyzed the AI applications in glaucoma.

Name of study	Software used	Conclusion on AI performance
Li et al.—GON detection from color fundus photographs[30]		• High sensitivity and specificity using DL systems • About half of false positives were due to large physiological cupping in image • Half of the false negatives was due to pathological myopia
Rogers et al.—The European Optic Disk Assessment Study[31]	Pegasus (v1.0, Visulytix Ltd., London, UK)	Accuracy of 83.4% comparable to that of ophthalmologists (80.5%) and optometrists (80%)
Emily Seo et al.—Evaluating optic disk images for manifest glaucoma detection using DL[32]	Pegasus-disk	• Categorized the disks in the 186 images as 0.00 to 1.00. • Specialist sensitivity 77.8% and specificity 93.3% • DL sensitivity 77.8% and specificity 81.9%
Phene et al.—Glaucoma detection by DL and glaucoma specialists. Features used to identify glaucoma in optic disk images.[33]		Higher sensitivity and specificity than eye care providers
Al Aswad et al.—Identifying glaucoma by DL from fundus images.[34]	Pegasus (v1.0, Visulytix Ltd., London, UK)	AUROC* 92.6% when compared to 69.6–84.9% for ophthalmologists
Fu et al.—Detection of glaucoma by DL from fundus images.[35]	M-Net and DENet	• *M-Net*: segmentation approach to calculate optic disk (OD) and optic cup (OC) values into a multi-label framework. • *DENet*: uses four deep streams on various levels
Cerentini et al.—Automatic identification of glaucoma using deep learning methods.[36]	GoogLeNet	Better detection of GON in poor quality images and subtle changes in ONH images
Kim et al.—Development and validation of a deep learning system for diagnosing glaucoma using OCT images.[37]	VGG-19**	Detecting glaucomatous damage with RNFL thickness maps and GCIPL*** analysis on par with human experts
Haleem et al.—Deformable model for automated optic disk and cup segmentation.[38]	Adaptive region based edge smoothing model (ARESM)	• Enabled automatic detection of optic disk and cup • Helps in analyzing different variations in the optic disk morphology
Muhammad et al.—Hybrid deep learning classifies glaucoma suspects from OCT scans.[39]	Hybrid deep learning method (HDLM)	Better differentiation between healthy suspect and early glaucoma with SS-OCT scans compared to traditional OCT and visual field metrics.
Asaoka et al.—detecting early onset glaucoma from OCT images.[40]		Detects early glaucoma from SD-OCT images with trained DL showing AUROC* of 93.7% while untrained DL showed 76.6% and 78.8%

Contd...

Contd...

Name of study	Software used	Conclusion on AI performance
Christopher et al.—Prediction of glaucoma progression from RNFL features with OCT images.[41]	Principal component analysis method	Studies with SS-OCT, cpRNFL**** circle scans, SD-OCT, standard automated perimetry, frequency doubling technology (FDT) with unsupervised ML showed RNFL PCA was associated with mean deviation in SAP, visual field testing, and cpRNFL and RNFL PCA had better chances of predicting progression
Niwas SI et al.—Analysis of AS-OCT images for detecting angle closure glaucoma[42]		Detected angle closure with AS-OCT images with accuracy of 89.2%
Li F et al.—Automatic differentiation of glaucoma visual field from nonglaucoma visual field using deep convolutional neural network.[43]		Higher accuracy in differentiating glaucomatous visual fields compared to ophthalmologists
Christopher et al.—DL algorithms predict progression of visual field defects from OCT images.[44]		Detected eyes with glaucomatous field defects from SD-OCT and optic nerve head images with high accuracy.
Asoaka et al.—Detecting preperimetric glaucoma with perimetry images using DL classifier.[45]	Deep feed forward neural network (FNN)	• Differentiated preperimetric glaucoma and normal eyes with visual fields. • AUROC of FNN was larger than other neural networks predicting preperimetric glaucoma
Goldbaum et al.—Machine classifier to predict the progression of glaucoma from visual fields.[46]	Variational Bayesian independent component mixture model	Assessed the patterns of visual field progression in glaucomatous eyes
Jammal et al.—Comparing gradings by human graders and DL algorithm in detecting glaucoma from fundus images.[47]		Showed more accuracy than humans in detecting GON with repeatable visual field losses
Li F et al.—smartphone-based visual field deep learning system for glaucoma detection.[48]	iGlaucoma	• Detects glaucoma from visual fields with more accuracy than ophthalmologists by combined pattern deviation plots, numerical displays, and numerical deviation plots • May serve as a screening tool at the primary eye care level

(AS-OCT: anterior segment optical coherence tomography; DL: deep learning; GON: glaucomatous optic neuropathy; ML: machine learning; OCT: optical coherence tomography; ONH: optic nerve head; PCA: principal component analysis; RNFL: retinal nerve fiber layer; SAP: standard automated perimetry; SD-OCT: spectral domain optical coherence tomography; SS-OCT: swept source optical coherence tomography)
*AUROC: Area under the receiver operating characteristic curve
**VGG-19: Visual Geometry Group
***GCIPL: Ganglion cell-inner plexiform layer
cpRNFL****: circumpapillary retinal nerve fiber layer

delineates the optic disk, cup, measures the cup to disk (CD) ratio, neuroretinal rim thickness, disk damage likelihood scale (DDLS) ratio and detects the violation of ISNT (inferior > superior > nasal > temporal) rule.

In addition to detecting glaucoma, fundus images were also used to quantify the shape of the optic nerve head (ONH) by DL. In the previous methods, the exact reasons by which the DL algorithms predicts the glaucoma from the fundus images are obscure. In this study, the cup and disk are segmented into 24 cross-sections to create a cup/disk ratio profile (pCDR) and then shape of pCDR is analyzed with a spatial model to derive a disk deformation index and detection rule using predictive methods. This method showed a very high accuracy of area under the receiver operating characteristic curve (AUROC) 99.6% and 91% on ORIGA data set and RIM-ONE (Retinal IMage database for Optic Nerve Evaluation) images.[49]

OPTICAL COHERENCE TOMOGRAPHY

The current OCT machines uses segmentation technique to provide relevant details like disk size, cupping, neuroretinal rim (NRR), RNFL thickness, and ganglion cell layer thickness. Various studies that analyzed the DL algorithm tested with OCT images are also given in the **Table 1**. Many of these studies were able to demonstrate that AI had good accuracy in detecting glaucoma and in predicting the progression of the disease.[50-53]

While many of the DL algorithm needed human labeling of the training data, Medeiros et al. used spectral-domain-OCT (SD-OCT) data to train the DL algorithm to quantify glaucomatous damage (RNFL thickness) on the optic disk images. This reduced the discrepancy in diagnosis due to large or small disks and thereby reducing the variations by the human grader. Hence, these gradings were highly reproducible. In addition to this, the time required to classify by human graders is also substantially reduced in this system.[54]

Another novel method of detecting glaucoma in early stages is by a technique called detection of apoptosing retinal cells (DARC). It is a method of visualizing apoptotic retinal cells when they are highlighted with fluorescence dye. A CNN aided algorithm designed to predict the glaucoma progression from OCT retinal nerve fiber layer measurement with DARC showed an accuracy of 97%, sensitivity 85.7%, and specificity of 91.7%. This technique has been approved by FDA as "exploratory endpoint for testing a new glaucoma drug in a clinical trial." Further studies are needed to validate this technique.[55,56]

Anterior Segment-Optical Coherence Tomography

The AS-OCT images have been used to train DL algorithms to identify angle closure glaucoma by structure segmentation technique. Niwas et al. were able to develop algorithms with accuracy of 89.2% in detecting angle closure glaucoma from AS-OCT images.

VISUAL FIELD ANALYSIS
Detection and Interpretation
The visual fields can be interpreted with greater accuracy and shorter time with AI. Li et al. demonstrated that a CNN can distinguish a glaucomatous visual field from nonglaucomatous fields.[43] Unsupervised ML and variational Bayesian independent component analysis mixture model (vB-ICA-mm) were employed to study the visual defects in glaucoma.[46]

Another study that employed variational Bayesian independent component analysis-mixture Model (VIM), an unsupervised ML classifier showed satisfactory results when analyzing frequency doubling technology (FDT) perimetry data.[57]

Andersson et al. demonstrated 93% sensitivity and 91% specificity in detecting glaucomatous visual field changes with AI systems on par with the results from clinicians.[58]

Estimation of Progression
In addition to detect the glaucomatous field defects, the progression in visual defects was detected by the quantifying the change in the field defect pattern with archetypal analysis, an unsupervised AI method. This may aid the clinicians to arrive at accurate diagnosis of glaucoma progression.[59] Goldbaum et al. used progression of patterns (POP), a ML classifier algorithm to estimate the progression of visual defects.[46] A DL system, CascadeNet-5 trained with 32,443 visual fields, was able to predict the progression of visual field defects for up to 5.5 years with a single visual field input.[60]

Another clinical decision-making tool, Kalman filters, was able to produce individualized estimates for the progression of primary open-angle glaucoma (POAG) at different target IOP levels. This tool can be used to individualize target IOP based on each patient's risk for progression. The model was developed with visual field images and IOP measurements of 571 participants with moderate to severe POAG from the Collaborative Initial Glaucoma Treatment Study or the Advances Glaucoma Intervention study.[61]

In the studies above, the results of a single investigation modality were utilized to train AI in detecting glaucoma. In a study by Oh et al., ANN was trained with four nonophthalmologic factors (age, sex, menopause, and duration of hypertension) and five ophthalmic factors (IOP, spherical equivalent refractive errors, vertical CD ratio, presence of superotemporal RNFL defect, and presence of inferotemporal RNFL defect). This model was able to detect glaucoma with an accuracy of 84%, sensitivity 78.3%, and specificity of 85.9% without studying the visual field defects.[62]

Artificial Intelligence in Intraocular Pressure Measurement
Artificial intelligence was studied to automate IOP measurement and detect glaucoma. The IOP measurements from the contact lens sensor (CLS)

(SENSIMED Triggerfish®) based 24-hour profiles were studied for their potential use in discriminating healthy eyes from POAG. The study showed that AI algorithm trained with CLS parameters was able to discriminate POAG from healthy eyes with AUROC of 0.611 and CI of 0.493–0.722. The feature set combining CLS and start IOP detected POAG with more accuracy than each of these parameters separately.[63]

Automation of Intraocular Pressure Estimation by Goldmann Applanation Tonometry

A study by Spaide et al. attempted to automate the estimation of IOP by analyzing the videos recorded using a slit lamp microscope and GAT. In this unique attempt, a DL algorithm was trained to study the position of tonometer and mires in the recorded videos to estimate the IOP using Imbert-Fick formula. The preliminary study documented similar results (mean difference of 0.9 mm Hg) with both standard GAT and automated GAT thereby increasing the reproducibility and reducing interobserver bias.[64]

CURRENT LIMITATIONS

Artificial intelligence clearly holds great potential to act as a rapid, reliable, and cost-effective screening tool in ophthalmology. It can aid in reducing the workload of the ophthalmologists, reach the unreached population with telemedicine, and in early detection of patients thereby reducing the development of complications of glaucoma. However, the AI fraternity need to overcome certain challenges to ensure its successful implementation.

Adversarialization and Black Box Artificial Intelligence

Referred as Black Box AI, the processes involved in decision making in certain DL algorithms especially image-based algorithms are not visible for monitoring. When these systems were given images subtly altered at a pixel level (adversarialization), they seem to lack consistency in diagnosing the disease unlike the clinicians who were able to detect the disease in altered images.[65]

Detection of Multiple Diseases

The binary nature of the algorithms currently studied are designed to detect a particular disease. If the test image is of a patient with multiple conditions, the ability of the system to detect the disease drops significantly with each added condition to as low as 20–30%.[66]

Need for Standard Guidelines in Diagnosis of Glaucoma

Glaucoma is the diagnosis based on multiple parameters and lacks standard guidelines in diagnosis and treatment. AI processes depend on data based on set parameters, developing standard guidelines may aid in classifying and predicting disease progression in glaucoma. When designed accurately AI may ensure wide screening and good patient adherence.

Need for Quality Training Data

Artificial intelligence thrives in data and more data is needed to refine the learning pattern. The dearth of high-quality images is an issue to be addressed as the precision in identifying the disease conditions need more good quality data.

Another implication is that the machine is learning from the data given and hence the data given should be precise. If the training data was exclusively from a particular population, it may fail to detect the disease from a different population.[25] The training data set should contain a good mixture of variations to avoid this error.

Need for Human Intervention

Another challenge with AI is that although it shows promising results, human intervention is still necessary for deep analysis of the results as AI usually learns pattern of a specific disease and may miss subtle signs of others. Also, a minor error in the algorithm can lead to grave consequences. This must be taken into consideration in the initial days of implementation.

In the light of these limitations, the potential of AI needs to be weighed against its pitfalls in implementing.

The Future: Artificial Intelligence Aiding Ophthalmologists

With the recent developments in AI, the common concern of experts is whether AI will replace ophthalmologists. It is to be noted that AI like other diagnostic tool aids in diagnosis but with more precision and shall be incorporated in the many diagnostic machines used in day-to-day practice of ophthalmology. The management of diseases involves active interaction between the treating ophthalmologist and the patient regarding risks and benefits of different treatment options available and AI may be restricted to its role in diagnosis and prediction of progression.

Role in Telescreening

Artificial intelligence can augment screening patients in the community where the patient data and photographs are collected at the primary care center and referred to ophthalmologist for management advice. This initial step in triaging the patient may be easily carried out by AI through a Mobile App and can be used in reaching the unreached. This means more time is available for ophthalmologists to concentrate on activities that require their supervision and close monitoring.

Valuable Research Tool

The ability of AI to detect subtle features of disease from the images may play a role in analyzing new associations in glaucoma. This unsupervised learning may play a major role in identifying new risk factors, drug trials, and in other research activities.

CONCLUSION

Artificial intelligence can process information from multiple imaging techniques with great accuracy. This aids in identifying very early signs of disease that enables ophthalmologist to intervene and prevent the progression of disease process before the onset of symptoms. The ability of AI in grading the severity of the disease and predicting progression of disease helps ophthalmologists to analyze the best course management with little effort. Through all these steps, AI can ensure good patient compliance with timely reminders for treatment and follow-ups.

AI shows potential to transform glaucoma management through early diagnosis and individualized treatments and revolutionize screening with telemedicine. The advantages outweigh the challenges and ophthalmology is sure to benefit from AI. Nevertheless, human intervention will be an integral part in medicine, and AI serves to augment human effort in it.

REFERENCES

1. Hamet P, Tremblay J. Artificial intelligence in medicine. Metabolism. 2017;69S:S36-S40.
2. World Economic Forum. (2016). The fourth industrial revolution: What it means, how to respond. [online] Available from https://www.weforum.org/agenda/2016/01/the-fourth-industrial-revolution-what-it-means-and-how-to-respond/ [Last accessed March, 2021]
3. Poplin R, Varadarajan AV, Blumer K, Liu Y, McConnell MV, Corrado GS, et al. Prediction of cardiovascular risk factors from retinal fundus photographs via deep learning. Nat Biomed Eng. 2018;2(3):158-64.
4. Gulshan V, Peng L, Coram M, Stumpe MC, Wu D, Narayanaswamy A, et al. Development and validation of a deep learning algorithm for detection of diabetic retinopathy in retinal fundus photographs. JAMA. 2016;316(22):2402-10.
5. Brownlee J. [2016]. Supervised and Unsupervised Machine Learning Algorithms. [online] Available from: https://machinelearningmastery.com/supervised-and-unsupervised-machine-learning-algorithms [Last accessed March, 2021].
6. Fenner BJ, Wong RLM, Lam WC, Tan GSW, Cheung GCM. Advances in retinal imaging and applications in diabetic retinopathy screening: a review. Ophthalmol Ther. 2018;7(2):333-46.
7. American Academy of Ophthalmology. [2021]. AI Can Transform Medicine—But, First, Clinicians Have Homework to Do. [online] Available from: https://www.aao.org/eyenet/academy-live/detail/ai-can-transform-medicine-first-clinicians-have-ho [Last accessed March, 2021].
8. Abramoff MD, Folk JC, Han DP, Walker JD, Williams DF, Russell SR, et al. Automated analysis of retinal images for detection of referable diabetic retinopathy. JAMA Ophthalmol. 2013;131(3):351-7.

9. Abràmoff MD, Lou Y, Erginay A, Clarida W, Amelon R, Folk JC, et al. Improved automated detection of diabetic retinopathy on a publicly available dataset through integration of deep learning. Invest Ophthalmol Vis Sci. 2016;57(13):5200-6.
10. FDA approves marketing for first AI device for diabetic retinopathy detection. [online] Available from: https://eyewire.news/articles/fda-permits-marketing-of-ai-based-device-to-detect-certain-diabetes-related-eye-problems/ [Last accessed March, 2021].
11. Sosale B, Aravind SR, Murthy H, Narayana S, Sharma U, Gowda SGV, et al. Simple, Mobile-based Artificial Intelligence Algorithm in the detection of Diabetic Retinopathy (SMART) study. BMJ Open Diabetes Res Care. 2020;8(1):e000892.
12. Burlina PM, Joshi N, Pekala M, Pacheco KD, Freund DE, Bressler NM. Automated grading of age-related macular degeneration from color fundus images using deep convolutional neural networks. JAMA Ophthalmol. 2017;135(11):1170-6.
13. Campbell JP, Ataer-Cansizoglu E, Bolon-Canedo V, Bozkurt A, Erdogmus D, Kalpathy-Cramer J, et al. Expert diagnosis of plus disease in retinopathy of prematurity from computer-based image analysis. JAMA Ophthalmol. 2016;134(6):651-7.
14. Ambrósio Jr R, Lopes BT, Faria-Correia F, Salomão MQ, Bühren J, Roberts CJ, et al. Integration of scheimpflug-based corneal tomography and biomechanical assessments for enhancing ectasia detection. J Refract Surg. 2017;33(7):434-43.
15. Hidalgo IR, Rozema JJ, Saad A, Gatinel D, Rodriguez P, Zakaria N, et al. Validation of an objective keratoconus detection system implemented in a Scheimpflug tomographer and comparison with other methods. Cornea. 2017;36(6):689-95.
16. Li Z, Guo C, Nie D, Lin D, Zhu Y, Chen C, et al. Deep learning for detecting retinal detachment and discerning macular status using ultra-widefield fundus images. Commun Biol. 2020;3(1):15.
17. Yang J, Zhang C, Wang E, Chen Y, Yu W. Utility of a public-available artificial intelligence in diagnosis of polypoidal choroidal vasculopathy. Graefes Arch Clin Exp Ophthalmol. 2020;258(1):17-21.
18. Liu X, Jiang J, Zhang K, Long E, Cui J, Zhu M, et al. Localization and diagnosis framework for pediatric cataracts based on slit-lamp images using deep features of a convolutional neural network. PLoS One. 2017;12(3):e0168606.
19. Varadarajan AV, Poplin R, Blumer K, Angermueller C, Ledsam J, Chopra R, et al. Deep learning for predicting refractive error from retinal fundus images. Invest Ophthalmol Vis Sci. 2018;59(7):2861-8.
20. Almeida JD, Silva AC, de Paiva AC, Teixeira JAM. Computational methodology for automatic detection of strabismus in digital images through Hirschberg test. Comput Biol Med. 2012;42(1):135-46.
21. Habibalahi A, Bala C, Allende A, Anwer AG, Goldys EM. Novel automated non-invasive detection of ocular surface squamous neoplasia using multispectral autofluorescence imaging. Ocul Surf. 2019;17(3):540-550.
22. Ladas JG, Siddiqui AA, Devgan U, Jun AS. A 3-D "Super surface" combining modern intraocular lens formulas to generate a "Super formula" and maximize accuracy. JAMA Ophthalmol. 2015;133(12):1431-6.
23. Rajalakshmi R, Subashini R, Anjana RM, Mohan V. Automated diabetic retinopathy detection in smartphone-based fundus photography using artificial intelligence. Eye. 2018;32(6):1138-44.
24. Natarajan S, Jain A, Krishnan R, Rogye A, Sivaprasad S. Diagnostic accuracy of community-based diabetic retinopathy screening with an offline artificial intelligence system on a smartphone. JAMA Ophthalmol. 2019;137(10):1182-8.
25. Ting DSW, Cheung CYL, Lim G, Tan GSW, Quang ND, Gan A, et al. Development and validation of a deep learning system for diabetic retinopathy and related eye diseases using retinal images from multiethnic populations with diabetes. JAMA. 2017;318(22):2211-23.

26. Hwang DK, Hsu CC, Chang KJ, Chao D, Sun CH, Jheng YC, et al. Artificial intelligence-based decision-making for age-related macular degeneration. Theranostics. 2019;9(1):232-45.
27. Worrall DE, Wilson CM, Brostow GJ. Automated retinopathy of prematurity case detection with convolutional neural networks. Springer Int Publ. 2016:68-76.
28. Yousefi S, Goldbaum MH, Balasubramanian M, Jung TP, Weinreb RN, Medeiros FA, et al. Glaucoma progression detection using structural retinal nerve fiber layer measurements and functional visual field points. IEEE Trans Biomed Eng. 2014;61(4):1143-54.
29. Zheng C, Johnson TV, Garg A, Boland MV. Artificial intelligence in glaucoma. Curr Opin Ophthalmol. 2019;30(2):97-103.
30. Li Z, He Y, Keel S, Meng W, Chang RT, He M. Efficacy of a deep learning system for detecting glaucomatous optic neuropathy based on color fundus photographs. Ophthalmology. 2018;125(8):1199-1206.
31. Rogers TW, Jaccard N, Carbonaro F, Lemij HG, Vermeer KA, Reus JG, et al. Evaluation of an AI system for the automated detection of glaucoma from stereoscopic optic disc photographs: the European Optic Disc Assessment Study. Eye (Lond). 2019;33(11):1791-7.
32. Seo E, Jaccard N, Trikha S, Pasquale LR, Song BJ. Automated evaluation of optic disc images for manifest glaucoma detection using a deep-learning, neural network-based algorithm. Invest Ophthalmol Vis Sci. 2018;59(9):2080.
33. Phene S, Dunn RC, Hammel N, Liu Y, Krause J, Kitade N, et al. Deep learning and glaucoma specialists: The relative importance of optic disc features to predict glaucoma referral in fundus photographs. Ophthalmology. 2019;126(12):1627-39.
34. Al-Aswad LA, Kapoor R, Chu CK, Walters S, Gong D, Garg A, et al. Evaluation of a deep learning system for identifying glaucomatous optic neuropathy based on color fundus photographs. J Glaucoma. 2019;28(12):1029-34.
35. Fu H, Cheng J, Xu Y, Liu J. Glaucoma detection based on deep learning network in fundus image. Springer Int Publ. 2019.
36. Cerentini A, Welfer D, Cordeiro d'Ornellas M, Pereira Haygert CJ, Dotto GN. Automatic identification of glaucoma using deep learning methods. Stud Health Technol Inform. 2017;245:318-21.
37. Kim KE, Kim JM, Song JE, Kee C, Han JC, Hyun SH. Development and validation of a deep learning system for diagnosing glaucoma using optical coherence tomography. J Clin Med. 2020;9(7):2167.
38. Haleem MS, Han L, van Hemert J, Li B, Fleming A, Pasquale LR, et al. A novel adaptive deformable model for automated optic disc and cup segmentation to aid glaucoma diagnosis. J Med Syst. 2017;42(1):20.
39. Muhammad H, Fuchs TJ, De Cuir N, Moraes CG, Blumberg DM, Liebmann JM, et al. Hybrid deep learning on single wide-field optical coherence tomography scans accurately classifies glaucoma suspects. J Glaucoma. 2017;26(12):1086-94.
40. Asaoka R, Murata H, Hirasawa K, Fujino Y, Matsuura M, Miki A, et al. Using deep learning and transfer learning to accurately diagnose early-onset glaucoma from macular optical coherence tomography images. Am J Ophthalmol. 2019;198:136-45.
41. Christopher M, Belghith A, Weinreb RN, Bowd C, Goldbaum MH, Saunders LJ, et al. Retinal nerve fiber layer features identified by unsupervised machine learning on optical coherence tomography scans predict glaucoma progression. Invest Ophthalmol Vis Sci. 2018;59(7):2748-56.
42. Niwas SI, Lin W, Bai X, Kwoh CK, Jay Kuo CC, Sng CC, et al. Automated anterior segment OCT image analysis for Angle Closure Glaucoma mechanisms classification. Comput Methods Programs Biomed. 2016;130:65-75.
43. Li F, Wang Z, Qu G, Song D, Yuan Y, Xu Y, et al. Automatic differentiation of glaucoma visual field from non-glaucoma visual field using deep convolutional neural network. BMC Med Imaging. 2018;18(1):35.

44. Christopher M, Bowd C, Belghith A, Goldbaum MH, Weinreb RN, Fazio MA, et al. Deep learning approaches predict glaucomatous visual field damage from OCT optic nerve head en face images and retinal nerve fiber layer thickness maps. Ophthalmology. 2020;127(3):346-56.
45. Asaoka R, Murata H, Iwase A, Araie M. Detecting preperimetric glaucoma with standard automated perimetry using a deep learning classifier. Ophthalmology. 2016;123(9):1974-80.
46. Goldbaum MH, Lee I, Jang G, Balasubramanian M, Sample PA, Weinreb RN, et al. Progression of patterns (POP): a machine classifier algorithm to identify glaucoma progression in visual fields. Invest Ophthalmol Vis Sci. 2012;53(10):6557-67.
47. Jammal AA, Thompson AC, Mariottoni EB, Berchuck SI, Urata CN, Estrela T, et al. Human versus Machine: comparing a deep learning algorithm to human gradings for detecting glaucoma on fundus photographs. Am J Ophthalmol. 2020;211:123-31.
48. Li F, Song D, Chen H, Xiong J, Li X, Zhong H, et al. Development and clinical deployment of a smartphone-based visual field deep learning system for glaucoma detection. NPJ Digit Med. 2020;3:123.
49. MacCormick IJC, Williams BM, Zheng Y, Li K, Al-Bander B, Czanner S, et al. Accurate, fast, data efficient and interpretable glaucoma diagnosis with automated spatial analysis of the whole cup to disc profile. PLoS One. 2019;14(1):e0209409.
50. Barella KA, Costa VP, Gonçalves Vidotti V, Silva FR, Dias M, Gomi ES. Glaucoma diagnostic accuracy of machine learning classifiers using retinal nerve fiber layer and optic nerve data from SD-OCT. J Ophthalmol. 2013;2013:789129.
51. Bizios D, Heijl A, Hougaard JL, Bengtsson B. Machine learning classifiers for glaucoma diagnosis based on classification of retinal nerve fibre layer thickness parameters measured by Stratus OCT. Acta Ophthalmol. 2010;88(1):44-52.
52. Larrosa JM, Polo V, Ferreras A, García-Martín E, Calvo P, Pablo LE. Neural Network Analysis of Different Segmentation Strategies of Nerve Fiber Layer Assessment for Glaucoma Diagnosis. J Glaucoma. 2015;24(9):672-8.
53. Ran AR, Cheung CY, Wang X, Chen H, Luo LY, Chan PP, et al. Detection of glaucomatous optic neuropathy with spectral-domain optical coherence tomography: a retrospective training and validation deep-learning analysis. Lancet Digit Health. 2019;1(4):e172-e182.
54. Medeiros FA, Jammal AA, Thompson AC. From Machine to Machine: An OCT-trained deep learning algorithm for objective quantification of glaucomatous damage in fundus photographs. Ophthalmology. 2019;126(4):513-21.
55. Normando EM, Yap TE, Maddison J, Miodragovic S, Bonetti P, Almonte M, et al. A CNN-aided method to predict glaucoma progression using DARC (Detection of Apoptosing Retinal Cells). Expert Rev Mol Diagn. 2020;20(7):737-48.
56. Yousefi S, Kiwaki T, Zheng Y, Sugiura H, Asaoka R, Murata H, et al. Detection of longitudinal visual field progression in glaucoma using Machine Learning. Am J Ophthalmol. 2018;193:71-9.
57. Bowd C, Weinreb RN, Balasubramanian M, Lee I, Jang G, Yousefi S, et al. Glaucomatous patterns in Frequency Doubling Technology (FDT) perimetry data identified by unsupervised machine learning classifiers. PLoS One. 2014;9(1):e85941.
58. Andersson S, Heijl A, Bizios D, Bengtsson B. Comparison of clinicians and an artificial neural network regarding accuracy and certainty in performance of visual field assessment for the diagnosis of glaucoma. Acta Ophthalmol. 2013;91(5):413-7.
59. Wang M, Shen LQ, Pasquale LR, Petrakos P, Formica S, Boland MV, et al. An artificial intelligence approach to detect visual field progression in glaucoma based on spatial pattern analysis. Invest Ophthalmol Vis Sci. 2019;60(1):365-75.
60. Wen JC, Lee CS, Keane PA, Xiao S, Rokem AS, Chen PP, et al. Forecasting future Humphrey Visual Fields using deep learning. PLoS One. 2019;14(4):e0214875.

61. Kazemian P, Lavieri MS, Van Oyen MP, Andrews C, Stein JD. Personalized prediction of glaucoma progression under different target intraocular pressure levels using filtered forecasting methods. Ophthalmology. 2018;125(4):569-77.
62. Oh E, Yoo TK, Hong S. Artificial neural network approach for differentiating open-angle glaucoma from glaucoma suspect without a visual field test. Invest Ophthalmol Vis Sci. 2015;56(6):3957-66.
63. Martin KR, Mansouri K, Weinreb RN, Wasilewicz R, Gisler C, Hennebert J, et al. Use of machine learning on contact lens sensor-derived parameters for the diagnosis of primary open-angle glaucoma. Am J Ophthalmol. 2018;194:46-53.
64. Spaide T, Wu Y, Yanagihara RT, Feng S, Ghabra O, Yi JS, et al. Using deep learning to automate Goldmann applanation tonometry readings. Ophthalmology. 2020;127(11):1498-1506.
65. Lynch S, Shah A, Folk J, Wu X, Abramoff M. Catastrophic failure in image-based convolutional neural network algorithms for detecting diabetic retinopathy. Invest Ophthalmol Vis Sci. 2017;58(8):3776.
66. Choi JY, Yoo TK, Seo JG, Kwak J, Um TT, Rim TH. Multi-categorical deep learning neural network to classify retinal images: a pilot study employing small database. PLoS One. 2017;12(11):e0187336.

CHAPTER 6

Optical Coherence Tomography Angiography in Posterior Uveitis

Saba Ishrat, Panchmi Gupta, Jasmine Ge

ABSTRACT

Optical coherence tomography angiography (OCTA) is a novel technique that has enabled fast, noninvasive, and high-resolution visualization of vasculature within the eye. Intraocular inflammation can be associated with various vascular flow abnormalities in a wide spectrum of uveitis disorders. Recognizing patterns of disruption in the blood flow is integral to the diagnosis, treatment, and prognosis of these ocular disorders. The use of OCTA technology in patients with ocular inflammation is likely to reveal novel features that may help in advancing our understanding of pathophysiology and natural history of the disease.

Keywords: OCTA, optical coherence tomography, uveitis, intraocular.

INTRODUCTION

Optical coherence tomography (OCT) has revolutionized the practice of ophthalmology over the past 2 decades. The continuous advancement in OCT technology has led to the development of futuristic OCT-based methods. One of the first demonstrations of imaging the vascular network in the human eye was performed in 2006 by using a method known as *optical coherence tomography angiography*. It is a novel technique that has enabled fast, noninvasive, high-resolution visualization of vasculature within the eye. It helps in combining the structural assessment of the ocular tissues obtained via OCT images with visualization of blood flow within the vessels in the imaged area. It yields in vivo quasi-histological images of the ocular tissues with a resolution beyond that of any other noninvasive technology.[1]

The intraocular vascular networks are complex, multi-layered, and critical to ocular function. Intraocular inflammation can be associated with various vascular flow abnormalities in a wide spectrum of uveitic disorders. Recognizing patterns of disruption in the blood flow is integral to the diagnosis, treatment, and prognosis of these ocular diseases.[2]

Since their invention, fundus fluorescein angiography (FFA) and indocyanine green angiography (ICGA) have been the gold standard modalities for the imaging of retinal and choroidal vessel morphology,[2] but these procedures are invasive and require the injection of intravenous dyes that may be poorly tolerated and associated with rare serious side effects.[3] These disadvantages limit the routine use of dye-based angiography to monitor the disease progression and treatment effect during each clinical visit.

Optical coherence tomography angiography or angio-OCT has emerged as a noninvasive alternative technique for the imaging of retinal and choroidal vasculatures.[4] The basis of OCTA depends on the reflectance of a light source from the surface of moving particles (erythrocytes), eliminating the need for dyes. Angio-OCT analyzes the intensity of the reflected signal and the time changes in the reflection caused by the moving blood cells flowing through the vessels. These differences in the OCT signal, measured by continuously capturing OCT images (B-scans) at each point on the retina, allow the formation of an image contrast between the perfused vessels and the surrounding tissue, which is stationary and does not display any time changes in the OCT signal.[5,6]

INTERPRETATION OF ANGIO-OPTICAL COHERENCE TOMOGRAPHY

Optical coherence tomography angiography images incorporate the structural information of a standard OCT scan with blood flow visualization. OCTA allows for segmentation of retinal and choroidal layers and, therefore, precisely localizing the abnormalities.[7] The images display the vascular networks contained within the explored tissue at different depths. Hence, it is important to be aware of which tissue layer is being shown in the image while interpreting.[8]

The OCTA image is displayed, most commonly, as an *en face* map of the vasculature. This image can include all the vessels seen in the entire retina or can be used to isolate the vascular network in different retinal layers. OCTA allows for segmentation of the *superficial capillary plexus (SCP)* in the superficial retina which extends from the internal limiting membrane (ILM) to the inner plexiform layer (IPL), the *deep capillary plexus* (DCP) in the middle retina from IPL (inner boundary) to the outer plexiform layer (outer boundary), and the outer retina, which is avascular and shows the presence of vessels only in pathologies such as choroidal neovascularization (CNV). Further, superficial segmentation permits the visualization of the *radial network of vessels* in the peripapillary area. A deeper segmentation allows the visualization of the *choriocapillaris* though the reduced penetration of the spectral domain optical coherence tomography (SD-OCT) signal beyond the retinal pigment epithelium (RPE) causes a loss of resolution at this level. The use of a longer wavelength swept source OCT which has a better penetration past the RPE, helps in better visualization of the choriocapillaris and of the structures beneath the RPE.[9,10]

SPECTRUM OF ABNORMAL VASCULAR CHANGES IN UVEITIDES

The changes in the retinal and choroidal vascular networks play an important role in the pathophysiology of uveitis. Various pathologic processes such as inflammation, local ischemia, vascular occlusion, and release of different cellular mediators lead to a host of retinochoroidal vascular defects. It, thus, becomes vitally important to pinpoint such vascular changes and optimize the management and follow-up of patients with uveitis. The commonly encountered anomalous vascular changes in uveitis can be retinal vasculitis, retinal ischemia, retinal neovascularization, vascular telangiectasia and collaterals, and inflammatory CNV.

Retinal Vasculitis

Almost all forms of intermediate and posterior uveitis could possibly involve the retinal vessels. The endothelial cell is the primary target of attack in vasculitis and this endothelial cell specific immune response causes direct damage and infiltration of the vessel wall by inflammatory cells. In cases with active vasculitis, the perivascular infiltration is visible clinically as focal, multifocal, or diffuse fluffy white sheathing or cuffing of blood vessels.[8,11]

Broadly retinal vasculitis may be divided into two types—*exudative* and *occlusive*. In exudative retinal vasculitis, the inflammatory mediators lead to the breakdown of the inner blood-retinal barrier (BRB). On the other hand, in occlusive vasculitis, the inflammatory process prevents normal blood flow within the vascular lumen. Various other vascular changes may also manifest like telangiectasias, vascular anastomoses, macroaneurysm, microaneurysms, and optic disk or preretinal neovascularization. These varied presentations of the disease and the need to ascertain the presence of "active" inflammation of the retinal vessel wall make the assessment of vasculitis challenging.[12]

Fundus fluorescein angiography is an integral tool in the diagnosis of retinal vasculitis, especially exudative variety, showing staining of the blood vessel wall and leakage.[13] However, in cases of occlusive vasculitis, the visualization of areas of capillary nonperfusion might be limited by leakage of dye.

Optical coherence tomography angiography is more sensitive than FFA in the identification of ischemic changes as it enables the clinician to visualize and quantitate retinal ischemic areas in occlusive vasculitis. Unlike FFA, the images obtained with OCTA are not limited by the presence of leakage, pooling or window defects. OCTA can provide information regarding capillary perfusion of both superficial and DCP. In vasculitis, OCTA images show decreased capillary density and branching and these changes are more profound in SCP than DCP.[14,15]

OPTICAL COHERENCE TOMOGRAPHY ANGIOGRAPHY VERSUS FLUORESCEIN ANGIOGRAPHY IN UVEITIS

- Fundus fluorescein angiography is an important tool in the diagnosis of active retinal vasculitis. *Leakage* of dye due to breakdown of the inner BRB and staining of the blood vessel wall with fluorescein is essential in assessing inflammatory activity. While OCTA may not detect leakage, it can illustrate selective changes in the density of vessels in the superficial and/or deep retinal capillary plexus in patients with vasculitis.[16,17]
- In diseases such as birdshot chorioretinopathy (BSCR), recent studies have identified a significant *capillary flow deficit* in the deep retinal capillary plexus. This is better visualized using OCTA but is poorly picked up by FFA. Assessing the flow density of the deep vascular complex may provide an additional biomarker of inflammatory activity.
- Vascular *leakage* of dye or *window defects* in FFA may obscure the visualization of adjacent capillary perfusion. OCTA can overcome this limitation and provide microvascular morphological details of retina and choroid in presence of leakage.
- Fundus fluorescein angiography is currently the gold standard for identifying inflammatory CNV.[18] In various uveitic choroidal disorders such as multifocal choroiditis (MFC) or punctate inner choroidopathy (PIC), the major cause of vision loss may be direct inflammatory damage of the retina and RPE[19] or/and secondary inflammatory CNV (iCNV).[20] It is essential to distinguish inflammatory from neovascular CNV to optimize therapy. However, it is challenging to differentiate them by FFA. OCTA, nonetheless, has improved the sensitivity and specificity of detecting iCNV due to retinochoroidal inflammatory disorders.
- Fundus fluorescein angiography can distinguish between active and inactive/stable CNV, whereas the activity of CNV lesions cannot be reliably determined by OCTA.[20]

OPTICAL COHERENCE TOMOGRAPHY ANGIOGRAPHY VERSUS INDOCYANINE GREEN ANGIOGRAPHY IN UVEITIS

Two broad categories of choroiditis causing hypocyanescence on ICGA are choriocapillaritis and stromal choroiditis.[21]

- *Inflammatory choriocapillaritis* leads to nonperfusion and appears as irregular areas of hypocyanescence on ICGA. This pattern is best seen in placoid disorders such as acute posterior multifocal placoid pigment epitheliopathy (APMPPE) and serpiginous choroiditis (SC). OCTA of the choriocapillaris illustrates clearly demarcated areas of flow deficit that precisely colocalize with the hypocyanescent ICGA lesions and provide a noninvasive biomarker of choroidal inflammatory ischemic activity as well as response to therapy.
- The second main mechanism leading to hypocyanescense on ICGA is the presence of *inflammatory lesions in choroidal stroma*[21] that can occupy

space and block diffusion of the ICG molecule to these areas as a result of which they appear dark. These lesions are evenly distributed in the choroidal stroma in cases of Vogt–Koyanagi–Harada (VKH) disease and BSCR[22] and are irregularly distributed in secondary stromal choroiditis, such as sarcoidosis and tuberculosis. ICGA is more sensitive in identifying small sarcoid granulomas which cannot be picked up with OCTA. Only larger, full-thickness of choroidal granulomas can be visualized on OCTA as areas of choriocapillaris nonflow.[23]

- A third mechanism of hypocyanescence in uveitis, which is rare, has been described by Chang et al.[24] who noted that RPE normally absorbs ICG leading to the physiological background hyperfluorescence seen with ICGA. In disorders affecting RPE-like multiple evanescent white dot syndrome (MEWDS) ICG uptake may be disrupted. OCTA[25] has demonstrated completely normal choriocapillaris flow with no evidence of microvascular disruption even in the areas corresponding to ICG hypocyanescence. OCTA is, therefore, a valuable diagnostic modality in such diseases.

The difference between traditional angiography (FFA/ICGA) and OCTA is summarized in **Table 1**.

TABLE 1: Summary of differences between fundus fluorescein/indocyanine green angiography and OCT angiography.

FFA/ICGA	OCTA
Invasive	Noninvasive
More time consuming	Less time consuming
Requires skilled technician for administration of dye and capture of flow at appropriate time frames	Easy to perform
Difficult to repeat at each follow-up visits	Good repeatability at follow-up visits to monitor treatment response
FFA cannot image several important layers of retinochoroidal blood vessels and only the superficial vascular plexus can be seen	OCTA allows the segmentation of retinal and choroidal vasculature at different layers (superficial capillary plexus, deep capillary plexus, avascular outer retina, radial peripapillary network and choriocapillaris)
Can detect leakage	Leakage cannot be detected
Leakage/window defect obscures the visualization of adjacent capillary perfusion details	Provides accurate microvascular morphological details even in presence of leakage
Cannot distinguish between inflammatory lesions from iCNV	Able to differentiate between iCNV and inflammatory lesions
Activity of CNV can be determined	Cannot reliably point out between active and inactive CNV

(CNV: choroidal neovascularization; FFA: fundus fluorescein angiography; ICGA: indocyanine green angiography; OCTA: optical coherence tomography angiography)

APPLICATIONS OF OPTICAL COHERENCE TOMOGRAPHY ANGIOGRAPHY IN OCULAR INFLAMMATION

Several uveitis conditions such as MFC, PIC, MEWDS, APMPPE, BSCR, and VKH disease target the photoreceptors, the RPE, or the choroid and show characteristic features on OCTA. The use of OCTA technology in patients with ocular inflammation is likely to reveal novel features that may help in advancing our understanding of pathophysiology and natural history of the disease.[26]

Multifocal Choroiditis

Multifocal choroiditis is an uncommon, chronic, and recurrent disease which mostly affects women of 20–60 years of age and can involve both eyes.[27] The disease may be associated with varying degrees of vitritis and mild nongranulomatous anterior segment inflammation. The characteristic lesions of MFC appear as yellowish-white spots, more commonly seen in the peripapillary region, the posterior pole and mid periphery.[28] These lesions are seen at the level of the RPE or choriocapillaris and are small (50–100 μ) with varying amounts of subretinal fluid. Lesions may be arranged singly, in clusters, or in linear, or concentric streaks known as *Schlagel lines*. On resolution, they become punched out and atrophic with varying degrees of pigment and scarring.[23]

Visual prognosis in MFC may be guarded by disruption of the retina and RPE due to inflammation and/or iCNV.[29] Inflammatory lesions and iCNV must be distinguished for the sake of optimizing therapy. Inflammatory lesions require treatment with steroids and immunosuppressant therapy,[30] while iCNV is treated with intravitreal antivascular endothelial growth factor (anti-VEGF) agents. But, it is challenging to distinguish between both these lesions even with the use of advanced multimodal imaging since both can cause tissue disruption and breakdown of the BRB.[18,31]

Fundus fluorescein angiography is the gold standard for detecting CNV.[32] The typical presentation of CNV on FFA is early hyperfluorescence with late leakage, whereas the yellowish-white inflammatory dots seen in fundus of MFC patients appear hypo-/isofluorescent in early phase of FFA with late staining and leakage. Atrophic scar appears as an RPE window defect which shows early hyperfluorescence that decreases in the late phase. Hence, the classic findings on FFA are not always consistent and can vary with the type of CNV and the stage of inflammatory lesion during the course of disease.[33] It is, therefore, arduous to distinguish iCNV from the inflammatory lesions of MFC by FFA.

The spectral domain optical coherence tomography shows sub-RPE round-shaped drusen-like hyper-reflective deposits above the Bruch's membrane that break through the RPE and extend into the outer retinal layers. The break in RPE allows more OCT signal to penetrate the choroid resulting in choroidal hyper-reflectivity underneath the lesion. In addition, the ellipsoid zone overlying the MFC lesions is also disrupted.[29,31] In MFC, ICGA illustrates hypocyanescent spots which are otherwise not seen clinically or on FFA.[29,31,34,35]

Optical coherence tomography angiography, at the level of the choriocapillaris, demonstrates flow signal loss in MFC which is probably due to altered blood flow or frank loss of choriocapillaris, precisely corresponding to the hypocyanescent lesion seen in the late phase of ICGA.[36] It can remarkably distinguish the inflammatory lesions in MFC from iCNVs. MFC lesions do not show any internal flow on OCTA, in contrast to iCNV where blood flow is clearly visible within the neovascular network. OCTA demonstrates a higher sensitivity in detecting neovascular flow within MFC lesions but a lower specificity in differentiating active neovascularization versus an inactive scar.[20] However, FFA may provide insightful information in identifying active CNV. OCTA is, thus, a part of multimodal imaging methods to detect the presence of abnormal vasculature in subretinal hyper-reflective material seen on SD-OCT **(Table 2)**.

Punctate Inner Choroidopathy

Punctate inner choroidopathy is a subtype of MFC and a rare form of idiopathic posterior uveitis that occurs in otherwise healthy, predominantly, young adult myopic women.[37] Affected females may complain of blurred vision, floaters, scotoma, metamorphopsia, photophobia, and photopsia. An important distinguishing feature of PIC is the absence of anterior chamber or vitreous inflammation.[37] The funduscopic examination is characterized by multiple well-defined, punctate, yellowish-white lesions, measuring 100–300 µ at the level of outer retina, RPE and choriocapillaris,

TABLE 2: Characteristics of lesions in multifocal choroiditis (MFC) using multimodal imaging techniques.

FFA	ICGA	SD-OCT	OCTA
• Yellowish-white dots seen clinically in MFC appear hypofluorescent in early phase with gradual staining and leakage. Atrophic scar appears as an RPE window defect with early hyperfluorescene which decreases in the late phase • Early hyperfluorescence with late leakage is seen in iCNV	Hypocyanescent spots	• Sub-RPE round-shaped drusen-like hyper-reflective material. Choroidal hyper-reflectivity underneath the lesion • Ellipsoid zone disruption overlying the lesions	• Focal flow reduction in choriocapillaris • Network of tangled vessels in outer retina is seen in iCNV

(CNV: choroidal neovascularization; FFA: fundus fluorescein angiography; ICGA: indocyanine green angiography; OCTA: optical coherence tomography angiography; RPE: retinal pigment epithelium; SD-OCT: spectral domain-optical coherence tomography)

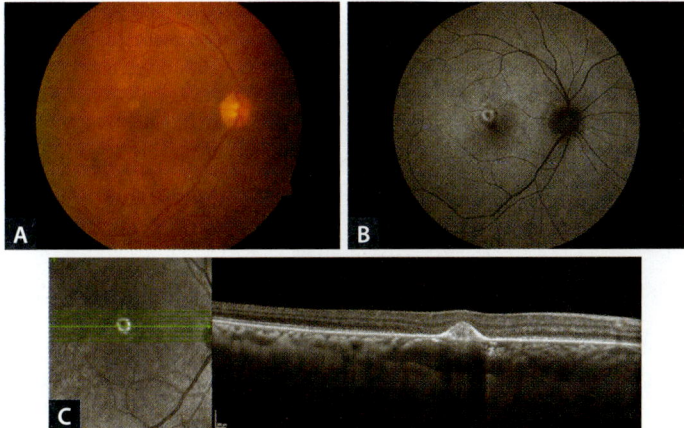

Figs. 1A to C: (A) Colored fundus photograph of punctate inner choroidopathy showing a yellow-white chorioretinal lesion at the posterior pole (juxtafoveal area); (B) Autofluoroscence image of the PIC lesion showing central hypoautofluorescence with a surrounding hyperautofluorescent ring; (C) OCT images showing a pigment epithelial detachment with hyper-reflective material under the retinal pigment epithelium with a fairly well-defined retinal pigment epithelium border.
(OCT: optical coherence tomography; PIC: punctate inner choroidopathy)

which may eventually become atrophic pigmented scars. These lesions characteristically cluster in the posterior pole and are generally not found in the peripheral retina. The most common and vision threatening complication of PIC is CNV[38] which has been reported in up to 69–75% patients. The current standard for imaging the lesions of PIC include SD-OCT, FFA, and ICGA. The findings of PIC lesions on aforesaid modalities are comparable to MFC lesions **(Figs. 1A to C)**.

Optical coherence tomography angiography provides a valuable insight into the characteristics of lesion in PIC. All eyes with punctate lesions reveal capillaries with crippled whitening, which may be indicative of erythrocyte accumulation in these areas. Areas of nonperfusion/hypoperfusion in the choriocapillaris are also detected **(Figs. 2 and 3)**. The type and morphology of CNV can also be characterized using OCTA. It is considered as a useful tool for monitoring and quantifying the response of CNV to treatment.

Vogt–Koyanagi–Harada Disease

Vogt–Koyanagi–Harada disease is a multisystem autoimmune inflammatory disorder characterized by bilateral granulomatous uveitis and neurologic, auditory and integumentary manifestation in its complete form.[39]

The disease typically manifests in four stages with characteristic ocular features that can be diagnosed using multimodal imaging **(Table 3)**. Systemic features including meningeal findings are most remarkable in the initial *prodromal stage*. This is followed by *acute ocular stage* and is associated with exudative retinal detachment. Next is *convalescent stage* in which there

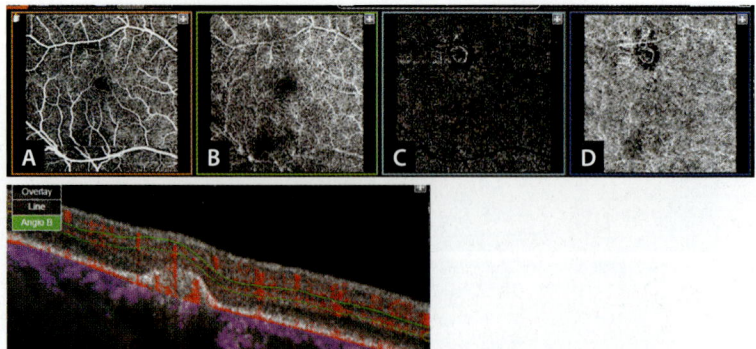

Figs. 2A to D: OCTA images of a 31-year-old myopic female with PIC showing: (A and B) Normal SCP and DCP at presentation; (C) Abnormal ring of vessel (choroidal neovascular membrane) in the avascular segment; (D) Vascular loop with surrounding hypoperfusion at the choriocapillaris level.
(DCP: deep capillary plexus; OCTA: optical coherence tomography angiography; PIC: punctate inner choroidopathy; SCP: superficial capillary plexus)

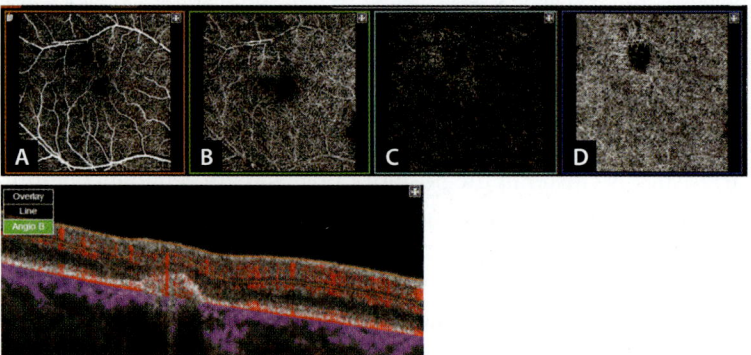

Figs. 3A to D: OCTA images (A to D) of the same patient after 3 monthly injections of anti-VEGF agent showing resolution in the size of CNV.
(CNV: choroidal neovascularization; OCTA: optical coherence tomography angiography; VEGF: vascular endothelial growth factor)

is pigment loss affecting various organs systems. Finally, the *last stage* is characterized by chronic anterior uveitis. There is considerable variation in this staging system and patients may present only with the acute ocular phase of VKH disease with classic exudative retinal detachment and signs of uveitis.

Histopathologically, VKH disease primarily affects the choroidal stroma with diffuse infiltration of inflammatory cells. Formation of large choroidal granulomas can compress the surrounding vasculature and impair the choroidal blood flow that appears as areas of flow void on OCTA. The inflammation may subsequently involve the RPE and outer retina.[40]

On OCTA, the choriocapillaris segment demonstrates multiple dark foci with loss of choriocapillaris representing severe hypoperfusion **(Figs. 4A to E)**. The edges of these lesions are discrete and clearly delineated. These

TABLE 3: Characteristic features of different stages of VKH disease on OCTA, EDI-OCT and ICGA.

Imaging modality	Acute	Convalescent	Healed/Chronic
OCTA	Multiple, large areas of flow void at the level of choriocapillaris	Size and number of choriocapillaris flow void areas decrease	Absence of choriocapillaris flow void areas. Restoration of normal vasculature
EDI-OCT	Exudative retinal detachment, undulations in inner retina, RPE folds and choroidal thickening	Resolution of subretinal fluid, decrease in choroidal thickening, decrease in RPE and inner retinal folds	Subretinal fluid resorbs, choroidal thickness becomes normal
ICGA	Early choroidal vessel hyperfluorescence, intermediate to late phase fuzziness of choroidal stromal vessels, disk hyperfluorescence and hypofluorescent dark dots	Decreased stromal and vascular hyperfluorescence, decrease in hypofluorescent dark spots	Normalization of stromal and vascular pattern, no evidence of disk hyperfluorescence and decrease in hypofluorescent dark spots

(EDI-OCT: enhanced depth imaging optical coherence tomography; ICGA: indocyanine green angiography; OCTA: optical coherence tomography angiography; VKH: Vogt–Koyanagi–Harada)

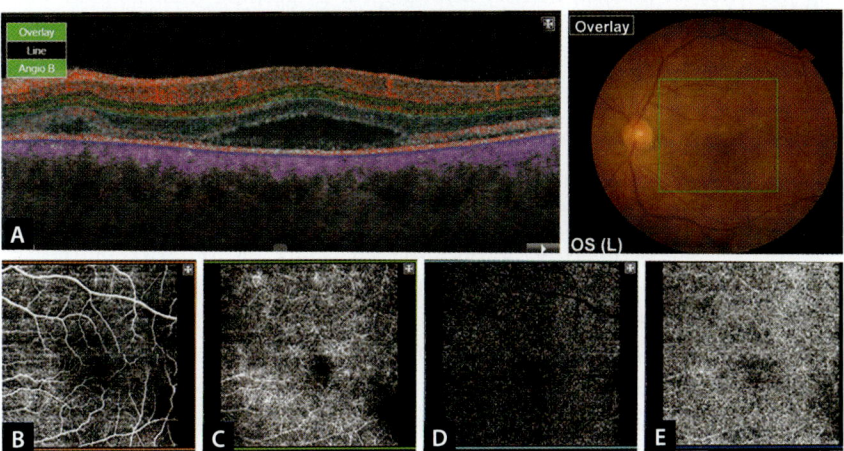

Figs. 4A to E: Acute stage of VKH disease showing: (A) Serous retinal detachment on OCT, and (B to E) OCTA of the same patient with corresponding flow void areas (dark) at the level of choriocapillaris (E).
(OCTA: optical coherence tomography angiography; VKH: Vogt–Koyanagi–Harada)

areas of choriocapillaris ischemia on OCTA colocalize with thickening and hyporeflectivity on enhanced depth imaging optical coherence tomography (EDI-OCT). On comparing OCTA with ICGA, the areas of flow void on OCTA correspond with the persistent hypocyanescent spots on ICGA. On follow-up, OCTA of patients with acute VKH disease depicts interval recovery in the choriocapillaris flow void areas **(Figs. 5A to E)** which correlate with the decrease in the subfoveal choroidal thickness displayed on EDI-OCT.[41]

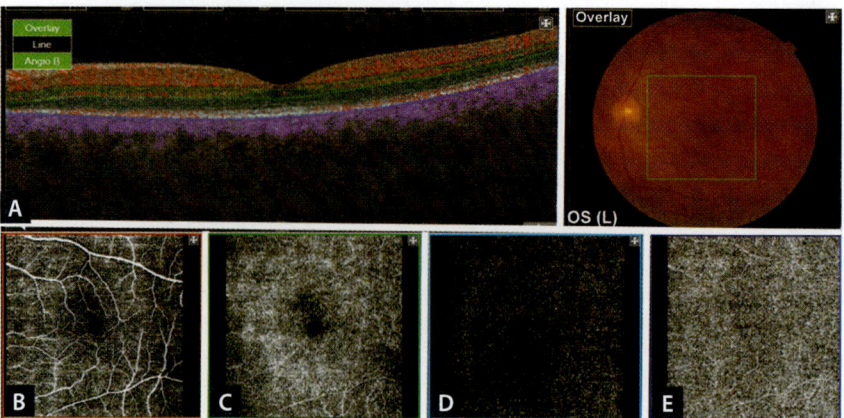

Figs. 5A to E: Same patient as in **Figure 4** showing: (A) Recovery with resolution of neurosensory detachment and flat OCT, and (B to E) Reperfusion of flow void area after treatment with steroids (E).
(OCT: optical coherence tomography)

Optical angio-OCT is an effective adjunct that may be sensitive in detecting the presence of disease activity and helpful in guiding treatment in VKH disease and equates well with imaging techniques, such as EDI-OCT and ICGA.

Acute Posterior Multifocal Placoid Pigment Epitheliopathy

Acute posterior multifocal placoid pigment epitheliopathy was first described by Gass in 1968.[42] Its pathogenesis has been controversial and the clinical features remain atypical for choroiditis including the rapid resolution of lesions and the near absence of damage to the choroid despite significant alterations in the RPE. In 1973, Deutman et al.[43] utilized fluorescein angiography and proposed that the RPE abnormalities in APMPPE were due to ischemia of the choriocapillaris. ICGA studies have supported choroidal involvement as a prominent feature **(Figs. 6A to G)**. Moreover, OCT illustrates increased inner choroidal hyporeflectivity in APMPPE.[44]

In 2017, Kklufas et al.[45] used *en face* OCT and OCTA technology to assess choroidal hypoperfusion in APMPPE. OCT images revealed circumscribed areas of hyporeflectivity at the level of the ellipsoid zone/RPE complex that is consistent with the area of reduced choriocapillaris flow on OCTA. The zone of choriocapillaris ischemia as visualized on OCTA was comparable to the area of hypofluoresence on ICGA. Moreover, careful assessment for signal attenuation revealed that the OCTA lesions were predominantly the result of a true inner choroidal flow void (presumably ischemia) rather than shadowing from the outer retinal placoid lesions. It was concluded that ICGA hypofluorescence was indeed the result of decreased choriocapillaris flow.

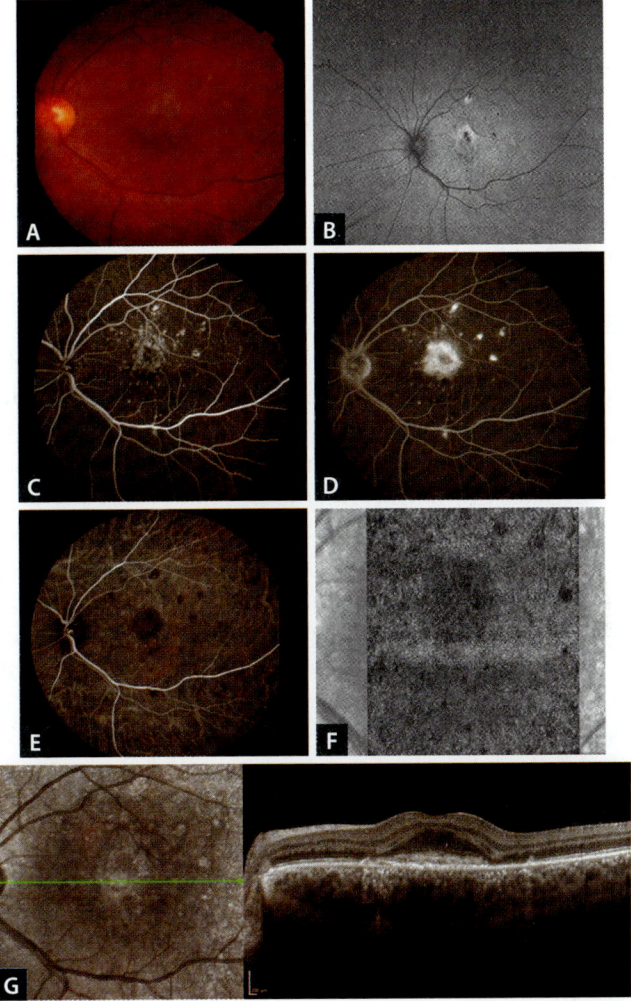

Figs. 6A to G: (A) Colored fundus photograph of left eye of a patient of APMPPE demonstrating multiple yellowish-white, subretinal, and placoid lesions of variable size located at the posterior pole; (B) Lesions showing hypoautofluorescence with some lesions showing hyperautofluorescent edges; (C) FFA images in early phase showing central hypofluorescence with surrounding hyperfluorescent borders (Christmas wreath-like appearance); (D) Late phase of angiogram showing staining of the lesions; (E) ICGA showing hypocyanescent lesions; (F) OCTA images at the level of choriocapillaris showing flow void areas which correspond with the areas of hypocyanescence seen on ICGA; (G) OCT showing hyper-reflective deposits over RPE corresponding to the lesion.
(APMPPE: acute posterior multifocal placoid pigment epitheliopathy; FFA: fundus fluorescein angiography; ICGA: indocyanine green angiography; OCTA: optical coherence tomography angiography)

On long-term follow-up, there is recovery of choriocapillaris flow and signs of vascular reperfusion with treatment or in the natural course of the disease. OCTA may provide an important tool to guide diagnosis, prognosis, and therapeutic response in patients with placoid-related disorders.[46]

Birdshot Chorioretinopathy

Birdshot chorioretinopathy (BSCR) is a type of idiopathic posterior uveitis with a strong association with human leukocyte antigen (HLA)-A29. The standardized diagnostic criteria for BSCR include presence of bilateral disease, at least three peripapillary "birdshot" lesions, low-grade anterior chamber inflammation, and low-grade vitritis.[47] In BSCR inflammation occurs independently, but simultaneously, in the choroid and the retina with retinal vasculitis being an important component. The course of the disease is long and insidious[48] with progressive deterioration of both central and peripheral retinal functions.[49] Due to this progressive nature of BSCR, it is vital to have accurate techniques for monitoring disease activity and measuring tissue damage else the chronic inflammation may lead to retinal atrophy.

Snellen visual acuity is an unreliable indicator of visual function and disease progression in BSCR. Alternative more reliable tests include visual field analysis and full field electroretinography.[22,50] Assessment of retinochoroidal vasculature is also important to accurately assess the severity and extent of intraocular inflammation.

Optical coherence tomography angiography can provide high-resolution imaging of retinochoroidal vascular changes in BSCR. The early birdshot lesions are inflammatory choroidal infiltrates which consist of epithelioid cells that surround the choroidal stromal melanocytes. These are partial thickness and do not affect the adjacent choriocapillaris resulting in normal OCTA analysis of choroid early in the course of disease. As the disease progresses the lesions show chronic granulomatous inflammation that can ultimately destroy uveal melanocytes. These inflammatory granulomas resolve with atrophy of choriocapillaris and the inner choroidal stroma. OCTA in advanced BSCR shows a complete loss or reduced choroidal blood flow.[25,51,52]

Optical coherence tomography angiography of the superficial retinal capillary plexus in BSCR depicts abnormal telangiectatic vessels, capillary dilatations, loops, and increased intercapillary space.[53] The most reliable finding among these is increased perifoveal intercapillary spaces.[23]

Pichi et al.[52] compared early frame fluorescein angiogram to the 3 × 3-mm OCTA segmented at the level of superficial retinal capillary plexus and found that foveal avascular zone (FAZ) of birdshot patients was better recognized and delineated using OCTA. The FAZ mean area on OCTA images was larger in eyes with BSCR compared to normal healthy eyes and this difference was statistically significant.

The findings on OCTA were compared to central retinal thickness (CRT) as measured by SD-OCT. Areas with hypoperfusion on OCTA demonstrated a statistically significant correlation with areas of decreased CRT on SD-OCT. It is speculated that flow reduction may be associated with ischemia that could lead to a decrease in retinal thickness on SD-OCT.

Phasukkijwatana et al.[54] found that there was more profound flow reduction at the DCP level, compared to the SCP, which may indicate that ischemia in addition to inflammation may play a role in the development of complications such as retinal neovascularization in BSCR.

Serpiginous Choroiditis

Serpiginous choroiditis is a rare form of uveitis (accounting for approximately 1% of posterior uveitis cases) which is categorized as a primary inflammatory choriocapillaropathy.[55] The SC group consists of four overlapping disorders that differ essentially in the pattern of placoid progression:

1. Classic SC
2. Macular SC
3. Serpiginous-like choroiditis (SLC)
4. Ampiginous choroiditis

Typically, all are rare, often bilateral, chronic, relapsing diseases associated with progressive inflammation and scarring of the RPE and inner choroid.

Serpiginous-like choroiditis differs from SC[56,57] by the presence of multifocal choroidal lesions. These lesions progress to confluent diffuse choroiditis finally resembling classic SC. Some patients may present with a progressive plaque-like ameboid pattern of choroiditis similar to ampiginous choroiditis. Remarkably, the macula is spared in most patients, thus, the visual outcome may be better than in classic SC which is associated with a poor visual prognosis. Patients with SLC usually have vitritis when the lesions are active.[58] SLC is an important manifestation of *Mycobacterium tuberculosis* associated posterior uveitis which is confirmed by polymerase chain reaction (PCR) analysis of vitreous and aqueous fluid.[59]

Optical coherence tomography angiography is useful in detecting choriocapillaris ischemia and atrophy as well as the development of CNV in SC. *En face* OCTA maps were compared with the EDI-OCT, FFA, and ICGA findings in SLC by Mandadi et al.[59] On OCTA, the superficial and deep retinal capillary plexus were normal in all eyes. The choriocapillaris showed reduced perfusion or "flow void" in the areas corresponding to both active and healed choroiditis lesions. During the active stage of the disease, the OCTA areas of flow-void correlated with the hypocyanescent lesions on ICG. In-between the active lesions healthy choriocapillaris and medium-sized choroidal vessels were seen. As the lesions healed, deeper medium-to-large choroidal vessels became more prominent and were better delineated on OCTA than on ICGA. The flow-void areas on OCTA were seen as "hyporeflective" areas of thickened choriocapillaris on EDI-OCT. However, during the healing stage, the prominent medium-to-large choroidal vessels visualized on OCTA corresponded to choriocapillaris atrophy on EDI-OCT.

At the initial evaluation, ICGA is preferable because it more clearly delineates choriocapillaris lesions. Nevertheless, OCTA replaces ICGA during subsequent follow-up visits because it is a noninvasive and easily performed imaging modality that reduces the number of angiograms needed.

Multiple Evanescent White Dot Syndrome

Multiple evanescent white dot syndrome, first reported by Jampol et al. in 1984,[60] is an acute-onset inflammatory syndrome characterized by 100–200 μm sized multiple yellow-white dots and spots that lie deep to the retina. The etiology is still unclear. However, photoreceptor dysfunction with decreased a-wave amplitude seen on electroretinographic analysis[61,62] indicates that the pathology resides in the outer retina and/or the RPE. Dell'omo et al. in 2010 described MEWDS as a choroidopathy based on ICGA findings.[63] In the late-phase of ICGA, MEWDS lesions show hypofluorescence suggestive of choroidal hypoperfusion.

Optical coherence tomography angiography was used by Pichi et al.[23] in acute cases of MEWDS. They found that superficial and deep retinal capillary plexus and the choroidal vasculature were entirely unremarkable and were analogous to normal capillary networks reported in healthy control eyes. Furthermore, in areas of ICGA hypofluorescence, OCTA demonstrated no evidence of vessel dilation or flow deficit with completely normal choriocapillaris flow.

The cause of choroidal hypofluorescence was intriguing given the normal choroidal findings on OCTA. Chang et al.[24] studied the ICGA absorption characteristics of the RPE and noted that the RPE normally absorbs indocyanine dye causing physiological background hyperfluorescence. However, in certain retinal disorders, such as MEWDS, the dysfunctional and disrupted RPE cells have reduced ICG uptake which may explain the late hypofluorescent lesions on ICGA. These dark spots on ICGA colocalize with the areas of disrupted RPE-photoreceptor complex seen on EDI-OCT.

Optical coherence tomography angiography supports the hypothesis that the choriocapillaris may not be involved in this disease and that MEWDS may be primarily the result of an abnormality at the level of the RPE-photoreceptor complex.

Inflammatory Cystoid Macular Edema

Cystoid macular edema (CME) is the most common cause of vision loss in uveitis patients. Any form of uveitis (anterior, posterior, or intermediate) can be complicated by CME.[64] The diagnosis of CME is made on clinical examination or imaging by OCT, FFA, or OCTA[65-67] as shown in **Table 4**. In addition, OCT is also important in the monitoring of treatment and determining the prognosis of CME in uveitis.[66,67] OCTA helps in detecting microvascular changes, and differential involvement of DCP versus SCP in uveitic CME.[68]

TABLE 4: Features suggestive of cystoid macular edema on different imaging modalities.

Imaging method	Features
OCT	- Cystoid spaces in inner retinal layers - Central macular thickening - Ellipsoid zone disruption in chronic cases
FFA	- Pooling of dye in cystic spaces - Perifoveal areas of capillary nonperfusion/hypoperfusion - Perifoveal capillary arcade disruption
OCTA	- Intraretinal cystoid spaces - Perifoveal capillary arcade disruption - Capillary abnormalities such as capillary dilatation and areas of rarefied capillaries - Areas of capillary nonperfusion/hypoperfusion - Disorganization of capillary network - Enlargement of FAZ - Reduction of capillary vascular density

(FAZ: foveal avascular zone; FFA: fundus fluorescein angiography; OCTA: optical coherence tomography angiography)

Optical Coherence Tomography Angiography Findings in Uveitic Cystoid Macular Edema

- *Cystoid spaces and hypoperfused areas*: This is the most common finding on OCTA in uveitic CME. The intraretinal cystoid spaces which are completely devoid of flow mainly affect the DCP and less commonly the SCP (<20% eyes).[68] The absence of flow signals is due to the peripheral displacement of retinal capillaries as well as the preferential development of cysts in nonperfused areas.[69,70] Similar location of cystoid spaces in the inner retinal layers is also reported in DME and pseudophakic CME.[69,70] However, areas of decreased retinal perfusion can also be seen in uveitis eyes without CME.
- *Capillary abnormalities*: Disorganized capillary networks involve more severely the DCP than the SCP.[68]
- *Reduced capillary vascular density (CVD)*: It is found in both the SCP and the DCP in uveitic CME.[68] This is also reported in pseudophakic CME.[70-72]
- *Enlarged FAZ*: Enlarged FAZ in uveitic CME is seen in the DCP but not the SCP.[68] This is reported in DME and retinal vein occlusion CME also.[73,74] Both a lower CVD as well as a larger FAZ can be explained by the displacement of capillaries by macular edema with or without capillary nonperfusion.

Overall, more severe DCP microvascular changes would be associated with a poorer VA at baseline, a longer duration to resolution (>6 months) and a higher central macular thickness (CMT).[68]

Optical coherence tomography angiography provides a deeper insight into the pathophysiological process of uveitic CME. The pathophysiology of uveitis

CME falls under a spectrum ranging from the nonischemic CME (similar to Irvine-Gass syndrome with induced capillary hyperpermeability) to severely ischemic CME (similar to DME or retinal vein occlusion). This suggests that both inflammatory factors and glial cells play a role in the development of uveitic CME as well as underlying retinal ischemic mechanisms.[68]

Optical coherence tomography angiography also aids in the monitoring of uveitic CME, assessing response to treatment and estimating the prognosis. After the complete resolution of uveitic CME, there is either a complete recovery of the capillary plexuses (as in nonischemic CME) or a persistence of areas of capillary rarefaction with poor perfusion (as in ischemic CME).

OPTICAL COHERENCE TOMOGRAPHY ANGIOGRAPHY FINDINGS IN INFLAMMATORY CHOROIDAL NEOVASCULARIZATION

Choroidal neovascularization is a sight-threatening complication of retinochoroidal inflammatory and infectious conditions.[75] This includes PIC,[20] MFC[76] and other white-dot syndromes,[77] SC,[78] and TB-associated choroiditis.[79]

Early diagnosis is imperative to institute timely anti-VEGF treatment to prevent visual loss.[80] However, these lesions are often difficult to detect clinically and on conventional imaging modalities such as OCT and FFA due to the presence of concomitant active or healed choroidal lesions with associated scarring and pigmentation that may confound the findings.[76,81,82] On FFA chorioretinal inflammatory lesions are commonly confused with iCNV since the leakage can be a characteristic feature of both lesion types (Watzke et al., 1984). ICGA may fail to identify very early stage of CNV when vascular changes are inconspicuous.[83]

Optical coherence tomography angiography is superior to other imaging modalities in diagnosis of inflammatory CNV.[84] It is quite sensitive in detecting iCNV even in the absence of fundus signs on clinical examination such as subretinal hemorrhages, exudation or peripapillary halo/fluid. The area and the density of inflammatory CNV can also be quantitated by OCTA.[85] Features of iCNV on various imaging modalities are summarized in **Table 5**.

Optical coherence tomography angiography can also be used to monitor the response of iCNV to treatment. Generally, small immature neovascular loops are VEGF sensitive and regress early with anti-VEGF treatment and remain stable even after treatment. The larger more intertwined net is more anti-VEGF-resistant. It may though shrink with treatment, but some can still show signs of vessel recanalization and remodeling post-treatment.[86,87]

Studies on the development of inflammatory CNV and use of OCTA in inflammatory conditions such as uveitis and choroiditis are fewer as compared to neovascular age-related macular degeneration (nAMD). Early studies have shown significant advantage of OCTA compared to other

TABLE 5: Inflammatory CNV findings on different imaging modalities.

Imaging method	Features
OCT	• Intraretinal or subretinal fluid along with subretinal pigment epithelial (RPE)/subretinal hyper-reflective material (SHRM) • Low-lying pigment epithelial detachments (PED) usually adjacent to an area of chorioretinal scarring • RPE and IS/OS disruption • Choroidal hyper-reflectivity
FFA	Early iso- or hyperfluorescence with late leakage
ICGA	Subtle ill-defined hypercyanescence
OCTA	Well-circumscribed neovascular complexes **(Figs. 7A to E)** with or without collaterals, vascular loops, intertwined nets, and feeder vessels • *"Lacy wheel shape"* and *"pruned large-trunk vessels"* found above RPE suggest active disease. • *"Dead tree aspect"* vessels are observed below the RPE and indicate inactive disease.

(CNV: choroidal neovascularization; FFA: fundus fluorescein angiography; ICGA: indocyanine green angiography; IS/OS: inner segment/outer segment; OCTA: optical coherence tomography angiography)

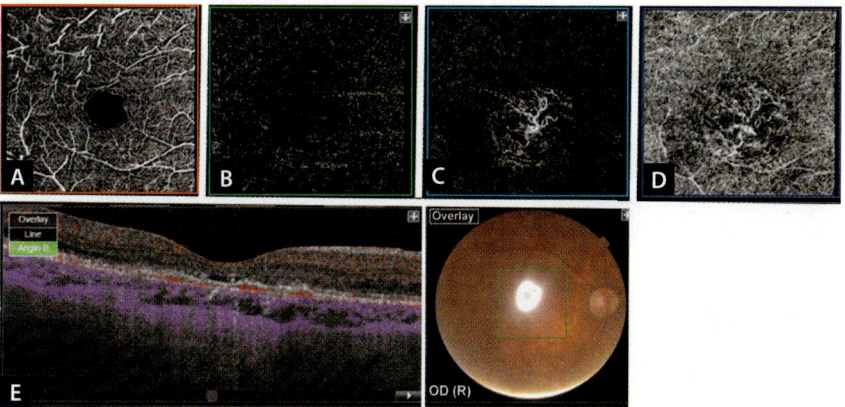

Figs.7A to E: OCTA showing iCNV. (A) Normal superficial capillary plexus; (B) Disruption of deep capillary plexus; (C and D) Network of tangled vessels (CNV) seen at the level of avascular and choriocapillaris segmentation; (E) OCT showing disruption of outer retinal layers with a sliver of subretinal fluid.
(CNV: choroidal neovascularization; OCTA: optical coherence tomography angiography)

investigations in distinguishing iCNV from inflammatory lesions, but it has limitation in distinguishing recurrent proliferating vessels from an old vascular scar.[32] Further studies in future may help to understand the OCTA features of inflammatory CNV in various retinochoroidal inflammatory conditions.

Common posterior uveitic entities with their characteristic features on different layers of OCTA are described in **Table 6**.

TABLE 6: OCTA findings in different uveitic entities.

Different layers seen on OCTA	Superficial capillary plexus: Superficial retina	Deep capillary plexus: Middle retina	Outer retina (avascular)	Choriocapillaris	Choroid
Inflammatory vasculitis	Reduced capillary density and branching				
Birdshot chorioretinopathy	Increased intercapillary spaces, enlarged FAZ and focal areas of abnormal tortuous vessels (telangiectasias)	Capillary density is decreased though less than SCP		Active lesions demonstrate normal flow while atrophic healed lesions show complete loss or reduced flow	
MEWDS		Reduced capillary density more intense than SCP		Normal flow	
VKH disease				Multiple flow void areas in acute stage	
PIC/MFC			Network of intertwined vessels present if complicated by CNV	Focal flow reduction	
APMPPE				Flow reduction and ischemia	Flow reduction and ischemia
Uveitic macular edema	Flow void areas, disorganized and decreased capillary networks and enlarged FAZ	More profound changes in DCP including flow void areas, disorganized capillary networks, reduced capillary vascular density and enlarged FAZ			
Inflammatory CNV			Neovascular network		

(APMPPE: acute posterior multifocal placoid pigment epitheliopathy; CNV: choroidal neovascularization; DCP: deep capillary plexus; FAZ: foveal avascular zone; FFA: fundus fluorescein angiography; MEWDS: multiple evanescent white dot syndrome; MFC: multifocal choroiditis; OCTA: optical coherence tomography angiography; PIC: punctate inner choroidopathy; SCP: superficial capillary plexus; VKH: Vogt–Koyanagi–Harada)

LIMITATIONS OF OPTICAL COHERENCE TOMOGRAPHY ANGIOGRAPHY

Despite all the advantages of OCTA and the continuous improvement in the technology, it does have several limitations. Awareness of these limitations is necessary for accurate interpretation of OCTA images.

- *Motion artifact*: It is caused by blinking or fixation loss resulting in dark horizontal bands across the image. Despite the innovations in eye-tracking techniques, defective fixation in patients with poor visual acuity may hamper the acquisition of a high-quality image. This makes the use of OCTA in vision-impairing maculopathies daunting.[88]
- *Media opacities*: Media opacities such as cataract or corneal scarring may degrade signal quality.
- *Segmentation errors:* Automated segmentation errors are common mainly in the presence of pathology that distorts the retinal architecture such as intraretinal or subretinal fluid. In such cases manual segmentation is required to obtain precise and correct OCTA image slabs.
- *Projection artifacts*: These occur from the shadowing of overlying signals from the superficial retinal layers being reflected on the deeper hyper-reflective structure (choriocapillaris layer). This causes confusion in interpretation of OCTA images.[88] New algorithms have been developed to remove these artifacts which improve visualization of the choriocapillaris.[89]
- *Imaging of deeper choroidal vessels*: In normal eyes, reflection and scattering of signal by the RPE is a barrier to visualization of flow signal of the deeper choroidal vessels, even with the use of swept-source OCTA. However, flow within the deeper choroidal vessels can be well appreciated in the presence of RPE atrophy.[90]
- *Subretinal hemorrhage or fluid* can also attenuate signal which can make detection of choroidal neovascular complexes more difficult.

SUMMARY

Optical coherence tomography angiography provides high-resolution and depth-resolved information that has never been before available with dye-based angiography. Nonetheless, one should be watchful while interpreting OCTA due to its limitations and it should preferably be used in association with other imaging modalities. With further advancement in technology OCTA is bound to make major impacts in the diagnosis and management of posterior uveitis.

ACKNOWLEDGMENTS

We would like to acknowledge Prof Chee Soon Phiak, Singapore National Eye Center, Singapore, Dr Jay Siak, Singapore National Eye Center, Singapore,

Dr Isuru Desilva (Fellow, Moorfields Eye Hospital, London), and Dr Nikita Gupta, Post Graduate Institute, Chandigarh, India for their contributions.

REFERENCES

1. Makita S, Hong Y, Yamanari M, Yatagai T, Yasuno Y. Optical coherence angiography. Opt Express. 2006;14(17):7821-40.
2. Gorczynska I, Migacz JV, Zawadzki RJ, Capps AG, Werner JS. Comparison of amplitude-decorrelation, speckle-variance and phase-variance OCT angiography methods for imaging the human retina and choroid. Biomed Opt Express. 2016;7(3):911-42.
3. Yannuzzi LA, Sorenson JA, Guyer DR, Slakter JS, Chang B, Orlock D. Indocyanine green videoangiography: current status. Eur J Ophthalmol. 1994;4(2):69-81.
4. Fingler J, Zawadzki RJ, Werner JS, Schwartz D, Fraser SE. Volumetric microvascular imaging of human retina using optical coherence tomography with a novel motion contrast technique. Opt Express. 2009;17(4):22190-200.
5. Wang RK, Jacques SL, Ma Z, Hurst S, Hanson SR, Gruber A. Three-dimensional optical angiography. Opt Express. 2007;15(7):4083-97.
6. Chen CL, Wang RK. Optical coherence tomography based angiography [Invited]. Biomed Opt Express. 2017;8(2):1056-82.
7. Fingler J, Schwartz D, Yang C, Fraser SE. Mobility and transverse flow visualization using phase variance contrast with spectral domain optical coherence tomography. Opt Express. 2007;15(20):12636-53.
8. Invernizzi A, Mapelli C, Viola F, Cigada M, Cimino L, Ratiglia R, et al. Choroidal granulomas visualized by enhanced depth imaging optical coherence tomography. Retina. 2015;35(3):525-31.
9. Fujimoto JG, Lumbroso B, Rispoli M, Huang D, Jia Y. Optical Coherence Tomography-Angiography: New Clinical Terminology. In: Lumbroso B (Ed) Clinical Guide to Angio-OCT (Non Invasive, Dyeless OCT Angiography). New Delhi: Jaypee Brothers Medical Publishers; 2015. pp. 10-43.
10. Musat O, Colta D, Cernat C, Boariu AM, Alexandru L, Georgescu R, et al. New perspectives in retinal imaging: angio-OCT. Roman J Ophthalmol. 2016;60(2):63-7.
11. Abu El-Asrar AM, Herbort CP, Tabbara KF. A clinical approach to the diagnosis of retinal vasculitis. Int Ophthalmol. 2010;30(2):149-73.
12. Park JJ, Soetikno BT, Fawzi AA. Characterization of the middle capillary plexus using optical coherence tomography angiography in healthy and diabetic eyes. Retina. 2016; 36(11):2039-50.
13. Walton RC, Ashmore ED. Retinal vasculitis. Curr Opin Ophthalmol. 2003;14(6):413-9.
14. Leder HA, Campbell JP, Sepah YJ, Gan T, Dunn JP, Hatef E, et al. Ultra-wide-field retinal imaging in the management of non-infectious retinal vasculitis. J Ophthalmic Inflam Infect. 2013;3(1):30.
15. Lee J, Rosen R. Optical coherence tomography angiography in diabetes. Curr Diabetes Rep. 2016;16(12):123.
16. Kim AY, Rodger DC, Shahidzadeh A, Chu Z, Koulisis N, Burkemper B, et al. Quantifying retinal microvascular changes in uveitis using spectral-domain optical coherence tomography angiography. Am J Ophthalmol. 2016;16(12):123.
17. Bessete AP, Levison AL, Baynes K, Lowder CY, Srivastava SK. Qualitative and quantitative analysis of optical coherence tomography angiography in patients with retinal vasculitis. Investig Ophthalmol Vis Sci. 2016;57(12):5504.
18. Kotsolis AI, Killian FA, Ladas ID, Yannuzzi LA. Fluorescein angiography and optical coherence tomography concordance for choroidal neovascularisation in multifocal choroidtis. Br J Ophthalmol. 2010;66(3):433-8.

19. Thorne JE, Wittenberg S, Jabs DA, Peters GB, Reed TL, Kedhar SR, et al. Multifocal choroiditis with panuveitis: incidence of ocular complications and of loss of visual acuity. Ophthalmology. 2006;113(12):2310-6.
20. Levison AL, Baynes KM, Lowder CY, Kaiser PK, Srivastava SK. Choroidal neovascularisation on optical coherence tomography angiography in punctate inner choroidopathy and multifocal choroiditis. Br J Ophthalmol. 2017;101(5):616-22.
21. Herbort CP, Mantovani A, Papadia M. Use of indocyanine green angiography in uveitis. Int Ophthalmol Clin. 2012;52(4):13-31.
22. Cao JH, Silpa-Archa S, Freitas-Neto CA, Foster CS. Birdshot chorioretinitis lesions on indocyanine green angiography as an indicator of disease activity. Retina. 2016;36(9):1751-7.
23. Pichi F, Sarraf D, Arepalli S, Lowder CY, Cunningham ET, Neri P, et al. The application of optical coherence tomography angiography in uveitis and inflammatory eye diseases. Prog Retin Eye Res. 2017;59:178-201.
24. Chang AA, Zhu M, Billson F. The interaction of indocyanine green with human retinal pigment epithelium. Investig Ophthalmol Vis Sci. 2005;46(4):1463-7.
25. Pichi F, Srivastava SK, Chexal S, Lembo A, Lima LH, Neri P, et al. En face optical coherence tomography and optical coherence tomography angiography of multiple evanescent white dot syndrome: New insights into pathogenesis. Retina. 2016;36(Suppl 1):S178-88.
26. Invernizzi A, Cozzi M, Staurenghi G. Optical coherence tomography and optical coherence tomography angiography in uveitis: a review. Clin Exp Ophthalmol. 2019;47(3):357-71.
27. Nozik RA, Dorsch W. A new chorioretinopathy associated with anterior uveitis. Am J Ophthalmol. 1973;76(5):758-62.
28. Crawford CM, Igboeli O. A Review of the inflammatory chorioretinopathies: the white dot syndromes. ISRN Inflamm. 2013;1(1):783190.
29. Vance SK, Khan S, Klancnik JM, Freund KB. Characteristic spectral-domain optical coherence tomography findings of multifocal choroiditis. Retina. 2011;31(4):717-23.
30. D'Ambrosio E, Tortorella P, Iannetti L. Management of uveitis-related choroidal neovascularization: from the pathogenesis to the therapy. J Ophthalmol. 2014;1(1):450428.
31. Haen SP, Spaide RF. Fundus autofluorescence in multifocal choroiditis and panuveitis. Am J Ophthalmol. 2008;145(5):847-53.
32. Cheng L, Chen X, Weng S, Mao L, Gong Y, Yu S, et al. Spectral-domain optical coherence tomography angiography findings in multifocal choroiditis with active lesions. Am J Ophthalmol. 2016;169:145-61.
33. Spaide RF, Klancnik JM, Cooney MJ. Retinal vascular layers imaged by fluorescein angiography and optical coherence tomography angiography. JAMA Ophthalmol. 2015;133(1):45-50.
34. Agrawal RV, Biswas J, Gunasekaran D. Indocyanine green angiography in posterior uveitis. Indian J Ophthalmol. 2013;61(4):148-59.
35. Kramer M, Priel E. Fundus autofluorescence imaging in multifocal choroiditis: beyond the spots. Ocul Immunol Inflamm. 2014;22(5):349-55.
36. Cerquaglia A, Lupidi M, Fiore T, Iaccheri B, Perri P, Cagini C. Deep inside multifocal choroiditis: an optical coherence tomography angiography approach. Int Ophthalmol. 2017;37(4):1047-51.
37. Watzke RC, Packer AJ, Folk JC, Benson WE, Burgess D, Ober RR. Punctate inner choroidopathy. Am J Ophthalmol. 1984;98(5):572-84.
38. Gerstenblith AT, Thorne JE, Sobrin L, Do DV, Shah SM, Foster CS, et al. Punctate inner choroidopathy: a survey analysis of 77 persons. Ophthalmology. 2007;114(6):1201-4.
39. Read RW, Holland GN, Rao NA, Tabbara KF, Ohno S, Arellanes-Garcia L, et al. Revised Diagnostic Criteria for Vogt-Koyanagi-Harada disease: Report of an International Committee on Nomenclature. Am J Ophthalmol. 2001;131(5):647-52.

40. Liu XY, Peng XY, Wang S, You QS, Li Y Bin, Xiao YY, et al. Features of optical coherence tomography for the daignosis of Vogt-Koyanagi-Harada disease. Retina. 2016;36(11):2116-23.
41. Aggarwal K, Agarwal A, Mahajan S, Invernizzi A, Mandadi SKR, Singh R, et al. The role of optical coherence tomography angiography in the diagnosis and management of acute Vogt-Koyanagi-Harada disease. Ocul Immunol Inflamm. 2018;26(1):142-53.
42. Gass JDM. Acute posterior multifocal placoid pigment epitheliopathy. Arch Ophthalmol. 1968;23(6):177-85.
43. Deutman AF, Boen Tan TN, Oosterhuis JA. Acute posterior multifocal placoid pigment epitheliopathy. Ophthalmologica. 1973;167(5):368-72.
44. Mrejen S, Sarraf D, Chexal S, Wald K, Freund KB. Choroidal involvement in acute posterior multifocal placoid pigment epitheliopathy. Ophthalmic Surg Lasers Imaging Retin. 2016;47(1):20-6.
45. Klufas MA, Phasukkijwatana N, Iafe NA, Prasad PS, Agarwal A, Gupta V, et al. Optical coherence tomography angiography reveals choriocapillaris flow reduction in placoid chorioretinitis. Ophthalmol Retin. 2017;1(1):77-91.
46. Dolz-Marco R, Sarraf D, Giovinazzo V, Freund KB. Optical coherence tomography angiography shows inner choroidal ischemia in acute posterior multifocal placoid pigment epitheliopathy. Retin Cases Br Reports. 2017;11(1):136-43.
47. Levinson RD, Brezin A, Rothova A, Accorinti M, Holland GN. Research Criteria for the Diagnosis of Birdshot Chorioretinopathy: Results of an International Consensus Conference. Am J Ophthalmol. 2006;141(1):185-7.
48. Touhami S, Fardeau C, Vanier A, Zambrowski O, Steinborn R, Simon C, et al. Birdshot retinochoroidopathy: prognostic factors of long-term visual outcome. Am J Ophthalmol. 2016;170:190-6.
49. Symes R, Young M, Forooghian F. Quantitative assessment of retinal degeneration in birdshot chorioretinopathy using optical coherence tomography. Ophthalmic Surg Lasers Imaging Retin. 2015;46(10):1009-12.
50. Minos E, Barry RJ, Southworth S, Folkard A, Murray PI, Duker JS, et al. Birdshot chorioretinopathy: Current knowledge and new concepts in pathophysiology, diagnosis, monitoring and treatment. Orphanet J Rare Dis. 2016;11(1):61.
51. Pepple KL, Chu Z, Weinstein J, Munk MR, Van Gelder RN, Wang RK. Use of en face swept-source optical coherence tomography angiography in identifying choroidal flow voids in 3 patients with birdshot chorioretinopathy. JAMA Ophthalmol. 2018;136(11):1288-92.
52. De Carlo TE, Bonini Filho MA, Adhi M, Duker JS. Retinal and choroidal vasculature in birdshot chorioretinopathy analyzed using spectral domain optical coherence tomography angiography. Retina. 2015;35(11):2392-9.
53. Pichi F, Srivastava SK, Levinson A, Baynes KM, Traut C, Lowder CY. A focal chorioretinal Bartonella lesion analyzed by optical coherence tomography angiography. Ophthalmic Surg Lasers Imaging Retin. 2016;47(6):585-8.
54. Phasukkijwatana N, Iafe N, Sarraf D. Optical coherence tomography angiography of A29 birdshot chorioretinopathy complicated by retinal neovascularization. Retin Cases Br Reports. 2017;11(1):S68-S72.
55. Nazari Khanamiri H, Rao NA. Serpiginous choroiditis and infectious multifocal serpiginoid choroiditis. Surv Ophthalmol. 2013;58(3):203-32.
56. Bansal R, Gupta A, Gupta V. Imaging in the diagnosis and management of serpiginous choroiditis. Int Ophthalmol Clin. 2012;52(4):229-36.
57. Bansal R, Gupta A, Gupta V, Dogra MR, Sharma A, Bambery P. Tubercular serpiginous-like choroiditis presenting as multifocal serpiginoid choroiditis. Ophthalmology. 2012;119(11):2334-42.
58. Vasconcelos-Santos DV, Rao PK, Davies JB, Sohn EH, Rao NA. Clinical features of tuberculous serpiginous-like choroiditis in contrast to classic serpiginous choroiditis. Arch Ophthalmol. 2010;128(7):853-8.

59. Mandadi SKR, Agarwal A, Aggarwal K, Moharana B, Singh R, Sharma A, et al. Novel findings on optical coherence tomography angiography in patients with tubercular serpiginous-like choroiditis. Retina. 2017;37(9):1647-59.
60. Jampol LM, Sieving PA, Pugh D, Fishman GA, Gilbert H. Multiple evanescent white dot syndrome: I. Clinical Findings. Arch Ophthalmol. 1984;102(5):671-4.
61. Moschos MM, Gouliopoulos NS, Kalogeropoulos C. Electrophysiological examination in uveitis: a review of the literature. Clin Ophthalmol. 2014;8:199-214.
62. Yamamoto S, Hayashi M, Tsuruoka M, Yamamoto T, Tsukahara I, Takeuchi S. S-cone electroretinograms in multiple evanescent white dot syndrome. Doc Ophthalmol. 2003;106(2):117-20.
63. Dell'Omo R, Wong R, Marino M, Konstantopoulou K, Pavesio C. Relationship between different fluorescein and indocyanine green angiography features in multiple evanescent white dot syndrome. Br J Ophthalmol. 2010;94(1):59-63.
64. Rothova A, Suttorp-van Schulten MSA, Frits Treffers W, Kijlstra A. Causes and frequency of blindness in patients with intraocular inflammatory disease. Br J Ophthalmol. 1996;80(4):332-6.
65. Cunningham ET, Rathinam SR, Tugal-Tutkun I, Muccioli C, Zierhut M. Vogt-koyanagi-harada disease. Ocul Immunol Inflam. 2014;22(4):249-52.
66. Fardeau C, Champion E, Massamba N, Lehoang P. Uveitic macular edema. Eye. 2016;30(10):1277-92.
67. Agarwal A, Pichi F, Invernizzi A, Gupta V. Disease of the year: differential diagnosis of uveitic macular edema. Ocul Immunol Inflam. 2019;222(3):261-3.
68. Khochtali S, Abroug N, Megzari K, Gargouri MA, Ksiaa I, Ben Amor H, et al. Swept-source optical coherence tomography angiography findings in uveitic cystoid macular edema. Ocul Immunol Inflamm. 2019;27(8):1211-23.
69. Coscas GJ, Lupidi M, Coscas F, Cagini C, Souied EH. Optical coherence tomography angiography versus traditional multimodal imaging in assessing the activity of exudative age-related macular degeneration: a new diagnostic challenge. Retina. 2015;35(11):2219-28.
70. Chetrit M, Bonnin S, Mané V, Erginay A, Tadayoni R, Gaudric A, et al. Acute pseudophakic cystoid macular edema imaged by optical coherence tomography angiography. Retina. 2018;38(10):2073-80.
71. Mané V, Dupas B, Gaudric A, Bonnin S, Pedinielli A, Bousquet E, et al. Correlation between cystoid spaces in chronic diabetic macular edema and capillary nonperfusion detected by optical coherence tomography angiography. Retina. 2016;36(1):S102-10.
72. Al-Sheikh M, Akil H, Pfau M, Sadda SR. Swept-source OCT angiography imaging of the foveal avascular zone and macular capillary network density in diabetic retinopathy. Investig Ophthalmol Vis Sci. 2016;57(8):3907-13.
73. Samara WA, Shahlaee A, Sridhar J, Khan MA, Ho AC, Hsu J. Quantitative optical coherence tomography angiography features and visual function in eyes with branch retinal vein occlusion. Am J Ophthalmol. 2016;166:76-83.
74. Gill A, Cole ED, Novais EA, Louzada RN, de Carlo T, Duker JS, et al. Visualization of changes in the foveal avascular zone in both observed and treated diabetic macular edema using optical coherence tomography angiography. Int J Retin Vitr. 2017;3:19.
75. Neri P, Lettieri M, Fortuna C, Manoni M, Giovannini A. Inflammatory choroidal neovascularization. Middle East Afr J Ophthalmol. 2009;16(4):245-51.
76. Amer R, Priel E, Kramer M. Spectral-domain optical coherence tomographic features of choroidal neovascular membranes in multifocal choroiditis and punctate inner choroidopathy. Graefe's Arch Clin Exp Ophthalmol. 2015;253(6):949-57.
77. Nozaki M, Hamada S, Kimura M, Yoshida M, Ogura Y. Value of OCT angiography in the diagnosis of choroidal neovascularization complicating multiple evanescence white dot syndrome. Ophthalmic Surg Lasers Imaging Retin. 2016;47(6):580-4.

78. Parodi MB, Iacono P, La Spina C, Knutsson KA, Mansour A, Arevalo JF, et al. Intravitreal bevacizumab for choroidal neovascularisation in serpiginous choroiditis. Br J Ophthalmol. 2014;98(4):519-22.
79. Yee HY, Keane PA, Ho SL, Agrawal R. Optical coherence tomography angiography of choroidal neovascularization associated with tuberculous serpiginous-like choroiditis. Ocul Immunol Inflam. 2016;24(6):699-701.
80. Rouvas A, Petrou P, Douvali M, Ntouraki A, Vergados I, Georgalas I, et al. Intravitreal ranibizumab for the treatment of inflammatory choroidal neovascularization. Retina. 2011;31(5):871-9.
81. Agarwal A, Invernizzi A, Singh RB, Foulsham W, Aggarwal K, Handa S, et al. An update on inflammatory choroidal neovascularization: epidemiology, multimodal imaging, and management. J Ophthalmic Inflam Infect. 2018;8(1):13.
82. Spaide RF, Goldberg N, Freund KB. Redefining multifocal choroiditis and panuveitis and punctate inner choroidopathy through multimodal imaging. Retina. 2013;33(7):1315-24.
83. Bansal R, Bansal P, Gupta A, Gupta V, Dogra MR, Singh R, et al. Diagnostic challenges in inflammatory choroidal neovascular membranes. Ocul Immunol Inflamm. 2017;25(4):554-62.
84. Tan ACS, Tan GS, Denniston AK, Keane PA, Ang M, Milea D, et al. An overview of the clinical applications of optical coherence tomography angiography. Eye (Basingstoke). 2018;32(2):262-86.
85. Aggarwal K, Agarwal A, Sharma A, Sharma K, Gupta V. Detection of type 1 choroidal neovascular membranes using optical coherence tomography angiography in tubercular posterior uveitis. Retina. 2019;39(8):1595-606.
86. Tang W, Guo J, Liu W, Xu G. Optical coherence tomography angiography of inflammatory choroidal neovascularization early response after anti-VEGF treatment. Curr Eye Res. 2020;45(12):1556-62.
87. Demirel S, Yalçındağ N, Yanık Ö, Batıoğlu F, Özmert E. The use of optical coherence tomography angiography in the diagnosis of inflammatory type 1 choroidal neovascularization secondary to tuberculosis: a case report. Ocul Immunol Inflamm. 2020;27:1-7.
88. Spaide RF, Fujimoto JG, Waheed NK. Image artifacts in optical coherence tomography angiography. Retina. 2015;44(5):367-8.
89. Zhang M, Hwang TS, Campbell JP, Bailey ST, Wilson DJ, Huang D, et al. Projection-resolved optical coherence tomographic angiography. Biomed Opt Express. 2016;7(3):816-28.
90. Diaz JD, Wang JC, Oellers P, Lains I, Sobrin L, Husain D, et al. Imaging the deep choroidal vasculature using spectral domain and swept source optical coherence tomography angiography. J Vitreoretin Dis. 2018;2(3):146-54.

CHAPTER 7
Serpiginous Choroiditis

GVN Rama Kumar

ABSTRACT

Serpiginous choroiditis (SC) is a chronic, progressive, usually bilateral, recurrent inflammatory condition which affects the choroid, choriocapillaries and retinal pigment epithelium. Initially diagnosed in patients with tuberculosis and syphilis, SC, nowadays, is predominantly considered as organ-specific autoimmune process that has centrifugal spread starting in juxtapapillary region. Serpiginoid or serpiginous-like choroiditis is the term given for the variant associated with infective etiology and variable grades of other signs of intraocular inflammation apart from choroiditis. Though diagnosis of SC is clinical, with the advent of newer imaging modalities such as autoflourescence, OCT and ICG-A, monitoring the patient with SC for early diagnosis of recurrences and identification of complications such as choroidal neovascular membrane have become much easier. Treatment includes corticosteroids and immunosuppressive therapy. Patients should be monitored closely for disease progression and complications, including CNV and CME. Adequate timely treatment of each recurrent episode preserves useful vision in many patients.

Keywords: Serpiginous choroiditis, Serpiginoid choroiditis, Tuberculosis, Fundus Autoflourescence, Corticosteroids.

INTRODUCTION

The word "serpiginous" is an adjective which means "with a wavy or indented margin". Serpiginous choroiditis (SC) shows the similar wavy or ameboid-like lesions in choroid as a result of inflammation of unknown etiology.[1] Serpinginous choroiditis is a posterior uveitis displaying a geographic pattern of choroiditis **(Fig. 1)**, extending from the juxtapapillary choroid and intermittently spreading centrifugally.[2]

Serpiginous choroiditis may be defined as a chronic, progressive, usually bilateral, and recurrent inflammatory condition which affects the choroid, choriocapillaris, and retinal pigment epithelium (RPE).[2]

A clinical description of SC was first available in 1900, when Hutchinson described a condition with the appearance of borders in a map of a continent in his article "Serpiginous Choroiditis in Scrofulous Subjects: Choroidal

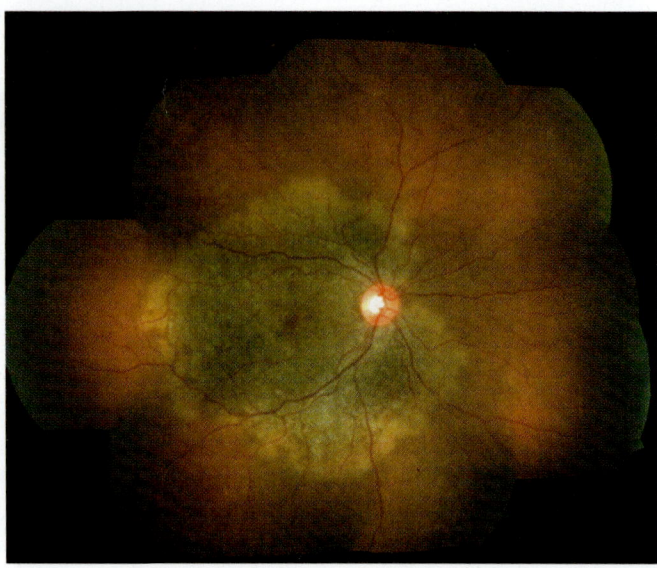

Fig. 1: Serpiginous choroiditis showing healed lesion near the optic disk with centrifugal extension.
Courtesy: Dr Sudarshan S, Senior Consultant, Uvea Services, Sankara Nethralaya, Chennai, Tamil Nadu, India.

Lupus."[3] In 1970, Gass coined SC to describe this entity with recurrences that usually begins in the peripapillary area and spread centrifugally over a period of months or years in a serpiginous or jigsaw puzzle-like distribution.[4]

The disease has been described by various other names in literature: peripapillary choroiditis, helicoid peripapillary choroidal sclerosis, helicoid peripapillary chorioretinal degeneration, geographic helicoid peripapillary choroidopathy, geographic helicoid choroidopathy, serpiginous choroidopathy and, recently, serpiginous-like choroiditis (SLC).

Serpiginous choroiditis is classified based on whether or not associated with any infective etiology into idiopathic SC and SLC or multifocal serpiginous choroiditis (MSC). In the middle of 20th century, tuberculosis was thought to be the cause, but later, it was described to present as SLC.[5,6]

EPIDEMIOLOGY

Serpiginous choroiditis is a relatively rare condition, prevalence ranging from 0.2 to 5% of all uveitis patients.[7] Prevalence in general population statistics is not available. A referral based epidemiologic study found SC represented 18.9% of posterior uveitis cases in India.[2] SC is recently classified as a distinct uveitis entity and because of varied nomenclature, many cases might have been diagnosed as other uveitis entities and thus, actual prevalence from uveitis clinics also may not be available.

Serpiginous choroiditis is a chronic, recurrent, and progressive disease that typically affects patients 30–60 years of age. There is a slight male predominance, but no racial predilection or consistent genetic factors have been associated with the disease.

ETIOLOGY

Serpiginous choroiditis typically occurs in otherwise healthy young individuals as a recurrent choroiditis with creepy serpentine progression.

Autoimmune Etiology

Idiopathic SC is supposed to be autoimmune.[2] Autoreactivity of circulating lymphocytes to retinal S antigen is observed in SC, but not in acute posterior multifocal placoid pigment epitheliopathy. The role of retinal photoreceptor protein-mediated damage is implicated in extensive damage to the retina in SC.[4] Occlusion of choriocapillaris has been attributed to the etiopathogenesis of SC.[1] The higher frequency of human leukocyte antigen (HLA)-B7, HLA-A2, HLA-B8, and HLA-Dw3 in patients with SC compared to the general population may suggest an underlying genetically predisposed autoimmune process.[8] SC can, therefore, be considered as an idiopathic intraocular inflammation with possible organ-specific autoimmune process as there is no proven association with any systemic autoimmune disease.

Infectious Etiology

Various organisms have been implicated in the pathogenesis of SC although treatment with specific antimicrobial agents did not show any significant positive clinical results.

Bacteria

Although pathogenesis, etiology, and differential diagnosis of SC, and the mimicking conditions remain a challenge, polymerase chain reaction (PCR) studies to detect microbial deoxyribonucleic acid (DNA) reveal that *Mycobacterium tuberculosis* (MTB) and herpes zoster infections play a role in the subset of patients with MSC.[9] MTB is the most common infectious organism implicated in etiopathogenesis of SLC. Association between SC and presumed tuberculosis was first described by Hutchinson.[1]

Viruses

Herpes viruses are proposed etiologic agents of SC.[1] A PCR study found DNA of herpes simplex virus (HSV) and varicella-zoster virus (VZV) in aqueous humor samples of eyes with SC. However, treatment with antivirals did not stop progression of disease.

Fungi

Intraocular fungal infections have a fulminant course and are unlikely to be confused with SC. A recent PCR study, although, has raised the possibility that *Candida* species may cause SC.[2]

CLINICAL FEATURES

Symptoms

Patients with SC typically present with the complaints of diminution of central vision, metamorphopsia, scotoma, difficulty in reading, visual field defects, or floaters. Visual acuity is typically 20/40 or less; however, it may range from 20/20 to counting fingers at 1–3 feet.

Tuberculous SLC predominantly affects younger adults of Asian-Indian origin. It is more likely to be multifocal, early in the course, with vitritis, has a relatively low complication and recurrence rates and is less commonly bilateral. It is usually associated with good visual outcome.[10] Patients remain asymptomatic until the macula is involved.

Signs

- Anterior chamber and vitreous reaction, if present, is low-grade and is mostly seen with SLC. Eye is quiet in idiopathic SC.
- Intraocular pressure remains normal.
- The new lesions are characterized by well-circumscribed patches of grayish-white or grayish-yellow discoloration at the level of the deep retina and RPE. These display a geographic pattern of choroidal atrophy associated with RPE changes that extend from the peripapillary area peripherally.
- Retina and RPE outside the margins of active or healed lesions appear normal. Examination of the fellow eye may show similar atrophic lesions in the juxtapapillary choroid.

Based on the morphology and characteristics of lesions, SC can be further subdivided into the following categories:

- *Peripapillary SC* is the most common type. Approximately 80% of the cases of SC reported are of peripapillary variety.[1] The lesion in peripapillary SC is usually unifocal and occurs around the optic disk and progresses in a serpentine pattern centrifugally to involve the macula. The average time between presentation in one eye and onset in the second eye is about 5 years.[1]
- *Macular SC* is relatively uncommon but a dreaded cause of vision loss because of early involvement of macula. It has a high risk of developing choroidal neovascularization (CNV). It may initially be confused with geographic atrophy, as seen in age-related macular degeneration, or with macular ischemia associated with various vasculopathies.[11]

Serpiginous-like Choroiditis

Serpiginous-like choroiditis is a distinct form of SC, characterized by multifocal choroidal lesions of varying shape and size. These lesions often coalesce to form diffuse choroiditis **(Fig. 2)** resembling SC in patients with presumed tuberculosis.[12]

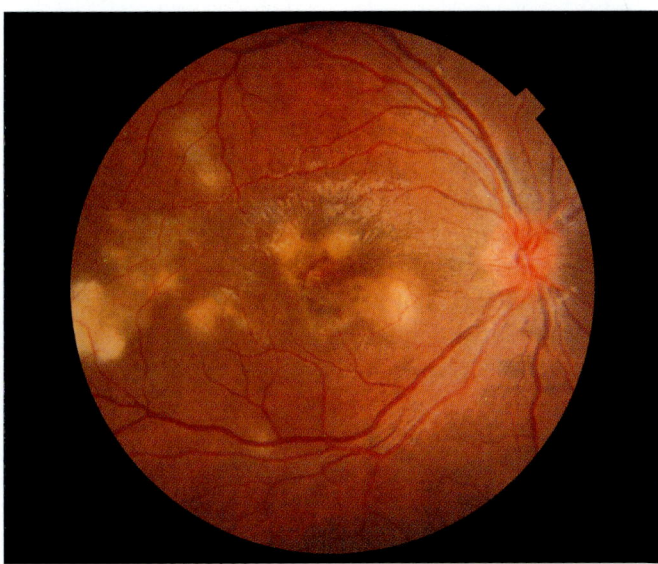

Fig. 2: Serpiginous-like choroiditis usually starts as multifocal choroiditis at macula and lesions progress and coalesce to form diffuse patch of choroiditis.

The term "serpiginoid" and "multifocal serpiginoid choroiditis" have also been used to refer these clinical entities. In contrast to patients with SC, patients with SLC are usually from tuberculosis endemic area and more likely to have unilateral presentation. They are relatively young and show multifocal lesions located in periphery of retina with frequent sparing of the juxtapapillary region. There occurs more inflammatory reaction in vitreous and the disease continues to show progression with development of new lesions despite effective corticosteroid therapy.[6,13]

HISTOPATHOLOGY

Histopathology findings in clinically inactive lesions of long-standing SC show a moderate mononuclear inflammatory cell infiltration of the choroid with focal aggregation of lymphocytes.[14] Fibrotic choroidal lesions are surrounded with variable degrees of RPE hyperplasia and defects in Bruch membrane with atrophic choriocapillaris, RPE, and photoreceptors.

DIAGNOSIS

The diagnosis of SC is based primarily on clinical examination. Imaging techniques and a thorough laboratory evaluation help in classifying the disease into idiopathic SC or SLC and plan the treatment. Imaging modalities that are helpful in confirming the diagnosis include fundus autofluorescence (FAF), fundus fluorescein angiography (FFA), indocyanine green angiography (ICGA), optical coherence tomography (OCT), and OCT angiography (OCTA).

Laboratory Tests

The diagnosis of idiopathic SC requires ruling out infective conditions, primarily tuberculosis, syphilis, and herpetic infections. In patients with typical SC who are from an area where tuberculosis is not endemic and who have no prior history of contact with tuberculosis, a negative tuberculin skin test, negative syphilis serology, and normal chest X-ray are usually sufficient.[2] Noninfectious choroiditis typically extends from the juxtapapillary area without significant vitritis or anterior chamber reaction. In contrast, atypical features, such as multifocal choroidal lesions, peripapillary choroid sparing, and significant anterior chamber or vitreous cellular reaction, mandate further investigations. In such patients, tuberculosis work up, syphilis serology, and anterior chamber or vitreous fluid analysis by PCR for MTB, VZV, and HSV may be required.

Imaging and Other Ancillary Diagnostic Tools

Fundus Autofluorescence

Being a noninvasive investigation, FAF has emerged as a valuable tool.

Active inflammation in SC is usually manifested as a hypoautofluorescent halo that surrounds the edges of hyperautofluorescent lesions, which probably represents edema of the deep retina or RPE.[15,16]

Subsequently, a sharp hypoautofluorescent border which represents a transitional zone of inactivity surrounds the hyperautofluorescent lesions.[17] The healed lesions of SC are characterized by totally hypoautofluorescent area with very sharp border, indicating the complete loss of fluorophores **(Figs. 3A and B)**.

Fundus autofluorescence can be useful in picking up subclinical reactivation of a previously healed lesion **(Figs. 4A and B)**. In contrast to

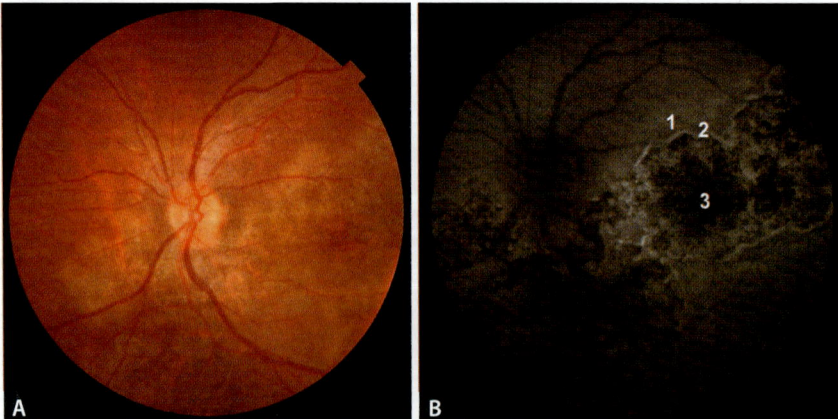

Figs. 3A and B: Fundus autofluorescence imaging of serpiginous choroiditis showing: (1) Hypoautofluorescence at the margin of active choroiditis, (2) Hyperautofluorescence at the junction of healing edge, and (3) Total hypoautofluorescence at the central healed part.

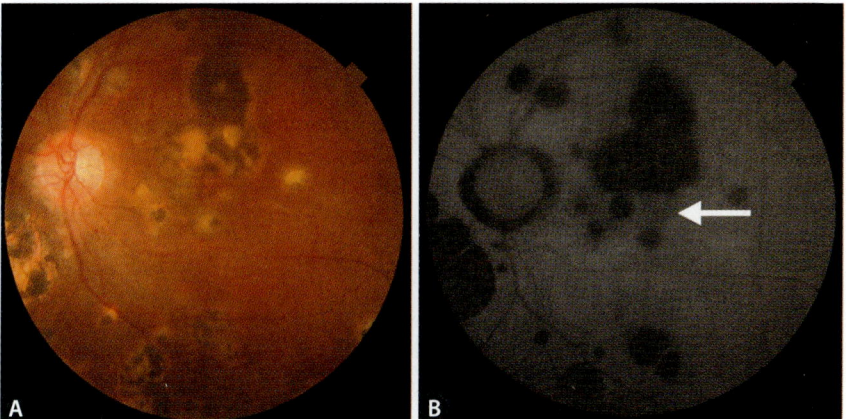

Figs. 4A and B: Fundus autofluorescence is useful to diagnose subtle reactivation of previously healed lesion which shows relative hypoautofluorescence at active edge (arrow).

diffuse, contagious pattern of hypoautofluorescence in SC, a complex, variegated pattern of hypoautofluorescence and hyperautofluorescence, has been described in patients with SLC.[15]

This difference was attributed to the direct involvement of RPE in eyes with SLC causing a greater damage to RPE in patients with SLC.

Fundus Fluorescein Angiography

Active SC lesions display hypofluorescent patches with irregular, poorly-defined borders **(Figs. 5A to C)** during the early phase of FFA. This hypofluorescence probably results from choriocapillaris hypoperfusion and blocked fluorescence as a result of edematous RPE and retina.[10]

In the mid-phase angiogram, a prominent hyperfluorescence may appear at the borders of the lesion. This is due to leakage from the bordering choriocapillaris. Focal areas of retinal vasculopathy may occasionally light up as retinal vessel wall staining. In late phases of FFA, the entire active lesion demonstrates a fairly uniform or spotty hyperfluorescence caused by leaking from the large choroidal vessels.

On the other hand, healed lesions show angiographic evidence of destruction of the RPE and choriocapillaris.[18] In clear contrast to the lesions of active choroiditis, these healed lesions demonstrate hypofluorescence with sharp margins in the early and mid-phase angiograms as a result of choriocapillaris damage and blockage from RPE hyperplasia **(Figs. 5B and C)**. In late phases, healed lesions show a variable amount of staining at the borders from leakage of the large choroidal vessels and surrounding choriocapillaris.[18-21]

Presence and severity of the pigment epithelial atrophy and hyperplasia, subretinal fibrosis, and choroidal atrophy modify the FFA appearance of the

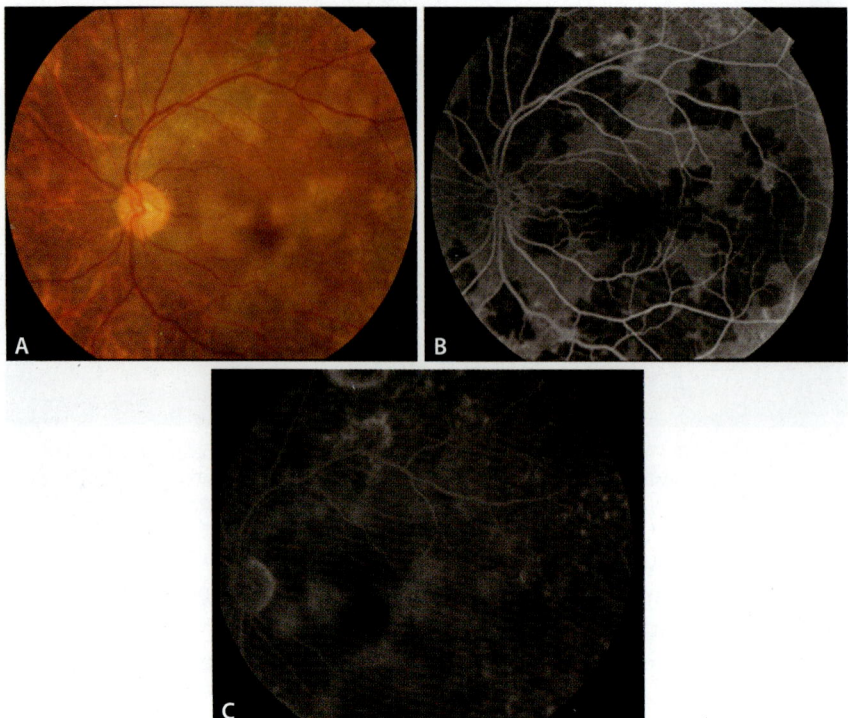

Figs. 5A to C: (A) Clinical photograph of active serpiginous choroiditis; (B) Fundus fluorescein angiography showing hypofluorescence of entire lesion in early phase; (C) Hyperfluorescence of active part and variable fluorescence of healed part of lesion in late phase of angiogram.

healed lesions. Fluorescein angiography is also helpful for detection of CNV, a complication of SC.[2]

Indocyanine Green Angiography

According to Giovannini et al.,[22] the ICGA-based classification of SC includes a subclinical or choroidal phase, an active phase, a subhealing phase, and an inactive healed phase.

In the subclinical or choroidal phase in which the inflammation is limited to the choriocapillaris and has not yet involved the overlying RPE and retina, fundus examination and FFA show no signs of choroiditis, however, ICGA reveals choriocapillaris nonperfusion as hypofluorescent patches. These hypofluorescent patches progress to active and visible choroiditis with an overlying yellowish-white retinal lesion that may show two patterns in ICGA. The more common pattern is characterized by early and late hypofluorescent patches with ill-defined margins that are larger than reciprocal FFA lesions. Margins of active lesions may show hyperfluorescence during the late phases. The less common pattern is early hypofluorescence with faint edges and late leakage and hyperfluorescence. With anti-inflammatory treatment, the size and intensity of ICGA lesions decrease.

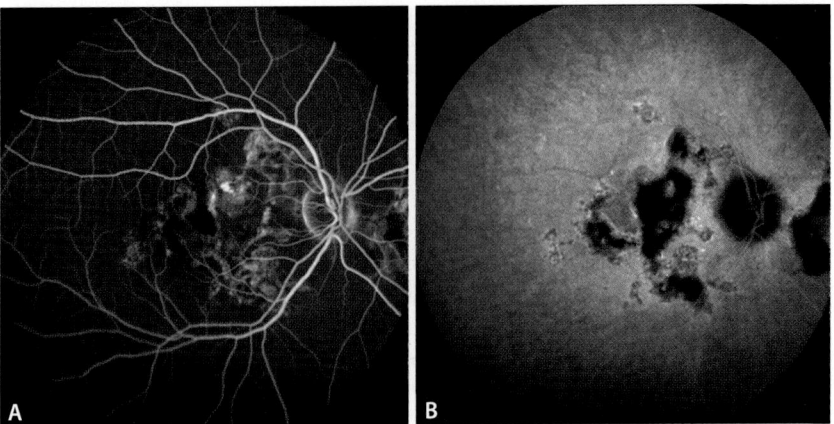

Figs. 6A and B: Simultaneous fundus fluorescein angiography (A) and indocyanine green angiography (ICGA) (B) imaging of serpiginous choroiditis. ICGA helps in diagnosing subclinical early activity or reactivation of disease.
Courtesy: Dr Sudarshan S, Senior Consultant, Uvea Services, Sankara Nethralaya, Chennai, Tamil Nadu, India.

In subhealing choroidal lesions, choroidal permeability alteration, usually adjacent to a recently healed active patch, can only be detected by ICGA as a slight, late hyperfluorescence **(Figs. 6A and B)**.

Optical Coherence Tomography

Characteristics of OCT features of active SC lesions include photoreceptor layer disruption associated with outer retinal and choriocapillaris hyper-reflectivity.[16]

In active choroiditis, the outer retina shows a uniform increased reflectivity, but the inner retina is usually spared. Outer retina may appear hyper-reflective in healed lesions also, but in contrast to the active phase, outer retinal hyper-reflectivity in healed lesions originates from RPE proliferation and migration. Consequently, outer retinal hyper-reflectivity in healed lesions is more granular and nonuniform. Retinal and RPE inflammation in active choroiditis is often associated with limited subretinal fluid overlying the area of choroiditis **(Figs. 7A and B)**.

Choroid may also appear hyper-reflective on OCT. This increased choroidal reflectivity is described as a "waterfall effect" and is attributed to inflammatory cell infiltration of the choroid.[23]

The choroidal hyper-reflectivity in healed SC lesions is attributed to enhanced light transmission through overlying RPE atrophy. Choroidal visualization is limited in contemporary time-domain and spectral-domain OCT methods. Novel-enhanced depth spectral domain-OCT imaging provides more details on the thickness and reflectivity of the choroid in active SC.

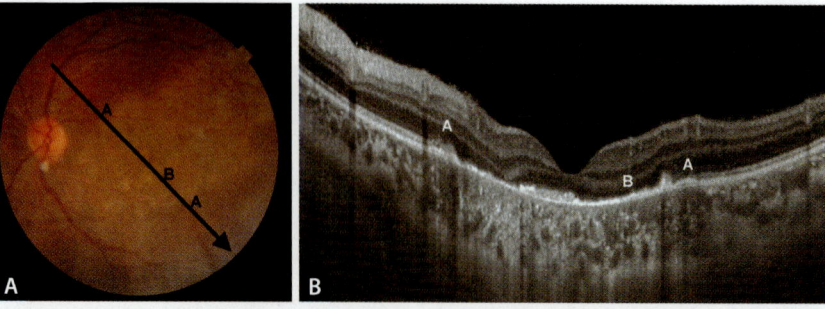

Figs. 7A and B: Optical coherence tomography showing: (A) Uniform hyper-reflectivity of outer retina and retinal pigment epithelium (RPE) of active part of lesion with adjacent hyporeflectivity; (B) Healed part of lesion showing granular hyper-reflectivity of RPE. Inner retina is spared.

Perimetry/Microperimetry

Dense scotomas related to both central and peripheral lesions have been well documented using Goldmann perimetry and Amsler grid testing. Visual field studies also confirmed the preservation of the inner retinal layers, including the nerve fiber layer, in the presence of severe outer retinal destruction. Even in the presence of serpiginous atrophic scars in the papillomacular bundle, the absence of foveal involvement leaves the central vision unaffected.[24]

However, if foveal function is compromised and the patient has unstable or extrafoveal fixation, conventional perimetry is not accurate enough to record the full functional impact of the inflammation and resultant scarring.[25]

Optical Coherence Tomography Angiography

Optical coherence tomography angiography is relatively a new noninvasive modality which can produce depth-resolved, high-resolution images of retinal and choroidal vasculature by detecting intravascular blood flow based on split-spectrum amplitude-decorrelation angiography without injecting the dye. OCTA in SC demonstrates decreased vascularity of choriocapillaris but intact retinal vascularity.[26]

COMPLICATIONS

Involvement of the fovea is the main vision-threatening concern in SC.[27] Central vision is usually affected when the foveal and parafoveal areas are directly involved by the lesion or when the extrafoveal lesions are complicated by CNV.

Choroidal neovascularization develops in up to 10–25% of eyes with SC usually at the surrounding boundaries of healed lesions.[28] Although the exact pathogenesis of CNV in SC is unknown, possibilities include ischemic injury to the choroid, Bruch membrane, and outer retina secondary to the choriocapillaris inflammation.[1] CNV development is not necessarily related to the disease activity and can be seen in both active and healed lesions.

Retinal vasculitis and ischemia are not constant features in SC, though there are reports of vascular occlusions and secondary neovascularization.[29-31] Such neovascularization might lead to retinal and vitreous hemorrhage. Optic nerve head neovascularization and combined retinal artery and vein occlusion may also occur in SC.[31,32] Strict inflammatory control usually decreases the incidence of such complications or even leads to spontaneous regression of the neovascularization.

Exacerbations of choroiditis might be accompanied by serous retinal detachment or pigment epithelial detachment in the absence of CNV.[33,34] These lesions usually resolve when the choroiditis subsides.

Review of FFA pictures as well as serial OCT examinations is crucial to rule out the presence of CNV, macular hole, and cystoid macular edema (CME).

MANAGEMENT

Treatment with systemic corticosteroids combined with immunosuppressive agents preserves central vision when used early in the disease course.[35] Possibility of tuberculosis and other infective etiology must be investigated before starting immunosuppressive therapy especially in tuberculosis endemic countries like India. Presence of an active systemic infection demands commencing its treatment prior to instituting immunosuppressive agents.

Systemic Treatment

Based on the presumed autoimmune pathogenesis of SC, the main approach has been the use of immunosuppressive therapy. The initial high dose of corticosteroids usually controls acute choroiditis, long-term treatment to prevent recurrences relies on immunomodulatory agents.

Corticosteroids

Corticosteroids alone or in combination with other immunosuppressive agents are the mainstay of therapy for SC.[36] Earlier moderate doses of corticosteroids (equal to 40 mg/day of prednisolone) were initially used, such treatment did not change the natural course of SC lesions.[37] Prompt treatment with 60–80 mg oral prednisolone or intravenous pulse methylprednisolone (1 g/day for 3 days) can limit choroiditis progression and prevent visual loss **(Figs. 8A and B)**. A clinical response to high-dose prednisolone (1 mg/kg) is usually evident within 24–36 hours.

Immunomodulatory Agents

Secchi et al.[38] described good outcomes in patients of SC where maximum patient showed significant recovery of visual acuity with cyclosporine therapy. Cyclosporine monotherapy was reported to be ineffective in another study[39] but when triple agent immunosuppression was given using

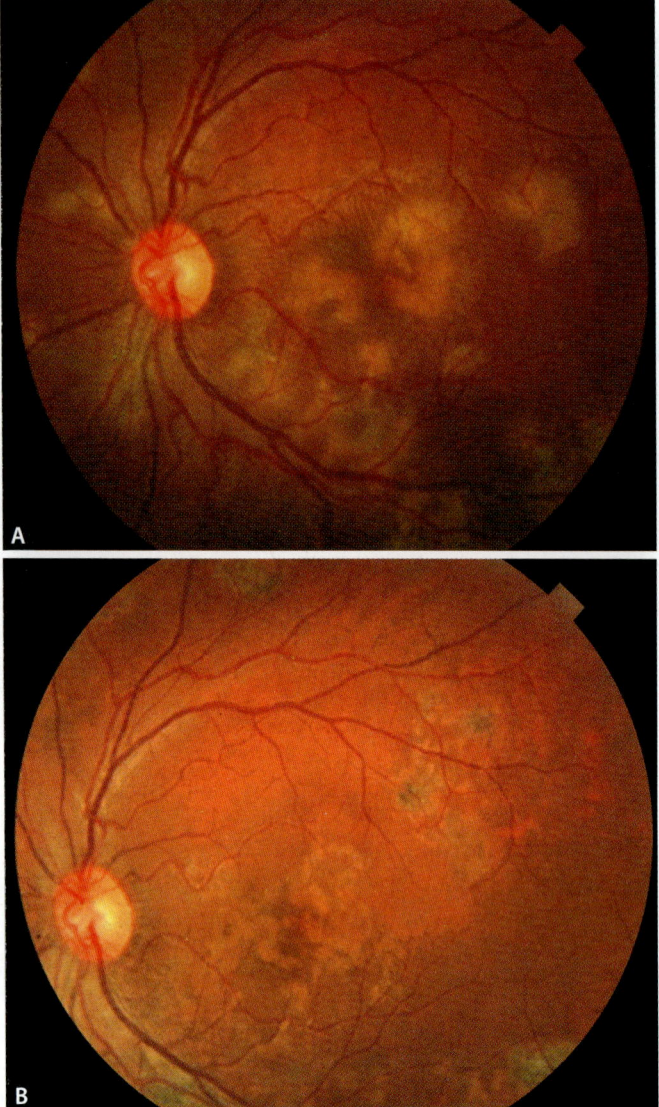

Figs. 8A and B: Active lesions of serpiginous choroiditis (A) usually respond well to systemic corticosteroid therapy and healing (B) starts within 1–2 weeks of starting therapy.

azathioprine, cyclosporine, and prednisolone[40] the inflammatory response got controlled. Looking at these conflicting reports immunosuppression is preferable in cases where center of macula is threatened or when the second eye is also affected by the disease. The ultimate aim of immunosuppression is to prevent progressive active lesions involving the macula by suppressing the inflammatory response. An immunomodulatory agent is usually required to prevent recurrence of choroiditis and to avoid or minimize corticosteroid side effects.[41]

- *T-cell inhibitor*: Cyclosporine is usually preferred in the treatment of SC with other immunosuppressive drugs.
- *Antimetabolites*: Azathioprine and mycophenolate mofetil are two antimetabolites used in SC patients. Azathioprine is a purine analog that has been effective for suppression of inflammatory bouts and induction of long-term remission in these patients. Azathioprine and cyclosporine synergistically modulate the immune response.
- *Alkylating agents*: Cyclosporine and chlorambucil may induce a sustained remission in vision threatening and refractory cases.
- *Biological agents*: Alternative treatment with biological agents such as interferon α-2a is a consideration for severe cases that require continued therapy with alkylating agents.

Local Treatment

Topical administration of corticosteroid may be necessary in patients with anterior segment inflammation. Intravenous,[32,40] peribulbar, subtenon, and intravitreal corticosteroid injections have also been used with variable success.[42]

Seth and Gaudio used intravitreal injection of triamcinolone to treat active SC threatening the fovea and reported immediate control of choroiditis.[43] The intravitreal corticosteroid injection might also have beneficial effects on CNV development in inflammatory conditions; however, the side effect profile, including cataract progression, increased intraocular pressure and a small possibility of endophthalmitis may limit its use.

Sustained-release intravitreal implants provide a theoretically ideal treatment mode for SC. In a study intraocular fluocinolone acetonide implant was placed in a case of SC and the authors found that choroiditis remained inactive during the follow-up period of 14 months.[43] Intravitreal steroid implants may be the preferred choice of treatment in near future because of encouraging case reports. Combined treatment with immunomodulators and biologics may be beneficial in preserving useful vision.

Combined Systemic and Local Treatment

Local drug delivery of corticosteroids in SC patients who are managed with systemic corticosteroids and/or additional immunosuppressive agents can reduce intraocular inflammation and minimize the required dose of systemic corticosteroids or immunomodulatory agents.[1]

DIFFERENTIAL DIAGNOSIS

Tuberculosis: *Mycobacterium tuberculosis* can cause SLC. It is important to differentiate SLC from SC as their treatment differs. Patients with SLC often present with multifocal lesions involving the periphery rather than peripapillary region. Anterior chamber cellular reaction and vitritis are also more common in SLC compared to SC. FAF may be helpful in distinguishing the two disease entities as SC has a homogeneous hypoautofluorescent pattern whereas SLC often demonstrates a more stippled appearance.

Acute posterior multifocal placoid pigment epitheliopathy (APMPPE): It can present a diagnostic challenge and may mimic SC early in the course of disease.

APMPPE lesions clinically appear similar to active SC as deep yellow-gray patches at the level of outer retina and inner choroid. They are typically multiple, discrete, and plaque like in appearance and predominantly involve the posterior pole.[44]

Acute posterior multifocal placoid pigment epitheliopathy lesions usually resolve on their own in a few weeks without treatment, with residual mild-to-moderate RPE changes. New lesions can develop over several subsequent weeks. Recurrent disease is uncommon and usually appears as new multifocal patches not associated with previously healed lesions. CNV is very rare in APMPPE.

Ampiginous choroiditis or relentless placoid chorioretinits: The ampiginous choroiditis lesions, as in APMPPE, develop at the level of RPE and choriocapillaris, but unlike APMPPE, the disease shows recurrences with severe pigment disturbance.[45] The lesions are usually widespread and may involve both the posterior pole and periphery.[46] OCT shows involvement of inner retinal layers also whereas in SC only outer retinal layers are involved.[47] The clinical course and multifocal appearance of the ampiginous choroiditis lesions distinguish it from SC, whereas the relentless progression of the disease differentiates it from APMPPE. Treatment of ampiginous choroiditis is similar to that of SC.

SUMMARY

Serpiginous choroiditis is a rare bilateral and idiopathic inflammatory disorder that causes geographic destruction of the retina and choroid in healthy middle-aged individuals. This chronic, recurrent, and progressive disease has a poor visual prognosis if the fovea is involved. Symptoms include blurred vision and central and paracentral scotomas. A thorough workup is necessary prior to initiating treatment to exclude other inflammatory or infectious etiologies that may mimic SC. Treatment includes corticosteroids and immunosuppressive therapy. Relentless progression of SC may occur over years with pigmentary retinal degeneration **(Figs. 9A to C)**. However, treatment of every recurrent episode preserves at least some useful vision. Patients should be monitored closely for disease progression and complications such as CNV and CME.

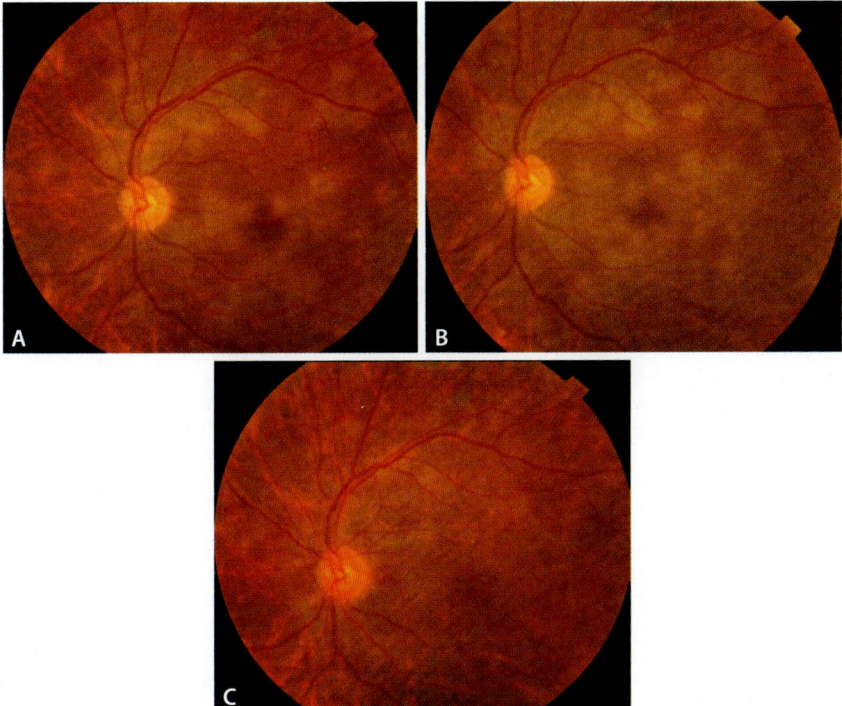

Figs. 9A to C: A case of relentless progression of serpiginous choroiditis showing: (A) Active choroiditis threatening fovea [with best-corrected visual acuity (BCVA) of 6/12]; (B) Progressive inflammation (deteriorated the vision to 6/36); (C) Resolved choroiditis patches with pigmentary degeneration (with visual improvement).

ACKNOWLEDGMENT

Dr Madhumita Prasad, MS, Consultant, Sankara Eye Centre, Indore helped in preparation of manuscript.

REFERENCES

1. Dutta Majumder P, Biswas J, Gupta A. Enigma of serpiginous choroiditis. Indian J Ophthalmol. 2019;67:325-33.
2. Nazari Khanamiri H, Rao NA. Serpiginous choroiditis and infectious multifocal serpiginoid choroiditis. Surv Ophthalmol. 2013;58(3):203-32.
3. Hutchinson J. Serpiginous choroiditis in scrofulous subjects: choroidal lupus. Arch Surg (Lond). 1900;11:126-35.
4. Gass JDM. Stereoscopic Atlas of macular diseases: a funduscopic and angiographic presentation. St Louis: CV Mosby Co; 1970. p. 66.
5. Witmer R. A specific form of recidivating choroiditis. Ophthalmologica. 1952;123: 353-4.
6. Vasconcelos-Santos DV, Rao PK, Davies JB, Sohn EH, Rao NA. Clinical features of tuberculous serpiginous like choroiditis in contrast to classic serpiginous choroiditis. Arch Ophthalmol. 2010;128:853-8.
7. Jones NP. The Manchester uveitis clinic: The first 3000 patients—epidemiology and case mix. Ocul Immunol Inflamm. 2015;23:118-26.

8. Cruz-Tapias P, Castiblanco J, Anaya JM. Chapter 17: HLA Association with Autoimmune Diseases. In: Anaya JM, Shoenfeld Y, Rojas-Villarraga A, Levy R, Cervera R (Eds). Autoimmunity: From Bench to Bedside [Internet]. Bogota (Colombia): El Rosario University Press; 2013. [online] Available from https://www.ncbi.nlm.nih.gov/books/NBK459459/ [Last accessed May, 2021].
9. Rao NA, Foster SC. Curbside consultation in uveitis: 49 clinical questions. 1. When should I be suspicious of tuberculosis and what testing is useful? Thorofare, NJ: SLACK; 2012. pp. 59-61.
10. Fraser-Bell S. Retina associates Serpiginous choroiditis and Tuberculous serpiginous-like choroiditis. [online] Available from: http://www.retina.com.au/retina-associates-case-of-the-month-april-2013/ [Last accessed May, 2021].
11. Schmitz-Valckenberg S, Sadda S, Staurenghi G, Chew EY, Fleckenstein M, Holz FG, et al. GEOGRAPHIC ATROPHY: Semantic Considerations and Literature Review. Retina. 2016;36(12):2250-64.
12. Gupta V, Agarwal A, Gupta A, Bambery P, Narang S. Clinical characteristics of serpiginous choroidopathy in North India. Am J Ophthalmol. 2002;134:47-56.
13. Gupta A, Bansal R, Gupta V, Sharma A, Bambery P. Ocular signs predictive of tubercular uveitis. Am J Ophthalmol. 2010;149:562-70.
14. Wu JS, Lewis H, Fine SL, Grover DA, Green WR. Clinicopathologic findings in a patient with serpiginous choroiditis and treated choroidal neovascularization. Retina. 1989;9(4):292-301.
15. Gupta A, Bansal R, Gupta V, Sharma A. Fundus autofluorescence in serpiginous-like choroiditis. Retina. 2012;32:814-25.
16. Cardillo Piccolino F, Grosso A, Savini E. Fundus autofluorescence in serpiginous choroiditis. Graefes Arch Clin Exp Ophthalmol. 2009;247:179-85.
17. Carreño E, Portero A, Herreras JM, López MI. Assessment of fundus autofluorescence in serpiginous and serpiginous-like choroidopathy. Eye (Lond). 2012;26:1232-6.
18. Gass JDM. Stereoscopic atlas of macular diseases: a funduscopic and angiographic presentation. St Louis: CV Mosby Co; 1997. pp. 158-65.
19. Baarsma GS, Deutman AF. Serpiginous (geographic) choroiditis. Doc Ophthalmol. 1976;40(2):269-85.
20. Hamilton AM, Bird AC. Geographical choroidopathy. Br J Ophthalmol. 1974;58(9):784-97.
21. Laatikainen L, Erkkilä H. A follow-up study on serpiginous choroiditis. Acta Ophthalmol (Copenh). 1981;59(5):707-18.
22. Giovannini A, Mariotti C, Ripa E, Scassellati-Sforzolini B. Indocyanine green angiographic findings in serpiginous choroidopathy. Br J Ophthalmol. 1996;80(6):536-40.
23. Gallagher MJ, Yilmaz T, Cervantes-Castañeda RA, Foster CS. The characteristic features of optical coherence tomography in posterior uveitis. Br J Ophthalmol. 2007;91(12):1680-5.
24. Schatz M, Maumenee AE, Patz A. Geographic helicoid peripapillary choroidopathy: clinical presentation and fluorescein angiographic findings. Trans Am Acad Ophthalmol Otolaryngol. 1974;78:747-61.
25. Pilotto E, Vujosevic S, Grgic VA, Sportiello P, Convento E, Secchi AG, et al. Retinal function in patients with serpiginous choroiditis: a microperimetry study. Graefes Arch Clin Exp Ophthalmol. 2010;248(9):1331-7.
26. Ahn SJ, Park SH, Lee BR. Multimodal imaging including optical coherence tomography angiography in serpiginous choroiditis. Ocul Immunol Inflamm. 2017;25:287-91.
27. Karagiannis DA, Sampat FV, Dowler J. Serpiginous choroidopathy with bilateral foveal sparing and good visual acuity after 18 years of disease. Retina. 2007;27(7):989-90.
28. Kuo IC, Cunningham ET Jr. Ocular neovascularization in patients with uveitis. Int Ophthalmol Clin. 2000;40:111-26.

29. Baglivo E, Boudjema S, Pieh C, Safran AB, Chizzolini C, Herbort C, et al. Vascular occlusion in serpiginous choroidopathy. Br J Ophthalmol. 2005;89(3):387-8.
30. Blumenkranz MS, Gass JD, Clarkson JG. Atypical serpiginous choroiditis. Arch Ophthalmol. 1982;100(11):1773-5.
31. Friberg TR. Serpiginous choroiditis with branch vein occlusion and bilateral periphlebitis. Arch Ophthalmol. 1988;106(5):585-6.
32. Masi RJ, O'Connor GR, Kimura SJ. Anterior uveitis in geographic or serpiginous choroiditis. Am J Ophthalmol. 1978;86(2):228-32.
33. Wojno T, Meredith TA. Unusual findings in serpiginous choroiditis. Am J Ophthalmol. 1982;94(5):650-5.
34. Hoyng C, Tilanus M, Deutman A. Atypical central lesions in serpiginous choroiditis treated with oral prednisone. Graefes Arch Clin Exp Ophthalmol. 1998;236(2):154-6.
35. Jabs DA, Rosenbaum JT, Foster CS, Holland GN, Jaffe GJ, Louie JS, et al. Guidelines for the use of immunosuppressive drugs in patients with ocular inflammatory disorders: recommendations of an expert panel. Am J Ophthalmol. 2000;130(4):492-513.
36. Hardy RA, Schatz H. Macular geographic helicoid choroidopathy. Arch Ophthalmol. 1987;105(9):1237-42.
37. Chisholm IH, Gass JDM, Hutton WL. The late stage of serpiginous (geographic) choroiditis. Am J Ophthalmol. 1976;82(3):343-51.
38. Secchi AG, Tognon MS, Maselli C. Cyclosporin A in the treatment of serpiginous choroiditis. Int Ophthalmol. 1990;14:395-9.
39. Laatikainen L, Tarkkanen A. Failure of cyclosporin A in serpiginous choroiditis. J Ocul Ther Surg. 1984;3:280-3.
40. Hooper PL, Kaplan HJ. Triple agent immunosuppression in serpiginous choroiditis. Ophthalmology. 1991;98:944-51.
41. Akpek EK, Baltatzis S, Yang J, Foster CS. Long-term immunosuppressive treatment of serpiginous choroiditis. Ocul Immuno lInflam. 2001;9(3):153-67.
42. Adigüzel U, Sari A, Ozmen C, Oz O. Intravitreal triamcinolone acetonide treatment for serpiginous choroiditis. Ocul Immunol Inflamm. 2006;14(6):375-8.
43. Seth RK, Gaudio PA. Treatment of serpiginous choroiditis with intravitreous fluocinolone acetonide implant. Ocul Immunol Inflamm. 2008;16(3):103-5.
44. Lyness AL, Bird AC. Recurrences of acute posterior multifocal placoid pigment epitheliopathy. Am J Ophthalmol. 1984;98(2):203-7.
45. Nussenblatt RB. Serpiginous choroiditis. In: Nussenlatt RB, Whitcup SM (Eds). Uveitis, Fundamentals and Clinical Practice, 4th Edition. Edinburgh: Mosby/Elsevier; 2010. pp. 373-82.
46. Lim WK, Buggage RR, Nussenblatt RB. Serpiginous choroiditis. Surv Ophthalmol. 2005;50(3):231-44.
47. Amer R, Florescu T. Optical coherence tomography in relentless placoid chorioretinitis. Clin Exp Ophthalmol. 2008;36(4):388-90.

CHAPTER 8

Pachychoroid: The Disease Spectrum

*Anand Rajendran, Ritesh Chainani,
Bhanu Pangtey, MY Vishal*

ABSTRACT

With the advent of advanced imaging modalities, especially optical coherence tomography (OCT), our ability to study the choroid and its role in influencing retinal pathology has been significantly enhanced over the last decade. One of the key outcomes of this has been our cognizance of the "Pachychoroid" or thickened choroid as an entity encompassing a spectrum of subretinal pathologies that are causal to a range of macular exudative and hemorrhagic pathologies. The clinical features of pachychoroid are decreased fundus tessellation, increased choroidal thickness, presence of pachyvessels, choriocapillaris thinning and choroidal hyperpermeability. The spectrum is further comprised of six distinct clinical entities—pachychoroid pigment epitheliopathy (PPE), central serous chorioretinopathy (CSCR), pachychoroid neovasculopathy (PNV), polypoidal choroidal vasculopathy (PCV), peripapillary pachychoroid syndrome (PPS), focal choroidal excavation (FCE).

Keywords: Pachychoroid, OCT, ICG, central serous chorioretinopathy, polypoidal choroidal vasculopathy, neovascularization.

INTRODUCTION

Cutting edge advances in optical coherence tomography (OCT) such as enhanced depth imaging (EDI) with SD-OCT and swept-source OCT (SS-OCT) have enabled retina specialists to study the subretinal structures, especially the choroid with greater clarity. Several macular pathologies are now understood to have their pathophysiological basis in the choroid. This has, consequently, led to a better understanding of these pathologies and their therapy. Choroidal thickness is more accurately assessed now and its thickness as being relevant to retinal pathology has been well demonstrated. The term "pachychoroid" [pachy-(prefix): thick] was first coined by Warrow et al. to characterize an atypical and persistent increase in choroidal thickness.[1] They described the retinal pigment epithelial changes terming them "pachychoroid pigment epitheliopathy (PPE)" in patients with thickened choroid devoid of subretinal fluid, which resembled that seen in fellow eyes of patients with unilateral serous chorioretinopathy (CSCR). Since then, multiple diseases with choroidal findings similar to PPE have been demonstrated and are being referred as the "pachychoroid disease spectrum".

With the advent of EDI and SS imaging, greater information regarding choroid is becoming available. Yamashita et al. used three different SD-OCT machines and reported high intra-class coefficient and intraraster correlation coefficient in the assessment of choroidal thickness.[2] However, on comparing SD-OCT and SS-OCT, Matso et al. showed that choroidal thickness between these machines was not comparable and the choroid is measured thicker in SS-OCT.[3]

The thickness of the choroid thus far has been estimated, via automated software or manually, in the perpendicular from the external edge of the hyper-reflective retinal pigment epithelium (RPE) to the internal edge sclera (choroid–sclera junction) at 500 μm interval from the fovea. Such measurements are seen to be highly reproducible.[4] Copete et al. demonstrated that SS-OCT identified the choroido-scleral junction better and showed more reproducible results as compared to SD-OCT.[5]

Choroidal thickness is affected by age (6 μm decrease every decade), refraction value, axial length (thinner in myopes), gender (thinner in female), circadian rhythm (statistically significant variations in subjects with thick choroids compared to subjects with thinner choroids, especially in the mornings) and several other factors.[6,7] While choroid thickness varies in many different studies, subfoveal choroid thickness is reported to range from 191 ± 74.2 to 354 ± 111 μ. The choroid is thickest in the subfoveal area with the nasal zone being thinner than the temporal.[8,9] A choroid with a thickness of over 395 μm was defined as a thick choroid.[10]

Recent articles have suggested >300 μ as pathological choroidal thickness. Also pachychoroid may include eyes with normal subfoveal choroidal thickness (SFCT) but having extrafoveal foci of greater choroidal thickness (defined as thickness >50 μm of the SFCT).[11]

It has been demonstrated to have a critical role in the pathophysiology of several diseases such as age-related macular degeneration (AMD), CSCR, Vogt–Koyanagi–Harada (VKH) disease, pathologic myopia. OCT remains the most popular modality for the study of the choroid. Evidence of isolated pachychoroid in all generations suggested that pachychoroid could be a dominant inherited condition.[10] Indocyanine green angiography (ICGA) is used to highlight choroidal hyperpermeability.

PACHYVESSELS MORPHOLOGY

Choroidal veins invariably disappear close to the macula on ICGA. In pachychoroid patients, they may come in close proximity to the macula, often passing by it.

The pachychoroid phenotype features are:[12,13]
- Reduced fundus tessellation on clinical examination or white light photography.

- Relatively increased choroidal thickness which may be focal or diffuse.
- Pathological dilation of outer choroidal (Haller) vessels, referred to as "pachyvessels".
- Loss of choriocapillaris and Sattler layers overlying pachyvessels.
- Choroidal hyperpermeability.

The pachychoroid disease is understood to constitute a spectrum of six different pathologies. These pathologies are considered to be the stages of the disease itself, as the increased severity in the preceding group leads the patient to the succeeding group of disease. The spectrum comprises the following six diseases groups:
1. Pachychoroid pigment epitheliopathy (PPE)
2. Central serous chorioretinopathy (CSCR)
3. Pachychoroid neovasculopathy (PNV)
4. Polypoidal choroidal vasculopathy (PCV)
5. Peripapillary pachychoroid syndrome (PPS)
6. Focal choroidal excavation (FCE)

Pachychoroid Pigment Epitheliopathy

Pachychoroid pigment epitheliopathy encompasses changes that are considered to represent a precursor of CSCR as it shares the features of CSCR without the presence of any subretinal fluid or any history suggestive of prior collection of subretinal fluid.[1] Pigment epithelial detachments (PEDs) may then occur in areas of choroidal hyperpermeability, increasing the risk of local RPE disruption, eventually resulting in the leakage of serous fluid into the subretinal space with subsequent macular detachment.

The characteristic findings of PPE are:
- The presence of the pachychoroid phenotype
- Reddish orange hue of the fundus with decreased tessellation (choroidal vascular markings)
- Absence of subretinal fluid
- Absence of subretinal fluid history
- Absence of drusen

Pachychoroid pigment epitheliopathy is, therefore, commonly mixed up with other diseases such as AMD, pigment epitheliitis, and pattern dystrophy. Diagnosis of the disease may help in monitoring of the patient and avoiding unnecessary testing and intervention. The degenerative process may commence with RPE changes prior to the accumulation of subretinal fluid.

The pachyvessels lie close to the vicinity of the RPE-Bruch membrane complex signaling that they may be mechanically inciting pigment epitheliopathy. OCT also highlights sub-RPE drusen-like deposits and focal RPE hyperplasia represented by several scattered small elevations of the RPE. Occasionally, small serous PEDs may be found. Swept source and EDI-OCT have also additionally shown—greater choroidal thickening, pachy-veins within Haller's layer, thinning of the Sattler's layer and choriocapillaris, and outer nuclear layer thinning.[1]

Choroidal hyperpermeability, demonstrated by mid-phase hyperfluorescence on ICGA, underlies these areas of RPE disturbances. Foci of both hyperautofluorescence and hypoautofluorescence may be revealed on fundus autofluorescence imaging of these areas of retinal pigment epitheliopathy. Retinal pigment epithelial hyperplasia is shown up on OCT scans through hyperautofluorescent foci. PPE is never associated with signs of previous subretinal fluid, such as tear-drop tracts, zonal areas of hyperautofluorescence or focal areas of speckled hyperautofluorescence.[1]

Central Serous Chorioretinopathy

Central serous chorioretinopathy, one of the most common of retinal disorders, is now being ascribed to the pachychoroid spectrum. It manifests as a serous macular detachment, idiopathic and noninflammatory, that may or may not be associated with a PED. As it is now being increasingly recognized, choroidal hyperpermeability causes the effusion under the retina.[14,15] The predisposing factors for CSCR are—a Type A personality, hysteria, and hypochondria, steroid use/Cushing syndrome, systemic hypertension, pregnancy, Japanese/Southeast Asian racial characteristics, systemic lupus erythematosus (SLE), and psychopharmacological medication.[1] Chronic or recurrent CSCR can persist with atrophic and/or neovascular sequelae, beyond the sixth and seventh decades.[16] The typically seen ill-defined leakage is due to the progressive pathologic changes in the RPE.

Optical coherence tomography angiography is likely to demonstrate pachy-veins in the Haller's layer.[15,17] The fundus fluorescein angiogram features of the ink-blot leak or the smoke-stack leak are well documented. A typical feature on ICGA are dilated choroidal vessels that are oriented diagonally and are noted to communicate with the vortex ampullae. ICGA shows choroidal hyperpermeability in areas where fluorescein angiography (FA) shows leakage at the level of the RPE **(Fig. 1A)**. OCT highlights the diffuse subretinal fluid, significant subretinal fibrin and subretinal fibrin alongside a thickened choroid **(Fig. 1B)**. Focal areas of speckled hyperautofluorescence on fundus autofluorescence denote the chronic presence of fluid, and occasionally linear, descending tear-drop tracts with a mottled fluorescence.

Pachychoroid Neovasculopathy

Freund et al. described the development of a type 1 choroidal neovascularization (CNV) as a late complication of chronic CSCR and PPE.[17] In susceptible individuals, a hyperpermeable, chronically exuding pachychoroid may lead to long-term degenerative effects on the RPE, Bruch's membrane and choriocapillaris. This in turn may induce, subsequently, neovascularization of the pachy-veins at Haller's layer. A relative absence of

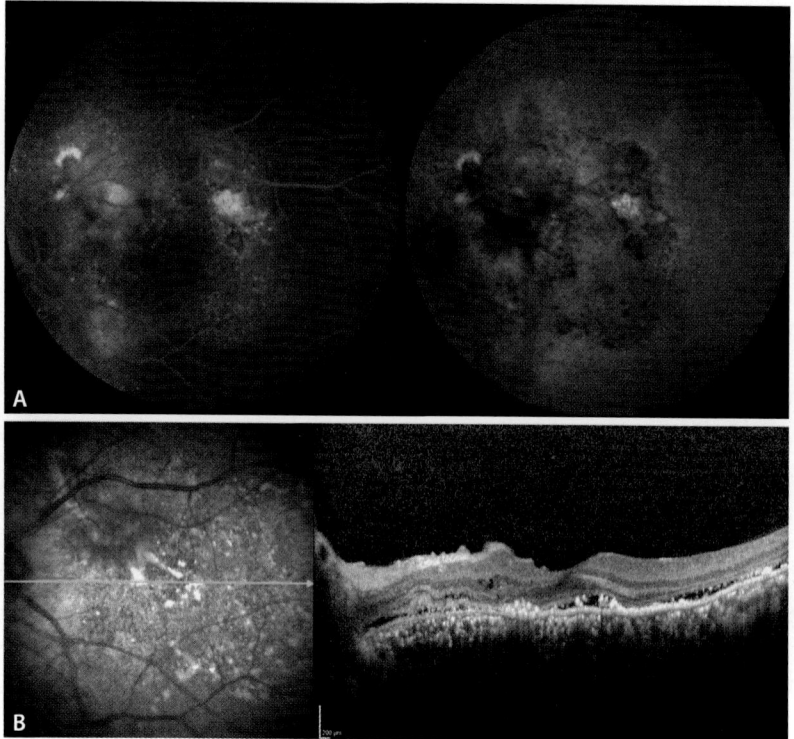

Figs. 1A and B: (A) FFA and ICGA images of a case of chronic CSCR showing the intense hyperfluorescence from leaking areas on the FFA with the corresponding choroidal hyperpermeable areas showing up as areas of hypercyanescence on the ICGA. A tear-drop tract is also evident; (B) The OCT shows the chronic CSCR with diffuse shallow subretinal fluid with extensive subretinal precipitates and fibrin alongside a thickened choroid.
(CSCR: central serous chorioretinopathy; FFA: fundus fluorescein angiography; ICGA: indocyanine green angiography; OCT: optical coherence tomography)

drusens, a younger age at onset of neovascularization, and a thick choroid with pachyvessels distinguish PNV from AMD and other degenerative conditions that lead to type 1 neovascularization.[12,16,17] Occasionally, the neovascular tissue of PNV in some eyes may evolve into polypoidal choroidal vasculopathy. OCT highlights its prime features—the presence of a wide minimal elevation of the RPE signifying neovascular proliferation within Bruch's membrane. This variety of type 1 neovascularization is characteristically found overlying an area of localized choroidal thickening with dilated choroidal vessels, seen on the OCT as the "double layer sign".[12,17] OCT angiography highlights the complex, tangled vein network under these irregular shallow PEDs. An ill-defined area of hyperfluorescence and/or late leakage of indeterminate origin on FA with a corresponding PED on cross-sectional structural OCT is often to be found. In these cases, ICGA often reveals both patchy areas of choroidal hyperpermeability in the mid-phases, and a discrete plaque of late hyperfluorescence reflective of the type 1 neovascular tissue[17] **(Figs. 2A and B)**.

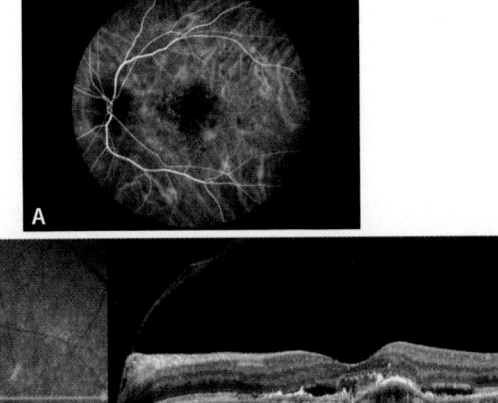

Figs. 2A and B: (A) Pachychoroid neovasculopathy (PCN) with areas of distinctive choroidal hyperpermeability seen as hypercyanescent zones on the indocyanine green angiography (ICGA); (B) Optical coherence tomography image of the PCN case with elevated retinal pigment epithelium (RPE) resembling a type I choroidal neovascular membrane (CNVM). A thickened choroid is also noted.

Polypoidal Choroidal Vasculopathy

Yannuzzi et al. asserted that PCV constituted 7.8% of the exudative AMD cases while studies from Asia placed that incidence in the range 25–50%.[18-20] Proliferation of the choroidal capillaries under the RPE with terminal aneurysmal development in the form of polyps is the hallmark.[18] These choroidal vascular polyps, the pathognomonic lesions, are clearly diagnosed by ICGA. ICGA helps to identify these polyps as early focal areas of intense hyperfluorescence that may reveal either late leakage or "wash-out" features depending on their degree of activity. These polypoidal structures cause leakage or hemorrhage beneath the RPE and neurosensory retina. The spectrum of clinical lesions ranges from serosanguinous PEDs and neurosensory detachments to bullous retinal detachments and vitreous hemorrhages with associated subretinal hemorrhage.[21] The OCT features of PCV cause it to be likened to a form of type 1 neovascularization and it remains a close differential to neovascular AMD.[22] In patients with PNV-essentially type 1 CNV secondary to CSC or PPE, this neovascularization develops polypoidal features. Hemorrhages and lipid exudation occurs through these polyps. Scrutiny of the morphology of the choroids of several patients diagnosed with PCV shows characteristics consistent with those of the pachychoroid phenotype: choroids thicker than are usual for AMD, minimal or absent drusen, pachyvessels with inner choroid thinning, and shallow irregular PEDs[1,12,20] (**Figs. 3A and B**).

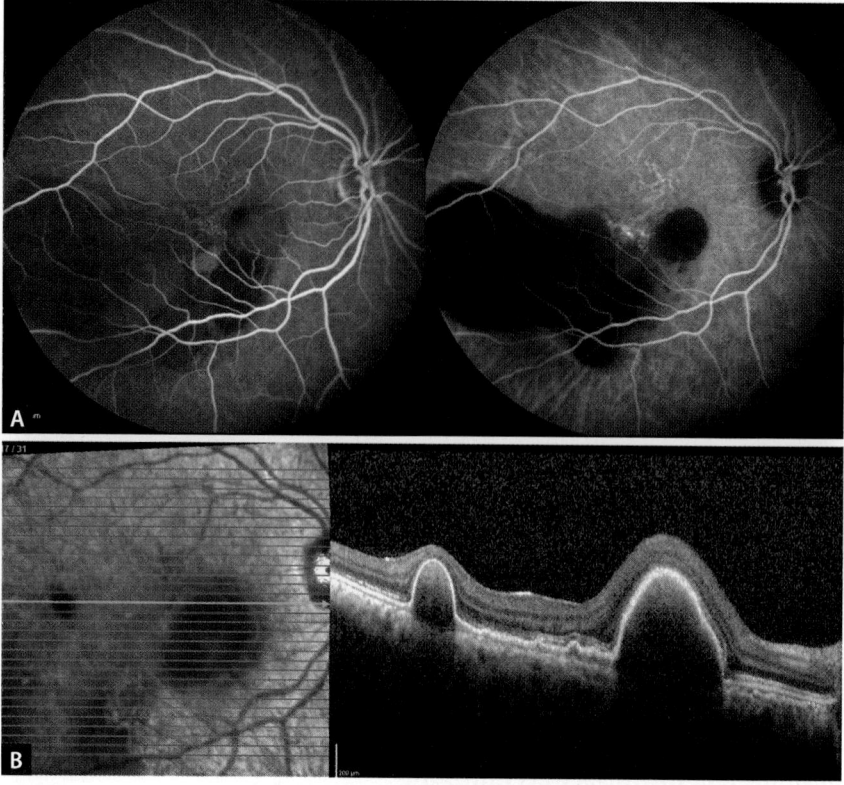

Figs. 3A and B: (A) A case of polypoidal choroidal vasculopathy (PCV) with massive subretinal hemorrhage seen as blocked fluorescence on FFA and ICGA. The ICGA additionally shows the branching vascular network terminating in the classic polyps seen as the hypercyanescent bulbs; (B) The tall peaked, thumb-shaped PEDs typical of PCV are noted on OCT with the thickened choroid.
(FFA: fundus fluorescein angiography; ICGA: indocyanine green angiography; OCT: optical coherence tomography; PEDs: pigment epithelial detachments)

Previously used terminology, aneurysmal type 1 neovascularization, is again being considered as a better term to define PCV (Recent advent of SS-OCT and EDI-OCT has confirmed that branching vascular network (BVN) and aneurysmal dilation are present between the basal lamina of the RPE layer and inner collagenous layer of Bruch's membrane). With more evidence of mechanisms that underlie aneurysm formation differ from those which promote neovascularization in AMD.[23]

Peripapillary Pachychoroid Syndrome

It has been a recently described entity by Phasukkijwatana et al. The greatest choroidal thickness is found close to the optic disk with intraretinal or subretinal fluid accumulation in the nasal macula. It may be associated with optic nerve head edema. Peripapillary serous PEDs, PPE or gravitating autofluorescent tracks may be seen.[24]

Focal Choroidal Excavation

The hallmark characteristics of FCE are localized area(s) of choroidal excavation without features of posterior staphyloma or scleral ectasia in patients who usually lack evidence of disease known to result in choroidal attenuation. Most commonly seen in 4th to 5th decade with no gender predilection. Most cases are seen in moderate myopes. OCT shows two types of FCE: photoreceptor tips directly in contact with RPE (conforming type) or detached from the RPE (nonconforming type). Eyes with FCE have been shown to have pachychoroid features including greater subfoveal choroidal thickness and choroidal vascular hyperpermeability in ICGA.[25]

Lim et al. reported FCV in eyes with PCV, CSCR, and CNV (both type 1 and type 2).[26] Most FCE remains stable or show minimal change with time. Some cases may rarely develop neovascularization.[27]

As advances in imaging modalities help to increase our capability in the assessment of the choroid, its thickness and vascularity, the spectrum of the pachychoroid phenotype is expanding. Further research on this topic is mandated to enhance our knowledge regarding this pachychoroid pathology and its many clinical ramifications in the posterior segment.

CONCLUSION

The study of choroidal morphology and its thickness profile, with the aid of advanced OCT and angiographic imaging capability has led to the recognition of the pachychoroid spectrum and the associated clinical entities. The role of the choroid in the pathophysiologic mechanisms of a variety of macular diseases had given us the opportunity to hone our diagnostic ability in terms of detecting them early as well as enhance our therapeutic strategies. It is envisaged that continued research of the choroid and its influence on retinal disease will further uncover such etiological relationships and help refine our management paradigms.

REFERENCES

1. Warrow DJ, Hoang QV, Freund KB. Pachychoroid pigment epitheliopathy. Retina. 2013;33(8):1659-72.
2. Yamashita T, Shirasawa M, Arimura N, Terasaki H, Sakamoto T. Repeatability and reproducibility of subfoveal choroidal thickness in normal eyes of Japanese using different SD-OCT devices. Invest Ophthalmol Vis Sci. 2012;53:1102-7.
3. Matsuo Y, Sakamoto T, Yamashita T, Tomita M, Shirasawa M, Terasaki H. Comparisons of choroidal thickness of normal eyes obtained by two different spectral-domain OCT instruments and one swept-source OCT instrument. Invest Ophthalmol Vis Sci. 2013;54:7630-6.
4. Rahman W, Chen FK, Yeoh J, Patel P, Tufail A, Da Cruz L. Repeatability of manual subfoveal choroidal thickness measurements in healthy subjects using the technique of enhanced depth imaging optical coherence tomography. Invest Ophthalmol Vis Sci. 2011;52:2267-71.
5. Copete S, Flores-Moreno I, Montero JA, Duker JS, Ruiz-Moreno JM. Direct comparison of spectral-domain and swept-source OCT in the measurement of choroidal thickness in normal eyes. Br J Ophthalmol. 2014;98(3):334-8.

6. Margolis R, Spaide RF. A pilot study of enhanced depth imaging optical coherence tomography of the choroid in normal eyes. Am J Ophthalmol. 2009;147:811-5.
7. Ikuno Y, Kawaguchi K, Nouchi T, Yasuno Y. Choroidal thickness in healthy Japanese subjects. Invest Ophthalmol Vis Sci. 2010;51:2173-6.
8. Wei WB, Xu L, Jonas JB, Shao L, Du KF, Wang S, et al. Subfoveal choroidal thickness: the Beijing Eye Study. Ophthalmology. 2013;120:175-80.
9. Bidaut-Garnier M, Schwartz C, Puyraveau M, Montard M, Delbosc B, Saleh M. Choroidal thickness measurement in children using optical coherence tomography. Retina. 2014;34:768-74.
10. Lehmann M, Bousquet E, Beydoun T, Behar-Cohen F. Pachychoroid: an inherited condition? Retina. 2015;35(1):10-6.
11. Dansingani KK, Balaratnasingam C, Naysan J, Freund KB. En face imaging of pachychoroid spectrum disorders with sweptsource optical coherence tomography. Retina. 2016;36:499-516.
12. Gallego-Pinazo R, Dolz-Marco R, Gomez-Ulla F, Mrejen S, Freund KB. Pachychoroid diseases of the Macula. Med Hypothesis Discov Innov Ophthalmol. 2014;3(4):111-5.
13. Akkaya S. Spectrum of pachychoroid diseases. Int Ophthalmol. 2017;1:1-8.
14. Spaide RF, Goldbaum M, Wong DW, Tang KC, Iida T. Serous detachment of the retina. Retina. 2003;23(6):820-46.
15. Imamura Y, Fujiwara T, Margolis R, Spaide RF. Enhanced depth imaging optical coherence tomography of the choroid in central serous chorioretinopathy. Retina. 2009;29(10):1469-73.
16. Fung AT, Yannuzzi LA, Freund KB. Type 1 (sub-retinal pigment epithelial) neovascularization in central serous chorioretinopathy masquerading as neovascular age-related macular degeneration. Retina. 2012;32(9):1829-37.
17. Pang CE, Freund KB. Pachychoroid Neovasculopathy. Retina. 2015;35:1-9.
18. Yannuzzi LA, Wong DW, Sforzolini BS. Polypoidal choroidal vasculopathy and neovascularised age-related macular degeneration. Arch Ophthalmol 1999;117:1503-10.
19. Maruko I, Iida T, Saito M, Nagayama D, Saito K. Clinical characteristics of exudative age-related macular degeneration in Japanese patients. Am J Ophthalmol. 2007;144(1):15-22.
20. Kwok AK, Lai TY, Chan CW, Neoh EL, Lam DS. Polypoidal choroidal vasculopathy in Chinese patients. Br J Ophthalmol. 2002;86(6):892-7.
21. Imamura Y, Engelbert M, Iida T, Freund KB, Yannuzzi LA. Polypoidal choroidal vasculopathy: A review. Surv Ophthalmol. 2010;55:501-15.
22. Squirrel DM, Bacon JF, Brand CS. To investigate the prevalence of Polypoidal choroidal vasculopathy in presumed age-related peripapillary subretinal neovascular membranes. Clin and Exp Ophthalmol. 2009;37:367-82.
23. Dansingani KK, Gal-Or O, Sadda SR. Understanding aneurysmal type 1 neovascularization (polypoidal choroidal vasculopathy): a lesson in the taxonomy of "expanded spectra": a review. Clin Exp Ophthalmol. 2018;46:189-200.
24. Phasukkijwatana N, Freund KB, Dolz-Marco R, Al-Sheikh M, Keane PA, Egan CA, et al. Peripaillary Pachychoroid Syndrome. Retina. 2018;38(9):1652-67.
25. Margolis R, Mukkamala SK, Jampol LM, Spaide RF, Ober MD, Sorenson JA, et al. The expanded spectrum of focal choroidal excavation. Arch Ophthalmol. 2011;129:1320-5.
26. Lim FP, Wong CW, Loh BK, Chan CM, Yeo I, Lee SY, et al. Prevalence and clinical correlates of focal choroidal excavation in eyes with age-related macular degeneration, polypoidal choroidal vasculopathy and central serous chorioretinopathy. Br J Ophthalmol. 2016;100:918-23.
27. Chung H, Byeon SH, Freund KB. Focal choroidal excavation and its association with pachychoroid spectrum disorders: a review of the Literature and Multimodal Imaging Findings. Retina. 2017;37(2):199-221.

CHAPTER 9

Glued Intrascleral Haptic Fixation of Intraocular Lens

Venkata Prabhakar G, Soosan Jacob

ABSTRACT

After cataract removal, intraocular lens (IOL) is placed inside the capsular bag. Problem arise when there is not enough capsular support to hold the IOL which can happen preoperatively such as in cases of lens subluxation secondary to trauma or pseudoexfoliation or iatrogenic during surgery. The options in such cases are scleral fixated IOL (SFIOL), iris fixated IOL (IFIOL), and anterior chamber IOL (ACIOL).

A conventional sutured SFIOL is a technique where sutures are used to fix IOL haptics to the sclera. Disadvantages of this technique include lack of stability and suture erosion which eventually leads to IOL decentration or dislocation. Glued IOL is an advanced technique of sutureless SFIOL where IOL haptics are fixed to the sclera through scleral tunnels. Sclerotomies are made under lamellar scleral flaps to externalize the haptics and scleral tunnels are made at the edge of the scleral flap into which the haptics are tucked. The flaps are finally closed with fibrin glue. This fixates the IOL in a stable manner to the sclera, thus solving problems of difficult centration, instability and suture erosion.

Keywords: Cataract surgery, IOL, cystoid macular edema, sutures, glue, scleral flaps, tunnels, zonulopathy, visual axis, pars plana.

INTRODUCTION

Placing an IOL after cataract surgery is a crucial step as it has a direct impact on the visual outcome. Situations can arise where there is a lack of adequate capsule to support an IOL which can be secondary to zonular weakness or posterior capsule rupture and can happen in up to 6.7% cases.[1,2] Surgeons should be well versed with alternative techniques to fix the IOL in case of any complication. In this situation, the surgeon generally has options of ACIOL, iris claw lens, and SFIOL.

Anterior chamber IOL has been reported to have complications of fibrosis of angle with subsequent glaucoma, endothelial loss leading to bullous keratopathy, pupil block, and cystoid macular edema (CME).[3] IFIOL needs a healthy iris, which makes it unsuitable in cases of trauma, congenital defects, or other iris pathology.

Sutured SFIOL has a steeper learning curve as it needs suture tracking and manipulation in the area of ciliary body which can lead to hemorrhage and macular edema. Sutures may be associated with complications of erosion[4] which can lead to long-term complications such as IOL tilt or dislocation. Blind ab interno needle pass may also increase the risk of retinal detachment and other posterior segment complications. This disadvantage of suture erosion is overcome by directly fixing the IOL haptic to the sclera. Intrascleral haptic fixation of a three-piece IOL was originally started by Gabor Scharioth.[5] This was further modified by Agarwal et al. to include scleral flaps and fibrin glue as part of the procedure. The recent advance is where glued IOL is done without disturbing the anterior hyaloid phase as described by one of the authors (Soosan Jacob).[6]

PRINCIPLE

Glued IOL works by using the concept of scleral flaps and intrascleral tunnels. Polymethylmethacrylate (PMMA) haptics are inserted in to scleral tunnels that are made parallel to limbus and scleral flaps are used to cover the sclerotomies, thus providing horizontal, vertical, and rotational stability to the IOL. Finally, using fibrin glue to close the flaps removes problems of exposure of any part of the IOL.

PREOPERATIVE EVALUATION

Cases with zonulopathy or cases taken up for secondary IOL implantation need careful thorough evaluation and careful management. Proper counseling, review of previous medical and surgical records as well as a comprehensive eye evaluation for zonulopathy, pupillary dilatation, specular count, thorough retinal examination, assessment of visual potential, etc., is a must. A B-scan is done if the cataract is dense. White-to-white (WTW) diameter should be measured as it correlates to the amount of haptic availability for tucking after haptic externalization. If WTW is >12 mm, the technique needs surgical modifications.

TECHNIQUE: STEP-BY-STEP APPROACH

First, a radial keratotomy marker or the Agarwal glued IOL marker is used to mark two points exactly 180° apart and centered on the visual axis. Then, the conjunctiva is dissected in the areas concerned. Two partial lamellar scleral flaps of 2.5 × 2.5 mm are created, centered[7] on these marks up to the limbus. Next, a conventional anterior chamber maintainer (ACM), a trocar ACM, or a 23-gauge pars plana sutureless trocar infusion cannula is fixed in the inferotemporal quadrant. If pars plana infusion is used, the tip of the pars plana infusion cannula should be seen within the vitreous cavity before turning the infusion on.

A 20-gauge needle is then used to create a sclerotomy 1 mm from the limbus under the scleral flap. The needle is directed posteriorly toward the center of the globe as parallel entry may cause the needle to push on the iris root. To release any vitreous adhesions or strands, an anterior and mid vitrectomy is performed via the sclerotomies. The infusion cannula prevents the globe from collapsing during all steps of surgery.

Inserting the IOL: A 2.8-mm keratome is used to make a corneal incision. This may be enlarged very slightly so as to allow easy insertion. A three-piece foldable IOL is loaded into the injector and the injector tip is introduced into the AC. The tip of the haptic is kept slightly outside the cartridge (lucky seven sign) so that it can be easily grasped with the forceps. Once the tip is grasped, the IOL is injected gently leaving the trailing haptic outside the wound in an "upright C" configuration. Wound-assisted injection of the three-piece IOL should be avoided as the IOL may drop into the vitreous accidentally.

Exteriorization: The exteriorization of the haptics is a key step in the glued IOL technique. Through the sclerotomy under the scleral flap, 23-gauge forceps are introduced. The tip of the haptic is caught with the forceps and exteriorized with the other hand while injection of the IOL continues very gently. The injector is then slowly withdrawn so that the trailing haptic passes through the wound outside the globe. The leading haptic should be grasped at its very tip so that it does not get caught or kinked at the sclerotomy during the withdrawal. The leading haptic, which has been grasped with the forceps, is thus exteriorized through the sclerotomy. It is then held firmly but gently by an assistant so that it does not get drawn back into the vitreous cavity during subsequent maneuvers. Alternatively, the haptic may be plugged into a hole made on a small silicon bit cut from intravenous tubing so that an assistant is not required to hold the haptic.

The handshake technique:[8] The technique utilizes two forceps, one of which holds one haptic. While the first haptic is held by an assistant, the tip of the trailing haptic is grasped by forceps and is flexed gently into the eye. Depending on ease of access, an end-gripping microforceps is introduced through the opposite sclerotomy or through the side-port. The first hand then transfers the haptic into the second forceps such that the first hand now becomes free. Handshake transfer of the haptic between two end-gripping microforceps is continued until the tip of the haptic is caught by the microforceps on the side where the haptic is to be exteriorized and is pulled out through the second sclerotomy. It is essential to hold the haptic at its tip before exteriorizing it so that it does not snag on the sclerotomy while being brought out. This technique allows for easy intraocular maneuvering of the entire haptic and IOL within a closed globe system. The leading haptic held by the assistant should not be released during this maneuver. Once both haptics are exteriorized on to the scleral surface, they can be released.

At this stage, the IOL remains firmly on the scleral surface without falling into the vitreous cavity. In addition to routine handshake transfer, the surgeon also needs to be familiar with the handshake technique as a means of transferring the haptic from one hand to the other, especially if one of the haptics is not caught or if it gets released accidentally into the vitreous.

Stabilizing the IOL: Vitrectomy is performed over the sclerotomy sites to remove any vitreous that may have prolapsed out through the sclerotomy. This is done by turning the cutting port toward the scleral surface. A bent 26-gauge needle is used to create a scleral tunnel at the edge of the scleral flap. This is created intrascleral parallel to the limbus and is done toward the direction of the exteriorized haptic on either side. A maker pen can be put on the needle while creating this so that the exact location of the tunnel is easily visualized. If the location of the tunnel is lost, one can recreate a new tunnel or use a simple rod to check its location by passing through the tunnel. The haptic is then tucked into the scleral pocket created. This secure tuck of the haptic within the pocket prevents any kind of movement of the IOL and provides great stability to the IOL.

At this stage, the degree of centration of the IOL is assessed and if decentration is noted, it is corrected. This is done simply by varying the degree of tuck of either haptic into the scleral pockets created on opposite sides.

Gluing the IOL: The infusion is then removed and the anterior chamber (AC) filled with air. This way the area of the sclerotomy, where the haptics are, is dry as there is no fluid coming out. Also, the air in the AC prevents collapse of the chamber and any hypotony in the postoperative period. The scleral bed is dried with a Weck-Cel sponge. Fibrin glue is then applied to the undersurface of the flap and the flap is glued down. The conjunctiva is also closed with glue and the corneal wound is hydrated and sutures applied if necessary **(Figs. 1 and 2)**.

NUANCES

Glued Intrascleral Haptic Fixation of an IOL in Large Eyes

In eyes with greater WTW diameter (>12 mm), certain adaptations, and modifications are adopted for adequate haptic externalization and subsequent tuck. The vertical diameter of the cornea is lesser than the horizontal diameter. So, in large eyes with WTW >12 mm, making vertical flaps[9] gives more haptic to externalize and so gives more tuck.

Performing an anterior sclerotomy at a distance of 0.5 mm from the limbus beneath the scleral flaps instead of 1.5 mm has an added advantage of allowing greater haptic externalization. A careful approach is essential as performing an anterior sclerotomy can lead to iridodialysis due to the 22-gauge needle entering the eye at a 0.5-mm distance from the limbus.

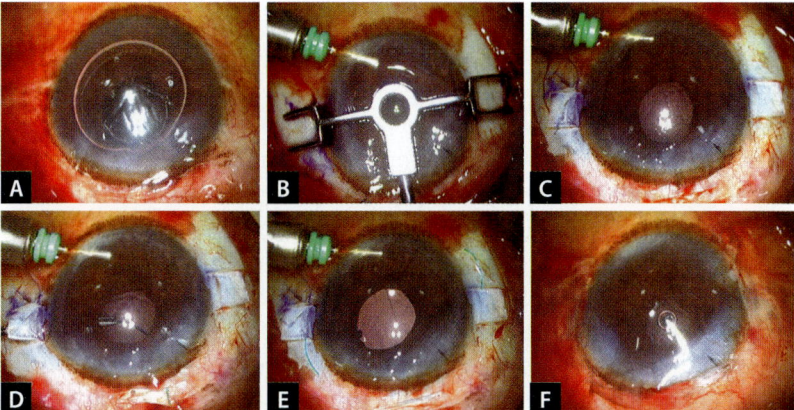

Figs. 1A to F: (A) Eye with posterior capsular rupture; (B) Glued IOL flaps are marked and TACM (Trocar Anterior Chamber Maintainer) inserted; (C) Glued IOL flaps are created; (D) Leading haptic is externalized with microforceps passed through first sclerotomy; (E) Trailing haptic is also externalized with microforceps passed through second sclerotomy; (F) Haptics are tucked into limbus parallel intrascleral Scharioth tunnels on either side and scleral flaps and conjunctiva are closed.

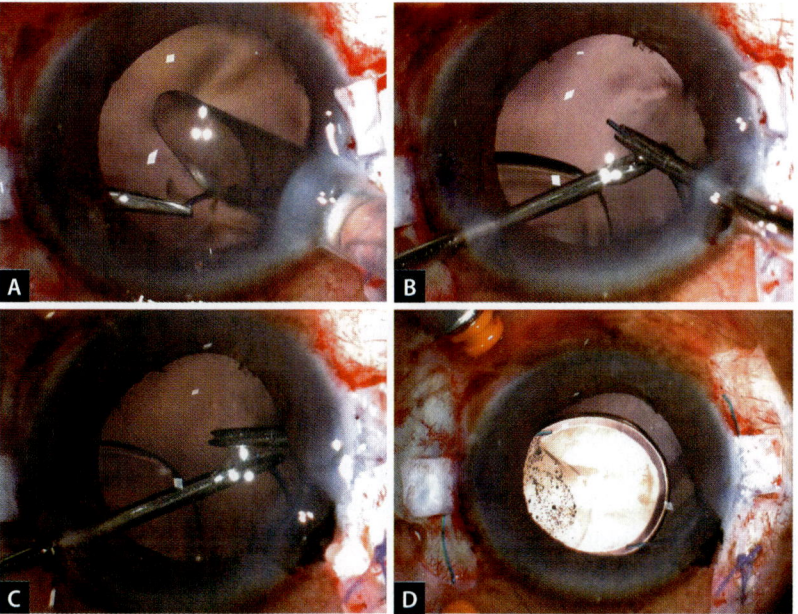

Figs. 2A to D: *Handshake technique:* (A) Leading haptic grasped with microforceps parallel to first sclerotomy; (B and C) Handshake transfer of trailing haptic from one hand to the other till the microforceps passed through the second sclerotomy is holding the haptic at its tip; (D) Both haptics are externalized.

The needle should be introduced vertically rather than horizontally to avoid hitting the iris root. Complications associated with hitting the base of the iris can also be avoided by performing a prior vitrector-assisted peripheral iridectomy (PI).[10] Although this avoids additional manipulation during the surgery, bleeding, and pigmentary disturbance can occasionally occur. If done vertically, the peripheral iridotomies are also hidden by the eyelids.

Supracapsular Glued IOL

This is the technique described by one of the authors (Soosan Jacob), in cases with zonular weakness or progressive subluxation, supracapsular glued IOL fixation[6] is done to retain an intact anterior hyaloid face and avoid vitreous disturbance while providing stable long-term IOL fixation. Phacoemulsification is followed by glued IOL implantation above intact anterior and posterior capsules. Sclerotomies are created ab interno or ab externo in a supracapsular plane under diametrically opposite lamellar scleral flaps without entering the vitreous cavity. Releasing capsular hooks and expanding the supracapsular space using viscoelastic helps do this safely and easily. Haptics are externalized in the supracapsular plane and tucked into intrascleral tunnels. Retention of intact zonule capsule complex maintains bicamerality of eye, thus leading to less CME and endophthalmodonesis which is important in cases which are predisposed to retinal detachment. Postoperative phimosis may be prevented by implanting a capsular tension ring in the primary surgery followed by optic capture into the rhexis. Alternately, anterior and posterior yttrium aluminum garnet (YAG) capsulotomy may be done in the early postoperative phase before phimosis becomes dense.

Combined Surgeries

Glued Intrascleral Haptic Fixation of an IOL as Scaffold

This technique essentially comprises the combination of the glued IOL with IOL scaffold procedure[11] and is adopted in cases with deficient sulcus support and retained nuclear material. Following a posterior capsule rupture, the nuclear fragments are pushed aside onto the iris, a three-piece IOL is injected beneath the fragments and over the iris. The IOL, therefore, plugs the pupil and acts as a scaffold preventing fragment drop as well as vitreous prolapse. Glued IOL flaps and sclerotomies are created. Intravitreal triamcinolone acetonide (IVTA) stained pars plana vitrectomy is done to cut vitreous strands. 360° access can be obtained by using both sclerotomies. The vitrector is also used alternating between cutting and aspirating modes to remove any cortex. The nuclear pieces are then emulsified with the phaco-probe introduced inside the AC. The tip of the haptics is then externalized through the sclerotomies as in a glued IOL procedure. If any fragments have dropped before the IOL scaffold could be placed, they should be removed from the vitreous cavity either at the same sitting or in a secondary surgery taking the help of a vitreoretinal surgeon. In case of large, dense fragments, instead of emulsifying the fragments, they may also be brought out through a small incision cataract surgery (SICS) tunnel.

Glued Capsular Hook

One of the authors (Soosan Jacob) has devised a device that allows fibrin glue-assisted sutureless transscleral fixation of the capsular bag and can be used for refixating subluxated cataracts and IOLs.

Glued Intrascleral Haptic Fixation of an IOL with Keratoplasty

In cases of endothelial pathologies, endothelial keratoplasty (EK) has many advantages over penetrating keratoplasty such as being a closed chamber technique with faster visual recovery, better quality of vision, lesser induction of irregular astigmatism, lesser chances of rejection, and less surface and suture-related problems. An important factor for the success of an EK is having a stable iris and IOL complex over which the graft is manipulated and attached to stroma. One option for providing such a platform is the glued IOL when the anterior and posterior capsule are not intact. Glued IOL can be combined with Descemet's stripping automated EK,[12] Descemet's stripping EK,[13] Descemet's membrane EK or pre-Descemet's EK.[14] It may also be done as a staged procedure performing the glued IOL first and the EK in a second sitting.

COMPLICATIONS

Intraoperative Complications

Scleral flaps should be 180° diagonally apart. Nondiagonal flaps about 5–10° also can affect the final positioning of the IOL. Surgery should not be proceeded with eccentric flaps as this eventually leads to decentration of the IOL. A fresh flap should be created diagonally opposite to the previous one. Alternately, if the original flap is large enough, a fresh sclerotomy may be created. This problem can be avoided by using Agarwal glued IOL sclera marker. Disproportionate flap size can give rise to disproportionate haptic tuck that can give rise to torsional instability.

An anteriorly placed sclerotomy can damage the iris base and lead to iridodialysis and hyphema. To prevent this, the 23-gauge needle should be introduced vertical rather than horizontal from the scleral site with the direction toward the mid-vitreous cavity. Sclerotomy placed >2 mm behind the limbus has the risk of having less haptic available for tucking that can lead to IOL destabilization and tilt.

Forceful sclerotomy entry at the limbus can lead to detachment of the iris from its root and hence an iridodialysis and hyphema. Any resistance encountered during the procedure of sclerotomy should be taken as a warning sign, and the needle should be withdrawn. Once resistance is felt at the entry site, it is better to withdraw the needle and re-enter in a more vertical plane or through a fresh sclerotomy. Large iridodialysis needs to be surgically repaired and sutured intraoperatively.

Incomplete vitrectomy and iris damage can happen during vitreous cutting. Triamcinolone can be used to stain the vitreous, this ensures that no vitreous strand is present in the AC and the pupil is totally free from vitreous. Improper vitreous removal can lead to pupil peaking and late retinal traction.

A haptic kink or break can be induced if the surgeon exerts undue pressure while holding the haptic during the various maneuvers that are performed intraocularly during the haptic externalization procedure. Haptic breakage might necessitate explantation of the IOL and replacement with another IOL.

Any error on the part of the surgeon during the handling of the IOL can lead to IOL drop. Sudden and uncontrolled unfolding of the IOL during injection can cause this, and therefore, unfolding of the IOL should always be gradual and slow. Improper handling of the haptics by a surgeon or failure of the assistant to hold the externalized haptic can cause the haptic to slip back in to the eye and lead to an IOL drop.

Postoperative Complications

Corneal decompensation usually results from excessive intraoperative manipulation and damage to the corneal endothelial cell resulting in pseudophakic bullous keratopathy. This can be prevented by using AC maintainer and good dispersive viscoelastic to coat the endothelium.

Improper haptic tuck and too thin scleral flaps can lead to haptic extrusion. Eyes with too thin flaps, excessive use of scleral cautery, and scleral thinning disorders such as rheumatoid arthritis are more prone for such complications. Under this situation, tucking has to be reperformed with proper conjunctival apposition.

Complicated cataract surgery and prolonged surgical manipulation with vitreous loss can predispose to the development of CME.[15] Gentle surgery with minimal manipulation and postoperative nonsteroidal anti-inflammatory drugs (NSAIDs) can help to avoid this complication.

Vitrectomy at the sclerotomy site is very crucial in preventing postoperative retinal traction. Eyes with congenital conditions with retinal degenerations, such as Marfan syndrome should undergo proper preoperative retinal screening and any predisposing conditions such as lattice or holes should be lasered. Supracapsular glued IOL fixation[6] described by one of us (Soosan Jacob) can prevent retina related problems in predisposed eyes.

Financial disclosure: Dr Jacob has a patent pending for modified versions of the glued capsular hook.

REFERENCES

1. Misra A, Burton RL. Incidence of intraoperative complications during phacoemulsification in vitrectomized and nonvitrectomized eyes: prospective study. J Cataract Refract Surg. 2005;31(5):1011-4.

2. Bhagat N, Nissirios N, Potdevin L, Chung J, Lama P, Zarbin MA, et al. Resident-performed phacoemulsification cataract surgery at New Jersey Medical School. Br J Ophthalmol. 2007;91(10):1315-7.
3. Dick HB, Augustin AJ. Lens implant selection with absence of capsular support. Curr Opin Ophthalmol. 2001;12(1):47-57.
4. Solomon K, Gussler JR, Gussler C, Van Meter WS. Incidence and management of complications of transsclerally sutured posterior chamber lenses. J Cataract Refract Surg. 1993;19(4):488-93.
5. Gabor SGB, Pavlidis MM. Sutureless intrascleral posterior chamber intraocular lens fixation. J Cataract Refract Surg. 2007;33(11):1851-4.
6. Jacob S, Narasimhan S, Agarwal A, Mazzotta C, Rechichi M, Agarwal A. Supracapsular glued intraocular lens in progressive subluxated cataracts: technique to retain an intact vitreous face. J Cataract Refract Surg. 2017;43(3):312-7.
7. Agarwal A, Narang P, Kumar DA, Agarwal A. Trocar anterior chamber maintainer: improvised infusion technique. J Cataract Refract Surg. 2016;42(2):185-9.
8. Agarwal A, Jacob S, Kumar DA, Agarwal A, Narasimhan S, Agarwal A, et al. Handshake technique for glued intrascleral haptic fixation of a posterior chamber intraocular lens. J Cataract Refract Surg. 2013;39(3):317-22.
9. Ladi JS, Shah NA. Vertical fixation with fibrin glue-assisted secondary posterior chamber intraocular lens implantation in a case of surgical aphakia. Indian J Ophthalmol. 2013;61(3):126-9.
10. Narang P, Agarwal A. Peripheral iridectomy for atraumatic haptic externalization in large eyes having anterior sclerotomy for glued intraocular lens. J Cataract Refract Surg. 2016;42(1):3-6.
11. Agarwal A, Jacob S, Agarwal A, Narasimhan S, Kumar DA, Agarwal A, et al. Glued intraocular lens scaffolding to create an artificial posterior capsule for nucleus removal in eyes with posterior capsule tear and insufficient iris and sulcus support. J Cataract Refract Surg. 2013;39(3):326-33.
12. Prakash G, Agarwal A, Jacob S, Kumar DA, Chaudhary P, Agarwal A, et al. Femtosecond-assisted descemet stripping automated endothelial keratoplasty with fibrin glue-assisted sutureless posterior chamber lens implantation. Cornea. 2010;29(11):1315-9.
13. Jacob S, Agarwal A, Kumar DA, Agarwal A, Agarwal A, Satish K, et al. Modified technique for combining DMEK with glued intrascleral haptic fixation of a posterior chamber IOL as a single-stage procedure. J Refract Surg. 2014;30(7):492-6.
14. Narang P, Agarwal A, Dua HS, Kumar DA, Jacob S, Agarwal A, et al. Glued intrascleral fixation of intraocular lens with pupilloplasty and pre-descemet endothelial keratoplasty: a triple procedure. Cornea. 2015;34(12):1627-31.
15. Kumar DA, Agarwal A, Packiyalakshmi S, Jacob S, Agarwal A. Complications and visual outcomes after glued foldable intraocular lens implantation in eyes with inadequate capsules. J Cataract Refract Surg. 2013;39(8):1211-8.

CHAPTER 10

Advances in Phacoemulsification

Shreesha Kumar Kodavoor, Tamilarasi S, Ramamurthy Dandapani

ABSTRACT

Cataract is an important cause of visual impairment worldwide. Cataract surgery and the expectations of the people having the surgery have changed drastically over years. Since phacoemulsification is already such a fast and efficient procedure, all of us are interested in new technologies that can expand our margin of safety. Recent advances in phacoemulsification techniques and technology have transformed the procedure to be less traumatic and more precise, ultimately increasing safety for patient. Here we give an overview of some of the advances in phacoemulsification which are geared to fulfill the unrelenting quest of surgical and refractive excellence.

Keywords: Phacoemulsification, FLACS, IntelliAxis-L, miLoop, Can Vac CCC, Zepto capsulotomy, NGENUITY 3D, ZEISS ARTEVO 800, image-guided cataract surgery, ORA, iOCT, PACS.

INTRODUCTION

Ever since Charles Kelman introduced phacoemulsification in 1967, phacomachines and technology have continued to evolve. Cataract surgery has transitioned into a refractive outcome-driven procedure over the last decade. Major advances in fluidics have continued to make procedures safer and more efficient. The storm of innovation and technological advances has made us to perform phacoemulsification with greater precision, effectiveness, safety and speed, and as surgeons we need to keep abreast of technology.

ADVANCES IN PHACOMACHINES

Centurion with Active Sentry® Handpiece

Active Fluidics (Alcon laboratories) of Centurion Vision System optimizes anterior chamber stability by allowing surgeons to proactively set and maintain a target intraocular pressures (IOP) during cataract removal. This has been made even more responsive with the addition of the Active Sentry® Handpiece,[1] which contains an integrated pressure sensor on it **(Fig. 1)**. Previously, pressure alterations at the tip of the phaco probe traveled to a sensor near the cassette. Now, the Active Sentry® Handpiece measures the

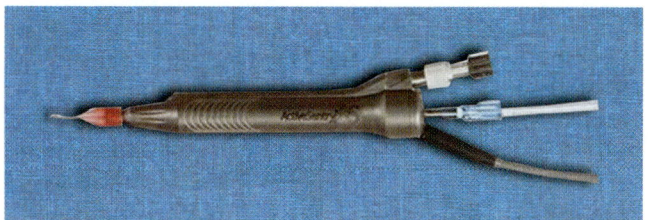

Fig. 1: Centurion Active Sentry® handpiece.

IOP very near the tip, eliminating that millisecond delay in adjusting the fluidics. This technology also automates the patient eye level (PEL) function and would also eliminate the persistent problem of setting the PEL. It also adjusts for an average leakage from incisions. All of these occur automatically engaging intermittently as needed to mitigate surge events and maintain chamber stability.

Balanced energy enhances phaco efficiency through OZil Intelligent Phaco (IP) and the Intrepid® Balanced Tip. Intrepid® Hybrid Tip, the polymer-ended phaco tip has no sharp or metal edges and this reduces the risk of capsular tears. The ultrasonic and fluidics performance are similar to the all-metal Intrepid® Balanced Tip except for the very brunescent cataract. When used together, Active Sentry® Handpiece with Intrepid® Hybrid Tip, phacoemulsification can be performed closer to the capsule and or with higher flow and vacuum levels even at more physiological IOP levels safely and efficiently.

Stellaris Elite™

Stellaris Elite™ (Bausch and Lomb) incorporates Adaptive Fluidics, which allows surgeons to maintain chamber stability at a high level of vacuum. This feature combines precise aspiration control with predictive infusion management. It is a pressurized fluid delivery system that modulates fluid pressure in response to the aspiration vacuum the surgeon commands. Attune energy management system, working synergistically with the chamber stability and vacuum efficiency of Adaptive Fluidics to deliver efficient, and low energy-controlled emulsification. The speed of 28.5 kHz provides the most efficient cavitation profile for efficient lens removal. The dual-linear foot pedal allows separate control of phaco, vacuum, and irrigation.

The Vitesse hypersonic vitrectomy system[2] (Bausch and Lomb) consists of a 23-gauge vitrectomy probe **(Fig. 2)** and a 33-mm long stainless steel needle with a 255 μm sized teardrop port at the tip, which oscillates with user-controlled amplitude (stroke length) of 0–60 μm, peak to peak. The Vitesse vitrectomy handpiece uses ultrasonic, harmonic needle tip movement at 28.5 kHz to generate fluidic and mechanical cutting action for fragmenting and removing vitreous. The hypersonic vitrectomy system uses low amplitude

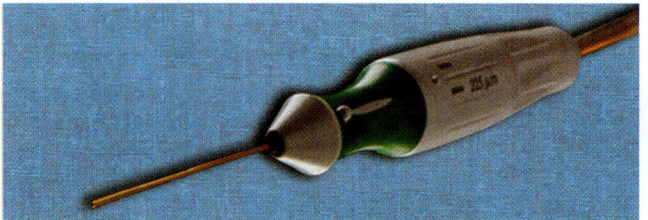

Fig. 2: 23-gauge Vitesse hypersonic vitrectomy probe.

motion of the tip to create oscillating high-speed flows near the port that "cut" vitreous. It also liquefies the vitreous in the vicinity of the port tip to the viscosity of water. This allows the hypersonic vitrector to address some of the limitations of the guillotine vitrector which include the turbulence created by the periodic opening and closing of the port, vitreous material being caught between the inner needle and the port edges, and the need for the outer needle port to be large enough to permit a reasonable amount of tissue to enter to achieve a cut. The hypersonic vitrector has a single needle instead of two needles, so there is no chance of trapping vitreous strands between the port edge and the needle. The port is continuously open, allowing the use of smaller port and larger inner-lumen diameters, which in turn lowers flow resistance with less dependence on infusion pressure. While most cataract surgeons are luckily not routinely performing vitrectomies, having access to this great technology could help improve our results when complications do occur.

Whitestar Signature® PRO

Whitestar Signature System (Abbott Medical Optic) and its recent upgrade, Whitestar Signature PRO, feature Fusion Fluidics, with the CASE (chamber stabilization environment) system. It has both peristaltic and venturi system and the surgeon can decide which system to use during the different parts of the surgery using the foot pedal on the fly to engage either peristaltic or venturi aspiration. It provides a very stable chamber and a really quick response when it comes to surge. It senses at a rate designed to provide the fastest compensation for any surge that may occur. It senses occlusion and when it feels like the occlusion is going to break, it automatically ramps down the vacuum to the preset lave (safe-landing level) so that you avoid surge (CASE mode).

FEMTOSECOND LASER PLATFORMS

Femtosecond laser-assisted cataract surgery (FLACS) potentially offers a paradigm shift in cataract surgery. The femtosecond laser can be used not only to create capsulotomies, corneal incisions, and fragment the lens, but also to produce penetrating corneal or intrastromal arcuate incisions **(Fig. 3)**

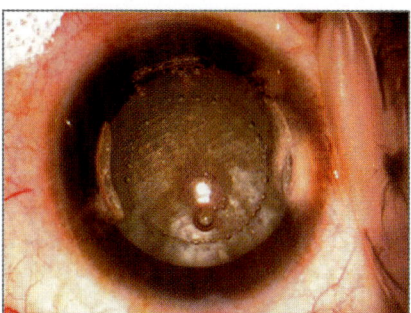

Fig. 3: Femtosecond-assisted arcuate keratotomy.

with high precision. The creation of arcuate incisions using a femtosecond laser gives surgeons the precision of image-guided technology.

Femtosecond laser platforms currently in use for cataract surgery include the LenSx Laser (Alcon, Fort Worth, Texas), Catalys (OptiMedica, Sunnyvale, California), LENSAR (LENSAR Inc., Orlando, Florida), and Victus (Technolas/Bausch and Lomb). All systems share common characteristics that include an anterior segment imaging system, patient interface, and femtosecond laser. All use either spectral-domain optical coherence tomography (OCT) or ray-tracing reconstruction [three-dimensional confocal structural illumination (3D CSI)] to image and map the treatment plan. However, all have differentiating factors, particularly in terms of patient interfacing systems and laser treatment algorithms. Lens fragmentation is performed in a cylinder pattern by some platforms; in a grid pattern by others; and some offer both. Anterior segment imaging is required to find anatomical landmarks for laser pattern mapping to optimize placement of the capsule opening. LenSx Laser and Catalys utilize fourier-domain OCT (FD-OCT), while LENSAR utilizes Scheimpflug imaging technology. LenSx Laser utilizes Circle Scan technology and its OCT has 8.5 mm depth. Patient-interface systems can be divided into contact (applanating) and noncontact (nonapplanating). The Catalys system features a noncontact liquid optical interface (LOI); the Victus has a curved patient interface; and the LENSAR has a noncontact fluid interface. The LenSx Laser has a curved hydrogel contact lens interface (CCL). The LenSx Laser system features a variable numerical aperture that is designed to deliver optimal beam performance to all parts of the anterior segment.

ADVANCES IN MICROSCOPES

NGENUITY® 3D

Three-dimensional digital visualization (NGENUITY® 3D-Alcon) **(Fig. 4)** is a newly developed technology in the domain of eye microsurgery. It consists of one 1080p camera, central processing unit (CPU), monitor, and polarized glasses. The camera is wired to the CPU, which processes the live image and displays overlapping stereo images on the widescreen HD monitor.

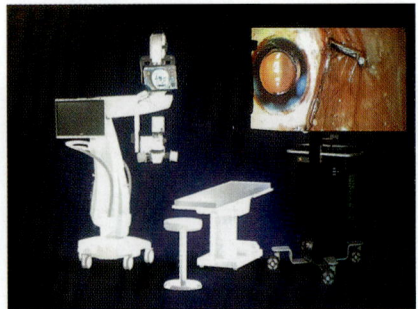

Fig. 4: Ngenuity® three-dimensional system.

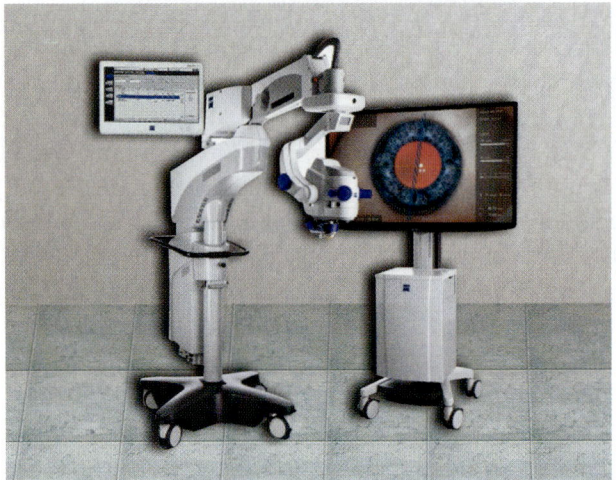

Fig. 5: Zeiss Artevo 800.

Three-dimensionality is then experienced by donning the circularly polarized glasses. Advantages of the system involve higher depth of field, improved field of view, and digital image filtering to enhance visualization without the use of vital dyes. One potential limitation of NGENUITY® 3D system may be the 0.09 second delay of the image shown on the monitor compared to the image seen directly under the microscope. However, it has been shown that this lag was not too noticeable and did not make much of a difference.[3]

ZEISS ARTEVO 800

Zeiss Artevo 800 is a completely integrated digital microscope **(Fig. 5)** and it produces a stereoscopic 3D image that is viewed using passive polarized glasses on a 55 inches 4K monitor. DigitalOptics allows for reduced light intensity, while providing outstanding depth of field and higher resolution images with natural colors. AdVision places essential data such as intra-operative OCT, cataract assistance functions, phaco vitrectomy values, patient information into the view of the surgeon without blocking the surgical field. The hybrid technology allows the surgeon to use oculars at any point, a sterile knob can redirect a portion of the light to them while rest of the crew watches on. In hybrid mode, 70% of the available light is sent to the oculars and the remaining 30% is sent to the 3D screen. There is a distinct advantage over previous iterations of 3D digital microscopes, in which switching between 3D visualization and ocular visualization was time-consuming. Auto-Adjust technology anticipates workflow and change settings automatically when switched between the anterior and posterior segment providing a great depth of focus.

Phenocaine-assisted Cataract Surgery

Stable mydriasis is one of the important prerequisite for safe cataract surgery. Phenocaine plus is a preservative-free intracameral injection containing phenylephrine 0.31%, lidocaine 1%, and tropicamide 0.02%. Injected during cataract surgery, it achieves rapid and stable pupillary dilatation without the use of preoperative dilating eye drops. It is a good alternative to topical mydriatics. It also provides sustained intraocular anesthesia for pain-free cataract surgery.

ADVANCES IN CAPSULORHEXIS

Can Vac Continuous Curvilinear Capsulorhexis

Continuous curvilinear capsulorhexis (CCC) enables safe phacoemulsification and in the bag implantation of intraocular lens. It is well known that the most difficult step in eyes with an intumescent cataract is obtaining a good capsulorhexis because of the tendency toward capsulorhexis extension and a wraparound capsule tear and the risk for nucleus drop. Capsulorhexis runoff or the Argentinean flag sign is common in cases of intumescent cataract because of the high intralenticular pressure, and it is imperative to prevent chamber fluctuations in these cases. Performing routine capsulorhexis with a cystotome in eyes with an intumescent cataract is difficult; even with a double capsulorhexis, there is a chance of runoff. Other capsulorhexis techniques, such as the femtosecond laser capsulotomy[4] and Zepto precision pulse capsulotomy (Mynosys Cellular Devices Inc.),[5] have been described; however, they are expensive. Authors (Shreesha Kumar Kodavoor, et al.[6,7]) have proposed a new capsulorhexis technique, Can Vac CCC (cannula vacuum-CCC), it has been found to be effective and safe in these cases.

Surgical Technique

After peribulbar anesthesia of lidocaine hydrochloride 2.0% (Xylocaine) is administered, the eye is prepared and draped. A side port is created 45° from the planned main port site, and the anterior capsule is stained with trypan blue (0.06%). The anterior chamber is filled with an ophthalmic viscosurgical

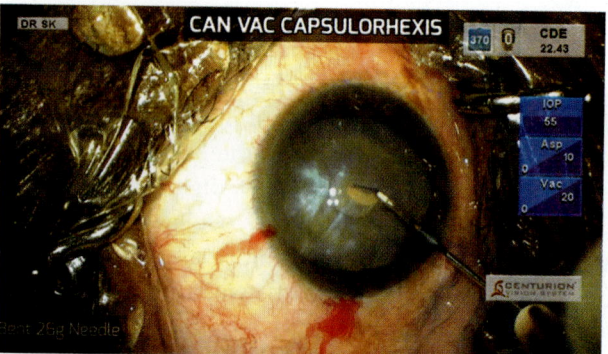

Fig. 6: Capsular tear using bent 26G needle.

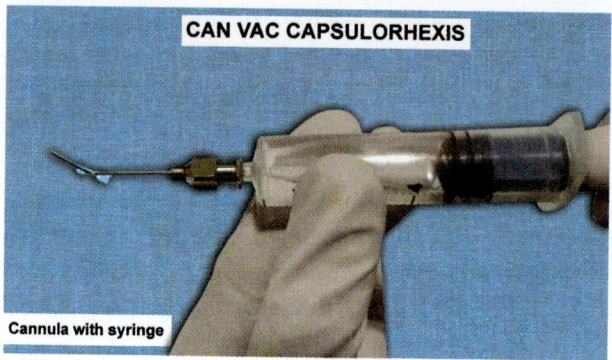

Fig. 7: A 25G cannula attached to 5-cc syringe with balanced salt solution (BSS). (Can Vac: cannula vacuum)

device (OVD). A 26-gauge needle is bent at the tip to make a cystotome, which is used to gently nick the center of the anterior lens capsule to raise a small flap **(Fig. 6)**.

A 25-gauge fine cannula with a flat tip is attached to a 5 mL syringe and then used to create the vacuum capsulorhexis. The cannula tip is used to hold the free flap of the capsulorhexis margin, and suction is manually created by withdrawing the syringe piston **(Fig. 7)**, while making a circular motion.

The vacuum is released by releasing the suction on the piston, and the capsule near the base of the tear is regrasped several times to complete the CCC, allowing for a more controlled capsulorhexis. Loose liquefied cortex released during the procedure can be removed using the cannula, providing better visualization and helping reduce intralenticular pressure **(Figs. 8 to 11)**.

Cannula vacuum continuous curvilinear capsulorhexis is an inexpensive technique for safe CCC creation in eyes with intumescent total cataract. It uses an affordable 25-gauge cannula. It allows the surgeon to create the capsulorhexis in a controlled manner and helps to remove liquefied cortex at the same time, which tends to obscure the surgical field. With this technique, the cannula is not withdrawn from the eye, preventing chamber collapse which is responsible for extension of rhexis to the periphery.

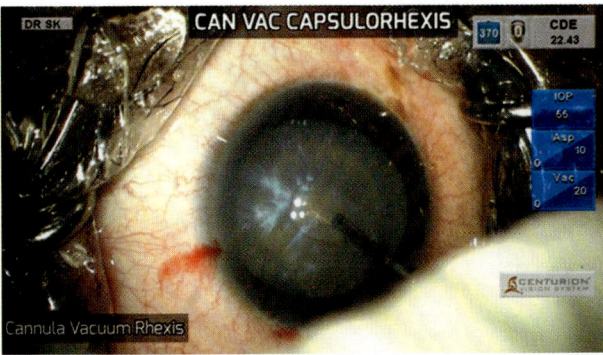

Fig. 8: Aspiration of loose cortex using 25G cannula.
(Can Vac: cannula vacuum)

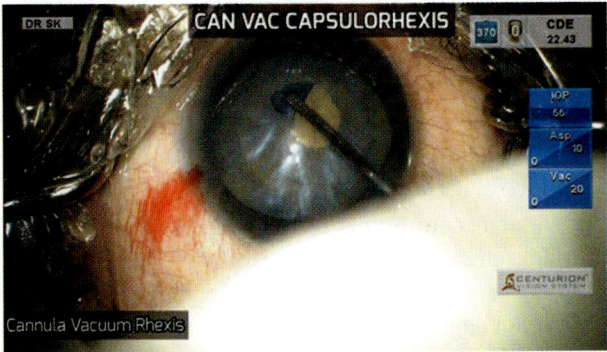

Fig. 9: Vacuum rhexis using 25G cannula.
(Can Vac: cannula vacuum)

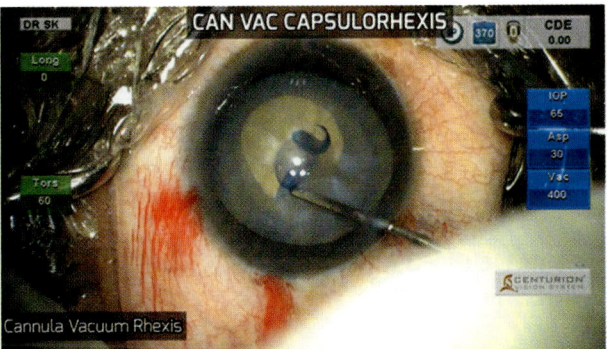

Fig. 10: Can Vac Rhexis in progress.
(Can Vac: cannula vacuum)

OTHER TECHNOLOGIES FOR CAPSULOTOMY

The precision pulse capsulotomy (Zepto) was Food and Drug Administration (FDA)-approved in June 2017. The device constitutes a control console with a disposable handpiece that inserts into a 2.2-mm clear cornea incision to deliver a transparent 6-mm silicone ring. The silicone ring suctions to

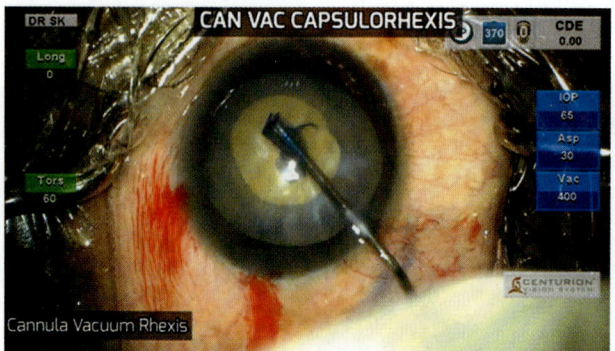

Fig. 11: Can Vac Rhexis completed.
(Can Vac: cannula vacuum)

the anterior capsule and surrounds a nitinol ring that transmits a 4 ms discharge of thermal energy to disrupt water molecules in the anterior capsule, instantaneously cleaving a complete 360° 5.2 mm capsulotomy. Like femtosecond laser capsulotomy, this technology creates reproducible, circular, centered capsulotomies with the important added advantages of portability, lower cost, ability to integrate directly into the standard surgical flow and intraoperative centration on the visual axis. The device does require adequate anterior chamber depth for insertion and manipulation, and initial learning curve challenges may occur with achieving complete 360° capsular suction and cleavage in nonstandard anterior chamber depths and subincisionally.[8]

Aperture continuous thermal capsulotomy (CTC) system (International Biomedical Devices) is a single-use precision pulse capsulotomy instrument without a suction ring that is currently in preclinical trials. It is inserted through a 1.8 mm incision to create capsulotomies between 4.5 and 6.5 mm. CAPSULaser (Excel-Lens) utilizes an orange-red wavelength laser mounted on a standard operating microscope to specifically cut a trypan blue-stained anterior capsule in a single, 1-s continuous, rather than pulsed, circular pass to create capsulotomies between 4.5 and 6.0 mm in diameter.

ADVANCES IN NUCLEUS MANAGEMENT IN PHACOEMULSIFICATION

miLOOP®

miLoop® (Iantech, Inc., Reno, NV, US) is an endocapsular new microsurgical device **(Fig. 12)** that uses a nitinol wire loop to dissect the cataract into multiple pieces, while it is still in the capsular bag. One of its unique advantages is that it truly bisects the cataract from equator to equator. It has the ability to make the surgery easier by dismantling the lens and mobilizing the fragmented pieces making them easier to aspirate. It decreases ultrasound energy levels[9] and apply minimal stress to capsule and zonules in denser cataracts.

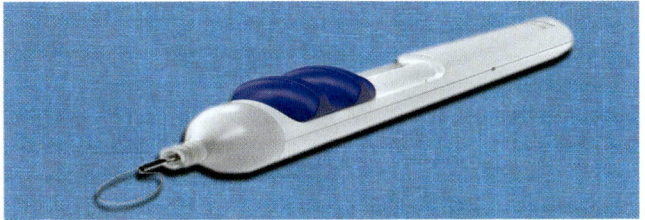

Fig. 12: miLoop.

ADVANCES IN TORIC ALIGNMENT DURING PHACOEMULSIFICATION

Popularity of toric intraocular lenses has increased and options to help align them accurately have proliferated. Using ink to mark the desired axis on the eye preoperatively has its own drawbacks of being broader rather than precise and it can fade or smudge. This can produce less-than-perfect results. Some of the more recent advances help surgeons achieve accurate toric alignment.

New IntelliAxis Refractive Capsulorhexis

One of the newest is IntelliAxis-L system, part of the latest upgrade to the Lensar Laser System (Lensar). IntelliAxis-L uses Lensar's diagnostic capabilities, iris registration software, and intraoperative imaging to precisely and "permanently" identify the location of the steep corneal axis at the capsular plane for toric intraocular lens (IOL) alignment. The system creates custom marks, which remain visible postoperatively to help identify any unexpected rotation and help guide any needed realignment of the toric IOL to its optimal position.

IMAGE-GUIDED CATARACT SURGERY

Intraoperative imaging can be used in capsulorhexis centration, wound and astigmatic keratotomy, IOL centration, and toric alignment. The utility of intraoperative imaging in correcting astigmatism and selecting IOL powers in routine cataract surgery remains an adjuvant to current preoperative keratometry and biometry.

Verion

The Alcon Verion System consists of the Verion Reference Unit and Verion Digital Marker that captures a reference image for use in intraoperative incisions, capsulotomies, and IOL alignment. This system utilizes real-time intraoperative imaging to display astigmatic axis and anatomic landmarks for toric IOL alignment while compensating for eye movement, zoom, instruments, and subconjunctival hemorrhage. Benefits of this system include its compatibility with platforms such as the LenSx® (LenSx Laser Inc., Aliso Viejo, CA, USA) and most surgical microscopes. The advantage of the

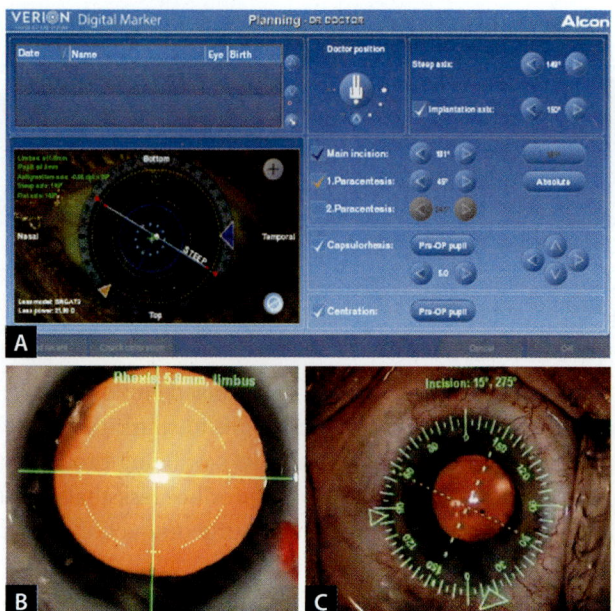

Figs. 13A to C: (A) Planning module of Verion; (B) Overlay for capsulorhexis; (C) Toric axis overlay for alignment of toric intraocular lens (IOL).

Verion System lies in the integration of preoperative imaging consisting of a reference image, keratometry readings, preoperative planning of the surgery including prediction of spherical and cylindrical IOL power, manipulating the lens calculations to determine whether arcuate incision alone, a toric IOL alone, or a combination of the two is the best option for astigmatism correction and intraoperative guidance with an overlay line view **(Figs. 13A to C)**. A randomized prospective clinical study demonstrated that the Verion System resulted in less postoperative deviation from target induced astigmatism and showed less postoperative toric IOL misalignment than using a manual marking technique.[10]

Callisto

The Zeiss Callisto is a component of the Zeiss Cataract Suite **(Fig. 14A)**, which consists of the IOL Master, Callisto Eye, and OPMI Lumera 700 Surgical Microscope. The IOL Master 500 and 700 obtain precise preoperative photographs that are matched to conjunctival markings and tracked intraoperatively, allowing for overlays of axis lines. Used in conjunction with the OPMI Lumera 700 Surgical Microscope, the Callisto Eye software allows for capsulorhexis centration, arcuate and main incision placement, multifocal IOL centration, and toric IOL alignment **(Fig. 14B)**. Tityal et al. compared manual marking and Zeiss Callisto-assisted toric IOL alignment and found that the deviation from target axis were 3.7 ± 2.8° to 5.8 ± 3.7°, respectively, at postoperative day one.[11]

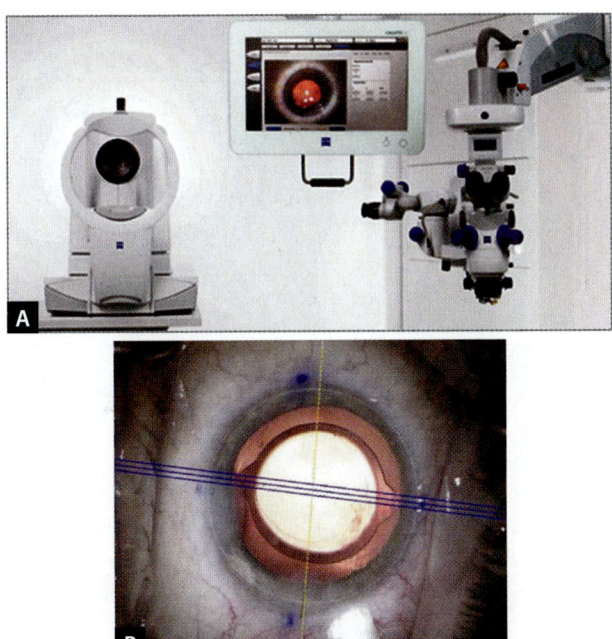

Figs. 14A and B: (A) Zeiss Cataract Suite Markerless; (B) Intraoperative toric intraocular lens (IOL) alignment using the Callisto.

INTRAOPERATIVE WAVEFRONT ABERROMETRY [OPTIWAVE REFRACTIVE ANALYSIS (ORA) SYSTEM]

The optiwave refractive analysis (ORA) System uses wavefront technology **(Fig. 15A)** to analyze the optical pathway of the eye and assists the surgeon by helping them make the best choices for IOL power and astigmatism correction. It is attached to the surgical microscope and has a wide dioptric range for both aphakic and pseudophakic measurements that are taken in the operating room to guide IOL power selection and lens placement **(Fig. 15B)**.[12] While consensus has not been reached on the role of intraoperative aberrometry on the uncomplicated eye, its utility in patients with prior refractive surgery and patients in need of astigmatism correction is more established. In postrefractive surgery eyes, it has been reported that the ORA System has the highest predictive accuracy of IOL power when compared to the Haigis L formula, Shammas formula, and clinical data bases of surgeon choices.[13] Extraneous factors such as eyelid pressure, eyelid speculums used in the pre- and intraoperative setting, and postsurgical changes can all add an element of variability with respect to astigmatism and spherical power to the overall measurements acquired during intraoperative aberrometry.

INTRAOPERATIVE OPTICAL COHERENCE TOMOGRAPHY

Intraoperative optical coherence tomography (iOCT) enables real-time visualization of ocular structures during surgery and enhances our

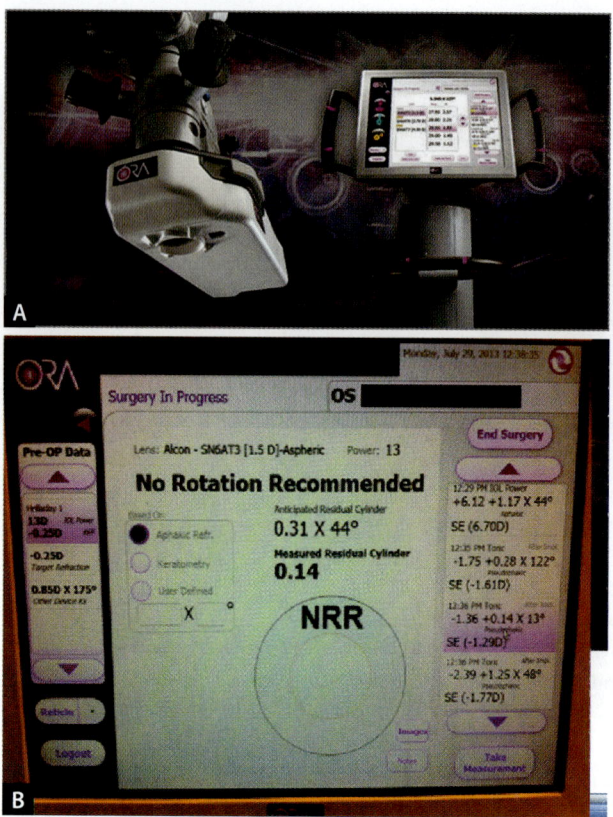

Figs. 15A and B: (A) Optiwave Refractive Analysis system; (B) Screen of optiwave refractive analysis (ORA) after toric intraocular lens (IOL) impantation showing "no rotation recommended".

understanding of intraoperative dynamics. It has evolved from a research idea to a clinically viable technology with microscope integration. In cataract surgery, iOCT is helpful in evaluating the corneal incision morphology, posterior capsule status, and postoperative intraocular lens position. Image quality, improved efficiency, OCT compatible surgical instrumentation, automated analysis software, instrument tracking systems, and enhanced visualization systems are all area of focus for improvement in future.

Cataract surgery is more like an extension of refractive surgery. Techniques and instrumentation for phacoemulsification have come a long way. With many advances made within the past few decades, the evolutionary and revolutionary changes have made our modern methods for surgery safer, more efficient, and less traumatic, with better visual outcome.

REFERENCES

1. Miller KM, Lubeck D, Woodard L, Cionni RJ, Berdahl JP. Key Insights: CENTURION with ACTIVE SENTRY Handpiece and INTREPID Hybrid Tip. Cataract Refract Surg Today. 2019.

2. Blinder KJ, Awh CC, Tewari A, Garg SJ, Srivastava SK, Kolesnitchenko V. Introduction to hypersonic vitrectomy. Curr Opin Ophthalmol. 2019;30(3):133-7.
3. Qian Z, Wang H, Fan H, Lin D, Li W. Three-dimensional digital visualization of phacoemulsification and intraocular lens implantation. Indian J Ophthalmol. 2019;67(3):341-3.
4. Gavriş M, Mateescu R, Belicioiu R, Olteanu I. Is laser assisted capsulotomy better than standard CCC? Rom J Ophthalmol. 2017;61(1):18-22.
5. Pandey SK, Sharma V. Zepto-rhexis: a new surgical technique of capsulorhexis using precision nano-pulse technology in difficult cataract cases. Indian J Ophthalmol. 2018;66(8):1165-8.
6. Kodavoor SK, Deb B, Ramamurthy D. Cannula-vacuum continuous curvilinear capsulorhexis: inexpensive technique for intumescent total cataract. J Cataract Refract Surg. 2019;45(7):899-902.
7. Kodavoor SK, Deb B, Soundarya B, Ramamurthy D. A Novel Inexpensive Rhexis Technique-Can Vac CCC for Immature and White Intumescent Cataract: our experience. Int J Ophthalmol Vis Sci. 2020;5(2):53-6.
8. Kelkar JA, Mehta HM, Kelkar AS, Agarwal AA, Kothari AA, Kelkar SB. Precision pulse capsulotomy in phacoemulsification: clinical experience in Indian eyes. Indian J Ophthalmol. 2018;66(9):1272-7.
9. Ianchulev T, Chang DF, Koo E, MacDonald S, Calvo E, Tyson FT, et al Micro-interventional endocapsular nucleus disassembly: novel technique and results of first-in-human randomised controlled study. Br J Ophthalmol. 2019;103(2):176-80.
10. Elhofi AH, Helaly HA. Comparison between digital and manual marking for toric intraocular lenses: a randomized trial. Medicine. 2015;94(38):e1618-4.
11. Titiyal JS, Kaur M, Jose C, Falera R, Kinkar A, Bageshwar LM. Comparative evaluation of toric intraocular lens alignment and visual quality with image-guided surgery and conventional three-step manual marking. Clin Ophthalmol. 2018;12:747-53.
12. Packer M. Effect of intraoperative aberrometry on the rate of postoperative enhancement: retrospective study. J Cataract Refract Surg. 2010;36(5):747-55.
13. Ianchulev T, Hoffer KJ, Yoo SH, Chang DF, Breen M, Padrick T, et al. Intraoperative refractive biometry for predicting intraocular lens power calculation after prior myopic refractive surgery. Ophthalmology. 2014;121(1):56-60.

CHAPTER 11

Recent Trends in the Management of Diabetic Retinopathy

Rajiv Raman, Sudipta Das, Ramachandran Rajalakshmi

ABSTRACT

Diabetic retinopathy (DR) is a devastating ocular complication of diabetes mellitus and is one of the leading causes of preventable blindness among working-age group population around the world. Despite the increased understanding of this disease, identification of successful treatment still remains a significant risk to global blindness. In this chapter, we have tried to review the existing ophthalmologic literature on treatment of DR to provide perspective on the relative prioritization of the various treatments in the contexts seen in present clinical practice. The newest classification incorporating the state-of-the-art technologies has made a paradigm shift in DR management. In general, laser photocoagulation continues to have a role though pharmacotherapy with the intravitreal anti-vascular endothelial growth factor (anti-VEGF) molecules have revolutionized present day DR management. Surgical intervention is reserved for advanced proliferative stages and in those situations that fail to respond to pharmacotherapy, laser, or combination therapy. Recent developments involving newer retinal diagnostics, novel pharmaceutical agents, and ocular drug delivery methods are proving beneficial in optimizing both initiation and maintenance of DR management. From surgical perspective, newer instruments, cutters, operating microscopes, viewing systems, and vitrectomy machines have started providing adequate surgical control, more precision, less surgical time, and complications resulting in better anatomical and visual outcome.

Keywords: Diabetic retinopathy, blindness, classification, anti-vascular growth factor, midvascular complication, vitrectomy.

INTRODUCTION

Diabetic retinopathy (DR) is the most common microvascular complication of diabetes, occurring in both type 1 and type 2 diabetes, caused by prolonged uncontrolled hyperglycemia and other risk factors. Cataract, glaucoma, ocular surface disorder (dry eye), ischemic optic neuropathy, cranial mononeuropathies/extraocular muscle palsy, retinal vascular disorders, and most importantly, DR are the common ocular associations of diabetes.

Diabetic retinopathy is the one of the leading causes of blindness in developing countries like India.[1] It is the ocular manifestation of end organ damage in patients with diabetes mellitus. It is associated with endothelial dysfunction and vascular occlusion leading to retinal hemorrhages, edema, and upregulated levels of vascular endothelial growth factor (VEGF) leading to new vessel formation which leak profusely.[2] DR is clinically staged into various types ranging from mild, moderate, and severe nonproliferative diabetic retinopathy (NPDR) and the proliferative stage depending on the extent of vascular abnormalities. Diabetic macular edema (DME) is a vision threatening complication of DR develops as a result of focal or diffuse vascular leakage in the macula. New vessel formation which occurs in the advanced stage of DR (PDR) gives rise to complications like vitreous hemorrhage, neovascular glaucoma (NVG), and tractional retinal detachment (TRD) which severely compromise visual acuity. A variety of investigation modalities like the fundus imaging, fundus fluorescein angiography (FFA), and optical coherence tomography (OCT) guide the clinician in determining the extent of progression and staging of the disease. Control of the systemic parameters can help to halt the progression of the disease in the early stages. Treatment modalities like focal laser photocoagulation, intravitreal anti-VEGF, and steroid injections are useful modalities to preserve and improve the vision in DME.[3] Progression to PDR requires treatment intervention in the form of panretinal photocoagulation (PRP) or surgical intervention in case of complications like nonresolving vitreous hemorrhage, TRD, or premacular hemorrhage.

EPIDEMIOLOGY

Epidemiological studies have described the natural history of DR. Studies done in the Western population have shown that the prevalence of DR increases with duration of diabetes, and nearly all persons with type 1 diabetes and >60% of those with type 2 diabetes have some retinopathy after 20 years of diabetes.[4]

A recent systematic review of 35 population-based studies conducted worldwide has reported the prevalence of DR and PDR, among individuals with diabetes, as 34.6% and 7.0%, respectively.[5] Men are at a higher risk of developing DR as opposed to women as reported in several studies.[6]

In the Indian scenario, the prevalence of DR is lower when compared to other ethnic populations. Prevalence studies have been carried out mostly in The Southern India to assess the burden of DR on the urban and rural population.[6,7] A study carried out in Chennai by Raman et al. has reported a prevalence rate of 18% in people with diabetes and 3.5 % in the general urban population above 40 years.[7] Gadkari et al. in a Pan India screening study carried out in 2014 have reported the prevalence of DR as 21.7% in people with diabetes in a predominantly urban population.[8] This shows that approximately 1 out of 5 people with diabetes in India can have DR.

Although urban Indian population-based studies suggest that the prevalence of DR is lower, given the large number people with diabetes in India (over 77 million) (IDF-2019 Atlas), even with the lower prevalence rates (18%), this would translate to over 14 million people with DR.[9]

Moreover, with the present change in lifestyle, diabetes strikes the Indians at a younger age.[10] Younger age of onset of diabetes implies that these people have a greater-risk of developing various complications due to diabetes during their prime productive life.[10,11]

Risk Factors

The onset and progression of DR may be influenced by many systemic factors. The major consistent risk factors for DR reported from various epidemiologic studies include the duration of diabetes, uncontrolled hyperglycemia, hypertension, dyslipidemia, diabetic kidney disease, anemia, and pregnancy. The most important nonmodifiable risk factor associated with DR is the duration of diabetes. Modifiable risk factors for DR include hyperglycemia, hypertension, and dyslipidemia. Other risk factors include ethnicity, genetic factors, etc.

The prevalence and incidence of retinopathy increase with increasing duration of diabetes. Duration of diabetes is the most important risk factor for development of DR. The proportion of persons with DR having more severe forms of retinopathy increases with increasing duration of diabetes. The Wisconsin Epidemiologic Study of Diabetic Retinopathy (WESDR) reported a high prevalence of DR of 50.3% and showed that a longer duration of diabetes is associated with an increasing 10-year incidence of any DR over duration up to 10 years in younger onset diabetes.[11] In the older onset diabetes taking insulin, longer duration of diabetes was associated with decreased risk of incidence of any DR, and progression of retinopathy.[11] Various studies report low prevalence of DR in South Asian Indians and Singapore Malay populations. Hispanic Caucasian populations have the highest reported prevalence across the world.[12] A few studies have reported that at the time of diagnosis of diabetes, prevalence rates of DR in type 2 are higher than in patients with type 1 diabetes.[13]

Studies report a higher incidence of DME in patients taking insulin.[14] However, this does not mean that there is an association between insulin and DR but it is due to the uncontrolled diabetes in patients that they require insulin. Prevalence of DME ranges from 0% in younger onset diabetes whose duration of diabetes is <5 years to 29% in patients whose duration of diabetes is 20 or more years.[14] Thus the occurrence of DME also depends on the duration of diabetes.[11,14]

The Singapore Eye Disease Study reported that Indian ethnicity, glycated hemoglobin (HbA1c), duration of diabetes, blood glucose, and systolic blood pressure are independent risk factors for any DR.[12] Blood sugar and blood pressure control are the key modifiable risk factors associated with the development of DR.[15] The American Diabetic Association recommends

HbA1c of 7% or lower as the target for glycemic control in most patients.[16] Chiefari et al. have reported that patients with type 2 DM who are carriers of high-mobility group A1 (HMGA1) variant have a low-risk of PDR in comparison to DM patients who do not carry this mutation. This explains the role of genetic factors in determining the progression of the disease.[17]

Increased duration of DM is also associated with increased prevalence of progression to PDR. The highest 10-year incidence of progression to PDR (49%) is when the duration of diabetes is between 10 and 14 years whereas its 10% when the duration of diabetes is <4 years. Progression also depends on the type of clinical features noted wherein patients with intraretinal microvascular abnormalities (IRMA) have a higher chance of progression to PDR as compared to patients with venous beading.[18] The Diabetic Retinopathy Clinical Research Network (DRCR.net) protocol S study has reported that worse baseline levels of PDR were associated with an increased risk of PDR progression, irrespective of the treatment modality used in patients with PDR.[19]

CLASSIFICATION AND CLINICAL FEATURES

The International Classification of Diabetic Retinopathy (ICDR) and DME disease severity scales have been developed by Wilkinson et al.[20] **(Table 1)**. These are based on the findings on routine clinical ophthalmic examination. There are five scales with increasing risk of retinopathy. The first level is no apparent retinopathy, and second level is mild NPDR that includes only microaneurysms (MA). The third and fourth levels are moderate and severe NPDR. The level of severe NPDR carries with it the most risk for progression to the fifth level PDR.

Nonproliferative Diabetic Retinopathy

Nonproliferative diabetic retinopathy is characterized by presence of MA, dot and blot hemorrhages, hard exudates, cotton wool spots, and vascular

TABLE 1: Diabetic Retinopathy Disease Severity Scale.

Proposed disease severity level	Findings observable on dilated ophthalmoscopy
• No apparent retinopathy (No diabetic retinopathy)	• No abnormalities
• Mild nonproliferative diabetic retinopathy (NPDR)	• Microaneurysms only
• Moderate nonproliferative diabetic retinopathy (NPDR)	• More than just microaneurysms but less than severe nonproliferative diabetic retinopathy
• Severe nonproliferative diabetic retinopathy (NPDR)	• *Anyone of the following*: (4:2:1 rule) – More than 20 intraretinal hemorrhages in each of 4 quadrants; – Definite venous beading in 2+ quadrants; – Prominent intraretinal microvascular abnormalities (IRMA) in 1+ quadrant and no signs of PDR
• Proliferative diabetic retinopathy (PDR)	• *One or more of the following*: – Neovascularization – Vitreous/preretinal hemorrhage

changes in the form of beading or looping, IRMA, and retinal edema in varying proportions. MA are the earliest detectable clinical signs in patients with DR. They are located in the inner nuclear layer of the retina but their presence can only be confirmed on FFA in which they appear as tiny hyperfluorescent spots mainly adjacent to the areas of capillary nonperfusion.[21] Retinal hemorrhages can either be of a flame shaped configuration in which they are located in the superficial nerve fiber layer or dot-blot hemorrhages in which case they are located in the middle retinal layers. Hard exudates are visible as yellowish white lesions located between the inner plexiform and inner nuclear layers. They occur secondary to chronic localized leakage from the retinal vessels. Progressive capillary nonperfusion is accompanied by development of cotton-wool spots, venous beading, and IRMA. IRMA are dilated micro vessels that seem to function as collateral channels mainly in areas of ischemia. Retinal edema is caused due to accumulation of fluid between the outer plexiform and the inner nuclear layers, which can later involve all layers of retina.[22] **Figure 1** shows the various stages of NPDR.

Proliferative Diabetic Retinopathy

Proliferative diabetic retinopathy that occurs with further retinal ischemia is characterized by the presence of new vessels either on the optic nerve head or within one disk diameter (DD) from it in which case its termed as neovascularization of the disk (NVD) or new vessel growth further than one DD away from disk along with the major vascular arcades termed as neovascularization elsewhere (NVE) **(Fig. 2)**. These fragile new vessels along with fibrous tissue grow along the posterior hyaloid and tend to rupture easily giving rise to vitreous hemorrhage or in case of a posterior vitreous detachment can get pulled anteriorly with the retina giving rise to tractional

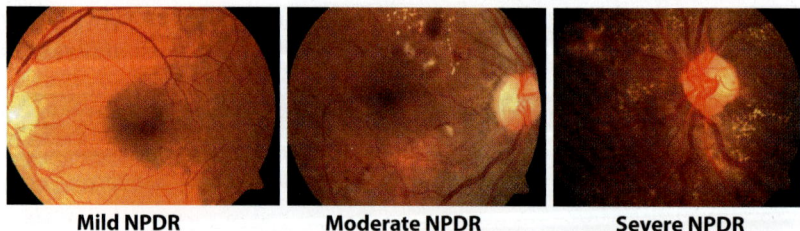

Fig. 1: Nonproliferative diabetic retinopathy (NPDR).

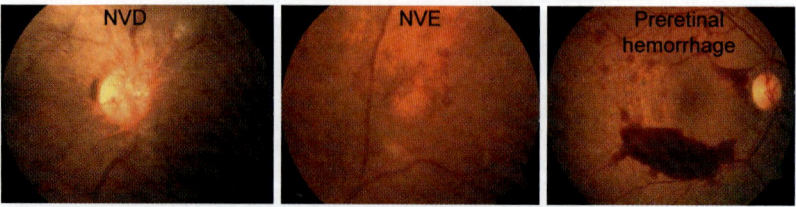

Fig. 2: Proliferative diabetic retinopathy (PDR).
(NVD: neovascularization of the disk; NVE: neovascularization elsewhere)

detachment of the retina.[21] If the neovascularization involves the anterior segment including angles of anterior chamber, it may lead to NVG, which may lead to severe unrelenting pain and irreversible blindness.

High-risk PDR is defined by the presence of one of the following:
- Neovascularization at the optic disk > 1/4–1/3 disk area
- Vitreous or preretinal hemorrhage, with less extensive NVD, or NVE-1/2 disk area or more in size
- Rubeosis iridis (abnormal blood vessels in the iris and the angles).

Diabetic Macular Edema

Diabetic macular edema is defined as retinal thickening at or within one DD of the center of the macula or the presence of definite hard exudates. DME occurs after breakdown of the inner blood-retinal barrier, resulting in accumulation of extracellular fluid in the macula.

Diabetic macular edema can be either being center involving DME (CIDME) or noncenter involving DME (NCIDME) based on OCT **(Table 2)**.[22] **Figure 3** shows the fundus images of CIDME and NCIDME.

TABLE 2: Classification of diabetic macular edema.

Diabetic macular edema (DME) classification by clinical appearance	
No apparent DME	No retinal thickening or hard exudates at macula
Mild DME	Some retinal thickening or hard exudates in posterior pole but distant from the center of the macula
Moderate DME	Retinal thickening or hard exudates approaching the center of the macula but not involving the center
Severe DME	Retinal thickening or hard exudates involving the center of the macula
DME classification by optical coherence tomography (OCT)	
Noncentral involving DME	Retinal thickening in the macula that does not involve central subfield zone in OCT (1 mm diameter)
Center involving DME	Retina thickening in the macula that involves the central subfield zone in OCT (1 mm diameter)

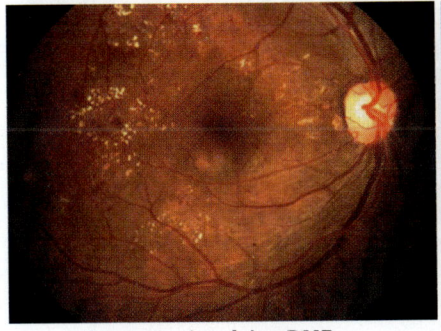
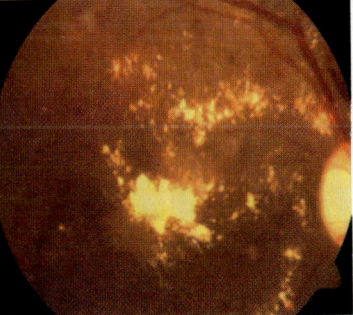

Noncenter involving DME   Center involving DME

Fig. 3: Diabetic macular edema (DME).

In CIDME, there is loss of foveal contour, cystic spaces involving center of fovea, neurosensory detachment involving the center of fovea, and retinal thickening in which the central subfield thickness on OCT >290 µm for women and >305 µm in men on spectral domain OCT (SD-OCT) (Zeiss Cirrus). In Heidelberg Spectralis, the central foveal thickness (CFT) parameters shows ≥305 µm in women and ≥320 µm in men.[23]

In NCIDME, there is definite retinal thickening within 3,000 µm of the center of the macula but not involving the center of the macula. On SD-OCT, it is seen as cystic spaces and/or retinal thickening in noncentral macular subfields.[24]

According to Wilkinson's classification, DME can be divided into mild, moderate, and severe based on the distance of the retinal thickening or hard exudates from the center of the macula. Tab earlier the term clinically significant macular edema (CSME) coined by Early Treatment of Diabetic Retinopathy Study (ETDRS) was used. CSME was defined based on slit lamp biomicroscopy as: "(1) thickening of the retina at or within 500 µm of the center of the macula; or (2) hard exudate at or within 500 µm of the center of the macula associated with thickening of adjacent retina; or (3) a zone of retinal thickening 1 disk area or larger, any part of which is within 1 DD of the center of the macula."[25] The ETDRS found that macular laser photocoagulation was effective in reducing visual loss from CSME.

In general, the type of leakage associated with DME can either be of a focal or a diffuse type. Focal diabetic edema is mainly caused due to leakage from MA and is associated with lipid exudates in a circinate pattern. Diffuse edema is the result of extensive capillary leakage.

Figures 4A and B demonstrates the stages and varying severity of nonsight threatening DR and sight-threatening DR (STDR).

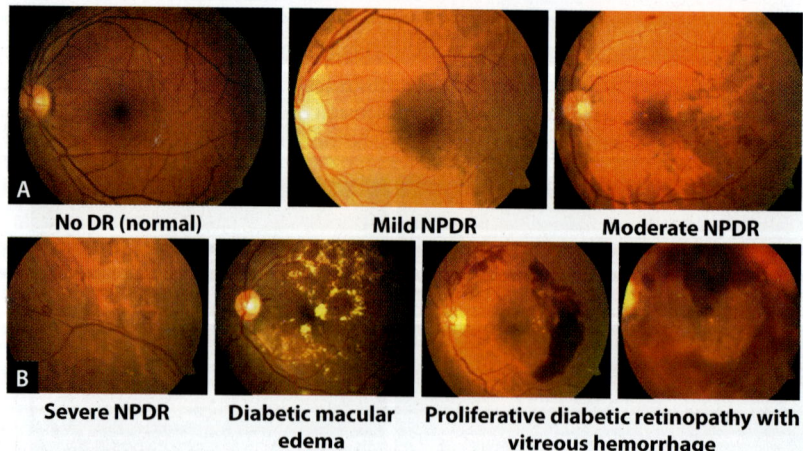

Figs. 4A and B: (A) Nonsight threatening diabetic retinopathy (DR); (B) Sight-threatening diabetic retinopathy (STDR).
(NPDR: nonproliferative diabetic retinopathy)

TABLE 3: Screening schedule for eye examination in diabetes.

Patient classification	Initial retinal examination	Follow-up retinal examination
Type 1 diabetes	Within 3–5 year after diagnosis	Annually; more frequently if indicated by ophthalmologist
Type 2 diabetes	At time of diagnosis of diabetes	Annually; more frequently if indicated by ophthalmologist
Pregnancy in pre-existing diabetes (but not in GDM)	Prior to conception or early in the during first trimester	• No retinopathy prior to conception or in early first trimester; every 12 months • Every 3 months, if mild NPDR • Every 1–2 months, if severe NPDR or worse or as advised by ophthalmologist

(GDM: gestational diabetes mellitus; NPDR: nonproliferative diabetic retinopathy)

Screening for Diabetic Retinopathy

All patients with a history of diabetes mellitus, irrespective of the type of diabetes need regular repetitive retinal examinations. Despite advancements in the delivery of ophthalmological care, DR remains a major cause of preventable blindness throughout the world. As individuals with even STDR may not have any symptoms, life-long evaluation by retinal screening of diabetic individuals is a valuable and necessary strategy. **Table 3** shows the frequency of retinal examination schedule. Fundus examination for DR assessment is done by direct ophthalmoscopy, indirect ophthalmoscopy, and slit-lamp biomicroscopy. Retinal color photography with a fundus camera is helpful in documenting the retinal lesions in DR. A wide range of fundus cameras are available for screening.

Telemedicine for Diabetic Retinopathy Screening

An advantage of technological advancements and digital retinal photography is the ability to transmit images to a centralized reading center for grading. The Joslin Diabetes Center in Boston is the pioneer in teleophthalmology, developing the Joslin Vision Network (JVN). Teleophthalmology is a diagnostic evaluation, which includes a remote digital retinal imaging done by trained technicians, using a digital fundus camera, transmission of images through internet to the centralized grading center for grading of DR, assessment and advice by the ophthalmologist/retina specialist. Telemedicine screening for early detection of DR, particularly of the rural population is being done by many major organizations in India.

Artificial Intelligence in Diabetic Retinopathy Screening

In the recent past, there has been an increasing interest in the development of automated analysis software using computer machine learning/artificial intelligence (AI) or deep neuronal learning for analysis of retinal images in people with diabetes by companies such as Google, Eyenuk, IDx, Microsoft, etc. The machine after being exposed to a lot of annotated images learns to grade DR by itself. These algorithms can automatically provide DR severity and referral recommendation to meet ophthalmologists. IDx is the first AI software to get US Food and Drug Administration (US-FDA) approval for DR screening in 2018.

INVESTIGATIONS

Early detection of DR is a key intervention, which can prevent vision loss. DR lesions can be detected using color fundus imaging, OCT, and invasive modalities such as FFA and appropriate treatment can be started. Following are some of the modalities, which can be used for screening of DR and investigations for management of STDR.

Color Fundus Photography

Stereoscopic color fundus photography (CFP) in seven standard fields (30°) are a gold standard method for detection of DR changes as stated by the ETDRS group.[25] CFP is an effective tool in demonstrating clinical signs of DR such as hemorrhages, cotton wool spots, hard exudates, and early neovascular tufts. Standard CFP provides a 30–50° image which includes the macula and optic nerve.[26] Two or three-fields fundus photography are currently recommended for screening instead of single field fundus photography as they provide better sensitivity and specificity in comparison.[27]

Nonmydriatic fundus imaging has emerged as a popular tool for screening DR, but has limitations including a higher technical failure rate resulting from small pupils and media opacities. Mydriatic fundus imaging gives a sensitivity of at least 80% in the detection of any grade of DR but caution has to be applied as there have been instances of mydriatic-induced angle closure.[28] Many models of low cost sleek hand-held and smartphone-based fundus camera are also in use for DR screening.

Color fundus imaging includes various subtypes including stereoscopic imaging, digital fundus photography, and confocal scanning laser ophthalmoscopy (CSLO). Stereoscopic fundus imaging provides a pseudo three-dimensional (3D) image formation from an ordinary two-dimensional fundus photograph by simply shifting the fundus camera a few millimeters between sequential photographs.[29]

Digital fundus photography can provide up to 100–200° field of view of the retina. Advent of ultra-wide field imaging using newer cameras such as Pomerantzeff camera,[30] Retcam (Clarity Medical Systems, Inc., Pleasanton, CA, USA), Optos Daytona Plus camera (Optos PLC, Dunfermline, UK) **(Fig. 5)**, and the Staurenghi lens (Ocular Staurenghi 230 SLO Retina Lens; Ocular Instruments Inc., Bellevue, WA, USA) have made a radical change in the way we view fundus now-a-days compared to what we used to do before.[31] CSLO uses a laser light and forms an image by a detailed point-by-point

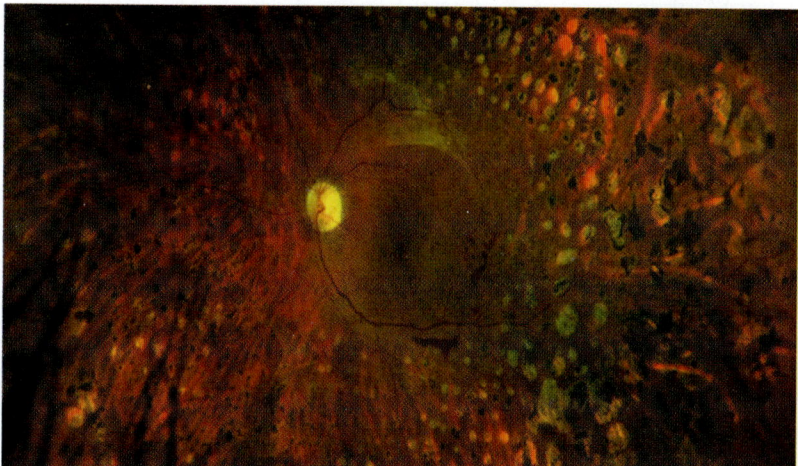

Fig. 5: Ultrawide fundus image of a post-PRP/PDR with fibrous proliferans with preretinal hemorrhage.
(PDR: proliferative diabetic retinopathy; PRP: panretinal photocoagulation)

scanning of the entire field and then capturing the reflected light through a small confocal pinhole, which in turn suppresses any scattered or reflected light outside the focal plane that could blur the image. The advantages include improved image quality, patient comfort, 3D imaging and video capability, and effective imaging of patients who do not dilate well.

Reports have shown that multicolor imaging of the fundus is superior to traditional color fundus photos in detecting and localizing foveal cysts, and helping in better delineation of clinical signs of DR.[32] Pece et al. have reported that DME eyes with higher fundus autofluorescence (FAF) at fovea had worse visual prognosis.[33] Multicolor imaging is thus a potential tool for screening DR in addition to CFP.

Fundus Fluorescein Angiography

Fundus fluorescein angiography (FFA) has been a major modality in detecting retinal ischemic changes and new vessel formation in various retinal vascular disorders including DR. It helps us to delineate areas of capillary nonperfusion and widening of foveal avascular zone (FAZ) in the macula. The landmark clinical trials of the DRS and ETDRS used fluorescein angiography (FA) in classifying disease severity, guiding laser therapy, and evaluating the response to therapy.[34,35] In DME, the macula on FFA shows MAs and IRMA interspersed between areas of focal or diffuse hyperfluorescence due to leakage from incompetent circulation. The ETDRS study used FFA as a guide for focal laser to leaking MAs and macular grid laser to areas of diffuse leakage and capillary nonperfusion with therapeutic benefit.[35,36] Wide field FFA is also critical in delineating peripheral ischemic areas as these areas have a role in central macular pathology due to liberation of growth factors and VEGF.[37] The European Society of Retina Specialists (EURETINA) recommend FFA to

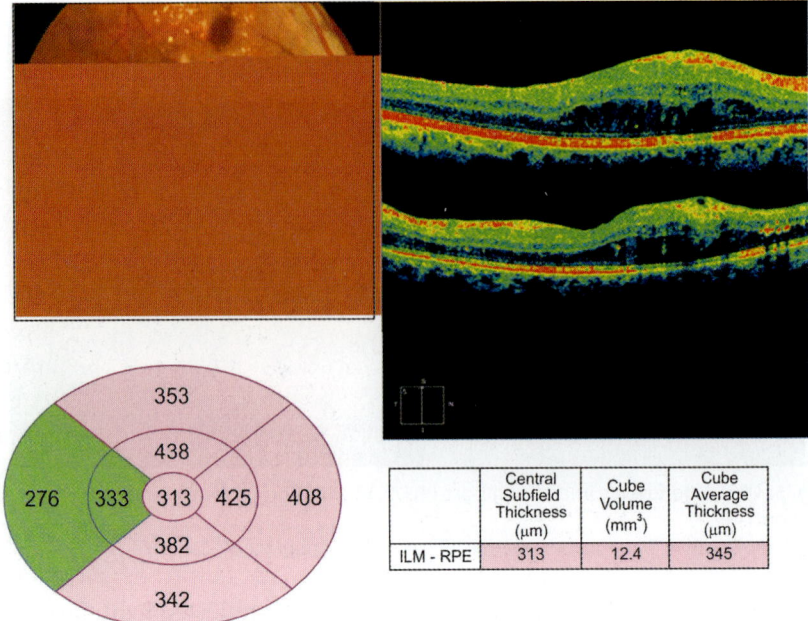

Fig. 6: Retinal color photography and optical coherence tomography (OCT) images of noncenter involving diabetic macular edema.
(ILM-RPE: internal limiting membrane-retinal pigment epithelium)

be an important diagnostic tool for assessing the function of the central and peripheral retina and it must be performed prior to the initiation of therapy to delineate and stage the DME and DR pathology.[3] FFA has contraindications such as renal failure, pregnancy, allergy to fluorescein dye, and must be used with caution in susceptible patients. A proper skin test of sodium fluorescein before FFA has become mandatory in almost all centers around the world.

Optical Coherence Tomography

Optical coherence tomography is used to obtain high-resolution cross-sectional images of the retina in a noninvasive manner. The use of SD-OCT has superseded the time domain OCT that was used in the past because of its faster scanning speed and improved axial and lateral scan resolution. OCT in DME has probably become the single most important tool as it helps in classification of DME and monitoring the progression and treatment evaluation in anti-VEGF for DME **(Fig. 6)**.[22] OCT also gives information regarding the CFT/central retinal thickness (CRT) which is affected by various parameters such as the presence or absence of subretinal fluid and intraretinal fluid. It also helps in prognosticating the disease severity by documenting the status of the inner retinal layers, external limiting membrane, and the ellipsoid zone. There are some landmark clinical trials based on OCT in DME. In RIDE/RISE studies, treatment was performed monthly with intravitreal anti-VEGF, but additional laser treatment was performed on as and when needed *pro-re-nata (*PRN) basis based on CRT in OCT.[38] CRT has also been used as the secondary efficacy end point in the VISTA/VIVID DME trials.[39] Along with best corrected visual acuity (BCVA), most major trials have considered increased CRT to be the re-treatment criteria. The finding that presence of subretinal fluid at baseline correlates with a better BCVA at the end of first year has been reported in the RESTORE study and has been confirmed by the RISE/RIDE trials.[38,40]

EURETINA guidelines recommend use of OCT in the diagnosis of DME along with a baseline FFA and fundus biomicroscopy.[3] Good baseline predictors for a good treatment response in terms of good BCVA are SRF and/or small intraretinal cysts and/or vitreomacular adhesion at baseline.[41,42] Factors that may predict worse visual gain after therapy include the disorganization or disruption of the inner retinal layers (DRIL), disruption of the inner and outer photoreceptor segments and/or ELM and subfoveal thin choroid at baseline.[42,43] EURETINA recommends that PRN (Pro-re-nata) treatment based only on CFT changes for the management of DME but individual OCT features have to be analyzed before making the retreatment decision.[3] **Table 4** provides the American Academy of Ophthalmology guidelines for the indication of use for FFA and OCT in DR management.[44]

Optical Coherence Tomography Angiography

Optical coherence tomography angiography (OCTA) is a noninvasive 3D imaging modality for visualization of the retinal and choroidal vascular networks at different depths **(Fig. 7)**. OCTA enables detection of areas of

TABLE 4: American Academy Guidelines for fundus fluorescein angiography (FFA) and optical coherence tomography (OCT).

Investigation	Situation	Usually	Occasionally	Never
FFA	Investigate unexplained vision loss	√	–	–
	Guide laser treatment for DME	√	–	–
	Identify clinically suspect NVE/NVD	√	–	–
	Identify area of capillary nonperfusion	–	√	–
	Screen for DR	–	–	√
OCT	Investigate unexplained vision loss	√	–	–
	Identify areas of vitreomacular traction	√	–	–
	Monitor response to treatment	√	–	–
	Evaluate patients difficult to examine	√	–	–
	Investigate other possible causes of macular edema	–	√	–
	Screen for DR	–	–	√

(DME: diabetic macular edema; DR: diabetic retinopathy; NVD: neovascularization of the disk; NVE: neovascularization elsewhere)

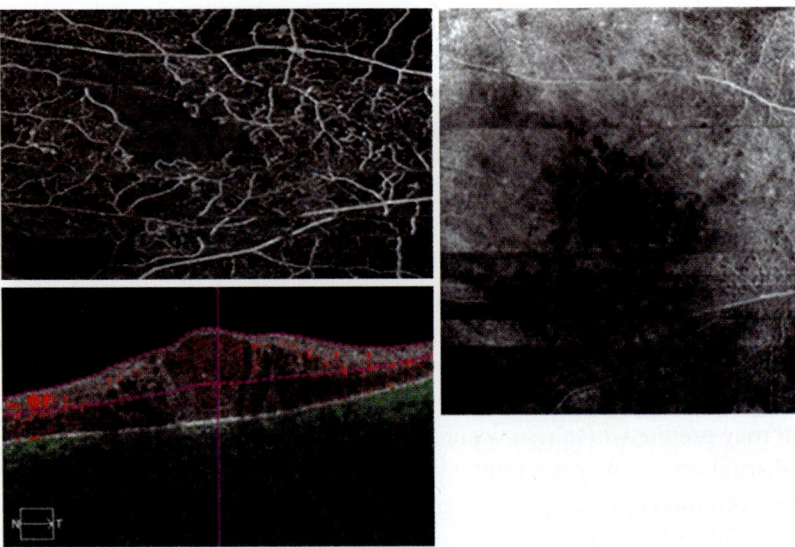

Fig. 7: Optical coherence tomography angiography (OCTA) in diabetic macular edema.

capillary nonperfusion, changes in FAZ and impairment of the choriocapillaris (CC) flow in people with diabetes with no apparent DR.[45] Takase et al. have reported that FAZ enlargement begins even before clinical changes of DR are apparent, and hence OCTA can also be used as a screening tool.[46] OCTA was comparable to clinical examination and FFA in demonstrating MAs, vascular loops, deep capillary plexus loss, IRMA, and new vessel (NV) formation.[47] OCTA also has added advantage of differentiating retinal NV from IRMA, which may not always be possible on clinical examination or FFA.[48] Thus, OCTA serves as an adjunct to distinguish between severe NPDR and PDR and may help in close follow-up of severe NPDR cases. Choi et al. have used ultra-high speed swept source OCTA and documented CC flow impairment in NPDR and PDR.[47] Dodo et al. reported that in the area of the disrupted ellipsoid zone, CC layer had greater areas of flow void further reiterating the fact that alteration of choroidal circulation has a role in the pathogenesis of DR.[49] Some major imitations of OCTA include projection and motion artifacts, segmentation errors, and inability to visualize leakage in contrast to FFA. Thus, OCTA can be used as an adjunct to FFA and OCT. EURETINA guidelines recommend OCTA alongside FFA to offer additional details regarding capillary loss and better delineation of the superficial or deep capillary plexus.[38]

TREATMENT

Systemic Considerations

Major clinical trials such as the Diabetes Control and Complications Trial (DCCT) and the United Kingdom Prospective Diabetes Study (UKPDS) have demonstrated the beneficial effects of intensive glycemic control in diabetic patients regardless of the type of diabetes.[50,51] The DCCT showed that the patients fared better than those on conventional therapy with regard to the progression of retinopathy despite the early worsening seen on induction of intensive therapy. Such patients had a lower-risk of progression to PDR and reduced need for laser and surgical intervention.

Hypertension is a major risk factor and plays an important role in the development and progression of DR.[52] Impaired autoregulatory capacity of the retinal vasculature in DR promotes macular edema when exposed to high blood pressure. The UKPDS demonstrated in their study that intensive blood pressure control helps to reduce the diabetic microvascular complications. The results observed were independent of glycemic control and regardless of the type of antihypertensive medications used. The WESDR study also has shown that the risk of progression to PDR increases in patients whose diastolic blood pressure at baseline were high.[15]

Proteinuria was a consistent finding reported by Klein et al. in half of all type 1 DM patients with PDR and 10 or more years of diabetes in the WESDR study.[53] The presence of gross proteinuria at baseline is associated with an increased risk of developing DME among type 1 patients in the WESDR. It is recommended that patients with early nephropathy with presence of microalbuminuria should be aggressively treated with diet modification and angiotensin-converting enzyme (ACE) inhibitors.[54] Retinopathy in patients with progressive renal dysfunction poorly responds to treatment and its necessary to keep a close watch with regular follows-ups.[53]

Progression of DR during pregnancy is usually a transient progression. Diabetes in early pregnancy study, a prospective study of 140 pregnant diabetic patients, found that women with the poorest glycemic control at baseline and the greatest reduction in HbA1c in the first trimester were at increased risk of retinopathy progression. Thus, a good glycemic control in patients contemplating pregnancy is critical. The treatment of high-risk PDR is same as in nonpregnant patients and PRP should be carefully considered in pregnant diabetic patients with PDR.[55]

Aspirin in diabetic patients is not associated with an increased risk of hemorrhage and has no demonstrated effect on retinopathy progression or DME.[56] Low hematocrit is an independent risk factor for the development of high-risk PDR and severe vision loss.[57] An association between the total cholesterol, high-density lipids (HDL) and retinopathy has been reported in few cross-sectional studies.[58] Cross-sectional analysis from the WESDR showed that cholesterol levels were associated with the severity of hard exudates but were not significant in predicting the severity of retinopathy in either type of diabetes.[59] The ACCORD (Action to Control Cardiovascular Risk in Diabetes) clinical trial of adults with established type 2 diabetes who are at a high-risk of cardiovascular disease (CVD) reported a higher mortality

TABLE 5: Management of diabetic retinopathy.

DR severity	Observe	PRP laser	Focal macula laser	IVI anti-VEGF	Vitrectomy
Mild NPDR	√	–	–	–	–
Moderate NPDR, no DME	√	–	–	–	–
NPDR-DME (noncenter involving)	–	–	√	–	–
NPDR-DME, center involving	–	–	–	√	–
Severe NPDR-large areas of nonperfusion*	–	√	–	√	–
PDR-flat NVE*	–	√	–	√	–
PDR-NVD	–	√	–	–	–
PDR-elevated NVE	–	√	–	–	–
PDR with center-involving DME**	–	√	–	√	–
PDR with nonresolving vitreous hemorrhage	–	–	–	–	√
Vitreomacular traction	–	–	–	–	√
Tractional or combined retinal detachment	–	–	–	–	√

*Option of PRP or anti-VEGF
**Anti-VEGF followed by PRP
(Anti-VEGF: anti-vascular endothelial growth factor; DME: diabetic macular edema; DR: diabetic retinopathy; IVI: intravitreal injection; NPDR: nonproliferative diabetic retinopathy; NVD: neovascularization of the disk; NVE: neovascularization elsewhere; PDR: proliferative diabetic retinopathy; PRP: panretinal photocoagulation; IVI: intravitreal injection)

rate in T2D patients who were randomized to intensive control of blood sugar compared to a standard control of blood sugar level. Hence, intensive control of blood sugar level is not recommended in such patients.[60]

Thus, there are many systemic factors that have an impact on the development and progression of diabetic eye disease and a multidisciplinary approach is required to stabilize the other systemic diseases in association with DR.

Table 5 provides brief management based on varying severity of DR.

Management of Diabetic Macular Edema

Conventional Laser Photocoagulation

Laser photocoagulation was a principal modality for the treatment of DME until the advent of intravitreal anti-VEGF injections. The ETDRS study demonstrated that focal laser photocoagulation reduces the risk of moderate vision loss in eyes with CSME, but less number of patients showed a visual acuity improvement of >3 lines.[61]

Protocol B of the DRCR net study demonstrated the beneficial effects of focal laser photocoagulation in phakic patients as compared to intravitreal triamcinolone at second and third year of follow-up.[62,63] The Ranibizumab for Edema of the mAcula in Diabetes-2 (READ-2) randomized patients with DME into groups receiving anti-VEGF therapy or laser alone, or focal/grid laser combined with anti-VEGF therapy and demonstrated a superiority in visual outcome in patients who received anti-VEGF alone or along with laser over the group treated with laser alone.[64] FFA done before planning focal laser helps to detect the leaking MA and areas of diffuse leakage to decide the areas of treatment. Currently, the modified ETDRS regimen is recommended which includes a less intense laser treatment, greater spacing than for a grid, targeting MA, avoiding foveal vasculature within at least 500 μm of the center of the macula.[65] EURETINA recommends use of laser in the vasogenic subform of DME, which is clinically characterized by the presence of focally grouped MA and in patients with CFT <300 μm with persisting vitreomacular traction. Subretinal fibrosis with choroidal neovascularization is a deadly complication of laser therapy, which may lead to permanent visual loss.[66]

Micropulse Diode Laser

The use of subthreshold laser photocoagulation has been gaining importance as it minimizes the destructive aspects of conventional grid laser photocoagulation and delivers low energy per pulse in the form of micropulses to the cells of the retinal pigment epithelium (RPE) and prevents lateral thermal spread of laser. Micropulse diode laser utilizes a wavelength of 811 nm and the deeper penetration spares the inner neurosensory retina. Beneficial effects of subthreshold micropulse laser have been demonstrated by Luttrull et al.[67] EURETINA recommends that subthreshold grid laser treatment may be helpful in eyes with better visual acuity affected by early diffuse DME.[3]

Intravitreal Anti-VEGF for DME

The DRCR.net protocol recognized that VEGF levels in the vitreous and retina were elevated in patients with ocular angiogenesis, including in eyes with PDR and it paved the way for treating DME using intravitreal anti-VEGF injections. Bevacizumab, ranibizumab, and aflibercept are the intravitreal anti-VEGF agents used to treat DME. Bevacizumab is a full-length humanized monoclonal antibody that inhibits all VEGF isoforms. It is FDA approved in the treatment of metastatic colon cancer but an off-label drug for ocular use.[68] Ranibizumab is a recombinant humanized Fab fragment of monoclonal antibody, which binds and inactivates all isoforms of VEGF-A and is approved for ocular use. The standard dose of intraocular ranibizumab is 0.5 mg in 0.05 mL. Aflibercept (Eylea) inhibits VEGF-A, VEGF-B, and placental growth factor and has shown efficacy and safety in the treatment of numerous ocular disorders.

DRCR.net Protocol-T[69] compared bevacizumab, ranibizumab, and aflibercept and demonstrated effectiveness for all three agents in eyes with central-involved DME (CI-DME). They concluded that aflibercept was superior to ranibizumab and bevacizumab at the end of first year with respect to BCVA gains and mean reduction in CFT in patients with a poor baseline visual acuity. However, at year 2, the mean visual acuity in the aflibercept group was superior only to the bevacizumab group. The RESTORE study demonstrated that ranibizumab monotherapy was superior to laser photocoagulation in patients with visual impairment due to DME.[70] They concluded that laser does not add any extra benefit for improving BCVA if given along with ranibizumab monotherapy. In RESTORE extension study ranibizumab was given to patients who underwent only laser monotherapy for 2 years. They recommend early initiation of ranibizumab treatment to reduce risk of vision loss as seen in the laser group compared to the ones who received ranibizumab from the beginning.[71] DRCR.net protocol 1 study showed that ranibizumab with deferred laser therapy (after 24 weeks) was more efficacious than ranibizumab with prompt laser in improving BCVA in patients with CI-DME.[72] The RISE and RIDE studies demonstrated superior visual gains in both the dosage groups of ranibizumab (0.3 mg and 0.5 mg) as compared to laser monotherapy at the end of 3 years.

Diabetic macular edema can be treated in a number of methods using intravitreal injections. Monthly injections are beneficial in the beginning of therapy, but the numbers of injections are seen to decrease after 1 year of treatment. A PRN approach after loading doses advocates use of intravitreal injections as and when needed based on retreatment criteria and is known to provide comparable visual gains. "Treat and extend" regimen stabilizes the disease process early in terms of BCVA gain and decrease in CFT thickness and then extends the interval between treatments until a new activity does not appear. Over treatment may be a disadvantage, as we may have to inject even after disease process has stabilized.

EURETINA guidelines recommend monthly regimen of ranibizumab in the initial phase of treatment. Monthly injections are recommended until visual acuity and/or OCT stability is reached. After the first year of monthly monitoring, interval of injections and monitoring visits can be extended upon visual acuity and/or anatomic stability. Treatment needs to be stopped if no anatomical or functional outcome is noted with two consecutive injections after initial BCVA and/or CFT improvement.

VISTA and VIVID clinical trials compared aflibercept (4 weekly and 8 weekly) and laser in patients DME-related vision loss.[73] They recommend the 8-weekly dose as the difference between the two-dosing regimens was statistically insignificant. Such as other major trials, VISTA and VIVID also showed that timely initiation with anti-VEGF injections are essential to prevent loss of letters in patients who were previously treated with laser.[73]

Aflibercept was approved in the US (in 2015) by the FDA for treatment of DME on basis of these trials. The approved dose is 2 mg per injection. It has the advantage of lesser number of injections required in the treatment of DME.[69,73]

The most serious complication of anti-VEGF injections is infectious endophthalmitis with rates between 0.019% and 0.09% in clinical trial settings.[74] Thromboembolic events may be a possible side effect of anti-VEGF therapy. A Cochrane Systematic Review in 2018 has reported that there is "moderate certainty evidence" of safety of anti-VEGF injections and as of 2019 no studies have shown a definite increased risk of thromboembolic events.[75]

Intravitreal Steroids for Diabetic Macular Edema

Corticosteroids produce an anti-inflammatory effect by decreasing the synthesis of various cytokines; interleukin IL-6, protein 10, monocyte-chemo attractant protein-1, platelet-derived growth factor-AA (PDGF-AA) and VEGF in the anterior chamber. After intravitreal injection of triamcinolone versus bevacizumab showed that all the mediators including VEGF were significantly decreased in triamcinolone-treated eyes, but only VEGF levels were decreased in the eyes treated with bevacizumab.[76]

DRCR.net protocol B[62] compared the role of intravitreal triamcinolone (1 mg) versus intravitreal triamcinolone (4 mg) versus focal/grid laser therapy in patients with DME. At the end of 2 years, vision was better in the laser group and patients who received triamcinolone developed complications including cataract and glaucoma. DRCR.net protocol 1 showed superior visual gains in patients receiving ranibizumab with laser as compared to the ones receiving triamcinolone or laser monotherapy at the end of 1 year of treatment. Cataract formation and glaucoma were the complications more commonly associated with triamcinolone group as compared to the other groups, which required treatment.[77]

PLACID trial randomized patients to receive either 0.7 mg ozurdex implant and laser at month 1 or laser monotherapy with a sham implant injection.[78] They reported superior visual gains in the ozurdex plus laser group as compared to the group, which received, only laser photocoagulation. Increased intraocular pressure (IOP) was more common in the ozurdex plus laser group however, no eyes required surgery to control IOP in contrast to trials involving triamcinolone in which some percentage of patients required surgery for glaucoma control. Cataract was more common in phakic patients who received ozurdex plus laser. The CHAMPLAIN study also demonstrated the efficacy of a single ozurdex implant in treatment of refractory DME with a history of pars plana vitrectomy (PPV).[79] The FDA approved ozurdex 0.7 mg in September 2014 for the treatment of adult patients with DME. The official product label in Europe recommends retreatment after approximately 6 months.

The Fluocinolone Acetonide in Diabetic Macular Edema (FAME) trials compared different dosages of fluocinolone (0.2 or 0.5 µg) versus sham injections in patients with DME and demonstrated superior visual gains in both fluocinolone groups in comparison to the sham group at the end of 2 years.[80] In a subgroup of patients they also reported higher BCVA gains in the chronic DME group as compared to the acute DME group who received the insert. There was a higher rate of complications such as cataract and glaucoma in both fluocinolone groups compared to the sham group. Fluocinolone (Iluvien) has been approved by the FDA in September 2014 for the treatment of DME in patients who have a history of being treated with corticosteroids and did not have a clinically significant elevation of IOP.[81]

The primary use of intravitreal steroids may be considered in patients who have a recent history of a major cardiovascular event, as anti-VEGF agents are to be avoided. It can be considered as secondary treatment in pseudophakic eyes, in cases of recalcitrant DME not responding to anti-VEGFs and in vitrectomized eyes. EURETINA recommends the use of dexamethasone as a first line agent among intravitreal steroids. The side effect profile must be explained to the patients before starting any intravitreal steroid. IOP monitoring is a must for all patients on intravitreal steroids. To date, no large randomized clinical trial has evaluated the use of intravitreal corticosteroid injection as a rescue treatment for eyes with persistent DME after anti-VEGF injection therapy.

MANAGEMENT OF PROLIFERATIVE DIABETIC RETINOPATHY

Proliferative diabetic retinopathy is an advanced stage of DR which, if not controlled by means of panretinal laser photocoagulation (PRP), may progress to complications such as vitreous hemorrhage and TRD requiring surgical intervention or advance diabetic eye disease, NVG, and optic atrophy which may lead to permanent loss of vision.

Laser Photocoagulation

Panretinal photocoagulation (PRP) or scatter laser photocoagulation reduces oxygen consumption at the outer retinal mitochondria focally and helps in improved oxygen delivery from the choroid to the ischemic retina.[82] ETDRS study report-3 recommends the use of peripheral scatter treatment to ablate ischemic retina to decrease the stimulus for neovascular growth.[83] The ETDRS compared the effect of early versus delayed PRP in earlier stages of DR and at the end of 5 years the rate of severe visual loss was slightly more in the delayed PRP group. The ETDRS protocol for full PRP included 1,200–1,600 spots of moderate burns of 0.1-second (100 ms) duration that is a one-half burn width apart and at least 2 DD from the fovea out to the equator. PRP is done usually with argon green laser can be delivered using slit lamp delivery using Mainster lens or Goldman 3 mirror contact lens.

It can be done using laser indirect ophthalmoscopy. There is increasing use of multispot laser machines like Pascal for PRP.

The number of sessions required was two or more for completion of treatment and it is preferable to keep the upper limit of burns as 900 in a single session thus avoiding overtreatment.[84] The anterior extent of scatter laser was recommended "to or beyond the equator" and the posterior extent of scatter laser was described as forming an oval around the macula and including the disk defined by a line passing two DD above, temporal to and below the center of the macula and 500 mm from the nasal one-half of the disk margin. Retreatment with supplemental or augmented scatter laser with a minimum of 500 scatter burns in untreated areas was indicated for the redevelopment of high-risk characteristics such as: (1) change in NV since last treatment, (2) appearance of NV in terms of vessel caliber or extent of fibrous tissue, (3) frequency and extent of VH since last treatment, (4) extent of fibrous proliferation/TRD and extent of laser scars. The ETDRS recommended against any PRP in patients with mild-to-moderate NPDR because of a low-risk of severe visual loss in these patients and there was a risk of moderate visual loss post-treatment. Re-examination visits at an interval of 2-4 months are recommended for patients with a higher-risk of progression such as severe NPDR and early PDR. Noncompliant patients are at increased risk of progressing to high-risk PDR.

The DRS study recommended a deferral of photocoagulation until high-risk characteristics develop for patients with severe NPDR and nonhigh-risk PDR as they had a reduced risk of severe vision loss with PRP.[85] DRS study recommended that patients with high-risk PDR should receive PRP expeditiously, as it usually induces regression of retinal neovascularization. Focal photocoagulation and/or anti-VEGF therapy prior to or along with PRPs should be performed when there is evidence that of associated DME or if PRP may increase the macular edema and increase the rate of moderate visual loss compared with untreated control eyes.[86] In patients with high-risk PDR, PRP should not be delayed and if anti-VEGF is to be given, both may be done one after the other.

Complications of laser photocoagulation in the anterior segment include corneal epithelial burns and lenticular burns. Posterior segment complications include macular edema, serous retinal detachment, and contraction of preretinal membranes, choroidal burns, choroidal detachment, and secondary glaucoma due to shallowing of AC. These complications were found to be less common in eyes which were treated using less extensive scatter laser by the ETDRS group. Avoidance of laser burns to the fibrous proliferative tissue is advocated so as to prevent traction which may lead to TRD in the future.[87] Photocoagulation of the long ciliary nerve is reported to have caused permanent mydriasis and loss of accommodation.[88] Inadvertent photocoagulation of the fovea results in a permanent scotoma. Thus, extreme caution is needed while setting the parameters before subjecting the patient to PRP and before deciding the areas of treatment. There is a significant body of evidence to demonstrate that short pulse PRP laser treatment will produce less laser burn scarring, less damage to the visual field and is less damaging to the retina than conventional long pulse 100 ms PRP treatment.

Intravitreal Anti-vascular Endothelial Growth Factor Injection

Patient compliance and follow-up are important factors for determining the use of anti-VEGF versus PRP. The DRCR.net protocol S study, which was a randomized controlled trial that compared PRP with ranibizumab in patients primarily with PDR with and without DME showed better visual acuity, less visual field loss, and less number of vitrectomy in the ranibizumab group but was associated with more treatments and visits.[89] As per Gross et al. rate of severe vision loss or serious PDR complications were uncommon with both PRP or ranibizumab; however, the ranibizumab group had lower rates of developing vision-impairing DME and less visual field loss.[90] Arevalo et al. stated that following anti-VEGF injection, cases with severe PDR may develop traction or pre-existing traction may progress.[91] However, Protocol S showed that there was no statistically significant difference between rates of TRD in PRP compared with anti-VEGF.

The DRCR.net protocol T had shown superior effect of aflibercept compared to bevacizumab and ranibizumab in improving DR severity at the end of first year. The RIDE and RISE trials reported that a lesser percentage of ranibizumab-treated eyes showed progression of DR compared with sham-treated eyes at 2 years.[92] Obeid et al. however, reported a higher rate of NVG in patients treated with anti-VEGF injections only and raised the questions regarding use of anti-VGEF in patients with PDR.[91]

Vitreoretinal Surgery

Vitrectomy in DR was mainly indicated for dense nonclearing vitreous hemorrhage >1-month duration and for TRD involving the center of the macula in early days before diabetic vitrectomy retinopathy study took place. Endophotocoagulation was not available until 1983 which created a major hurdle in developing vitreoretinal surgery.[93] Recent advancements in vitreoretinal surgery with small gauge valved cannulas and chandelier lighting systems have reduced the operating time and decreased the number of complications even with extensive fibrovascular proliferation (FVP).[94] Despite the advancements in vitreoretinal surgery, managing DR is a big challenge to the vitreoretinal surgeon.

Indications for Vitrectomy

The main indications for vitrectomy include persistent nonclearing vitreous hemorrhage, TRD threatening or involving the macula, combined tractional and rhegmatogenous retinal detachment (CRD) and dense premacular subhyaloid hemorrhage. Other indications include NVG, ghost cell glaucoma, and anterior hyaloidal FVP.[95]

Vitreous Hemorrhage

Vitreous hemorrhage (VH) should be observed initially with serial ultrasounds to evaluate for presence of FVP with traction in the macula or TRD threatening the macula. If there is no traction, observation, or bed rest with elevation of the head end of the bed can be advocated to the patient. The Diabetic Retinopathy Vitrectomy Study (DRVS) have demonstrated the benefit of early vitrectomy (1-4 months from onset) in severe vitreous hemorrhage in patients with type 1 diabetes mainly resulting in better visual recovery and visual outcomes at 2 and 4 years. However, patients with type 2 diabetes demonstrated a poorer postoperative visual outcome possibly due to greater severity of maculopathy in them.[93] The ETDRS reported progression of 20% patients with PDR to severe vision loss in spite of a good PRP.[96] In a retrospective study of 353 eyes operated for diabetic vitreous hemorrhage, improved visual outcomes were noted in 81% of the patients. Preoperative vision >5/200, minimal cataract, no neovascularization in the form of neovascularization in the iris (NVI)/NVG, and PRP in at least one quadrant were considered as favorable factors for a good visual outcome in this study.[97]

Presence and degree of activity of iris rubeosis is also an important factor which decides the timing of vitrectomy. Prompt vitrectomy is indicated to clear the media for PRP in cases of progressive rubeosis and NVG.[98]

Tractional Retinal Detachment

Tractional retinal detachment involving or threatening the macula has become the most common indication for vitrectomy since the ETDRS and DRS study. The DRVS described the course of extramacular TRD in the posterior pole over a period of 2 years. The rate of severe visual loss was greater in eyes with TRD more than four-disk areas than eyes with TRD less than four-disk areas. Risk of severe visual loss in eyes with active NV or new vitreous hemorrhage was more than in patients without these characteristics. Current consensus states that vitrectomy should be considered at an earlier stage prior to severe visual loss from TRD. In eyes with chronic macular detachment, there is atrophic retina beneath the tightly adherent fibrovascular membranes, and thus the chances of a successful surgery are low.[99]

Combined Tractional and Rhegmatogenous Retinal Detachment

Combined tractional and rhegmatogenous retinal detachment is different from a TRD and it often extends anteriorly to the ora serrata.[100] PDR may cause severe FVP resulting in progressive traction and posterior retinal breaks. The use of silicon oil and aggressive PRP after vitreous surgery is recommended in eyes with combined detachments as it reduces the incidence of postoperative rubeosis and prevents phthisis. Studies have reported a greater retinal reattachment rate and better visual outcomes in eyes in which silicon oil was used.[101] Anterior hyaloidial FVP.

Severe Fibrovascular Proliferation (FVP)

Severe FVP without any surgical intervention may lead to profound loss of vision. From the available literature it is seen that the cases with severe FVP are best treated with extensive PRP laser prior to early vitrectomy, which is preferably undertaken before the development of strong fibrovascular attachments.[102]

The growth of fibrovascular tissue on the anterior vitreous base in PDR is a severe complication following vitrectomy. This can lead to retinal detachment, ciliary body detachment, and NVG which lead to surgical failure and needs repeat vitrectomy.[103]

Premacular Hemorrhage

Dense premacular hemorrhage can cause profound loss of vision. If it does not clear, it may lead to FVP, preretinal membrane formation, and traction macular detachment. In a study with five patients reported excellent visual outcomes when treated with vitrectomy after identifying the location of sub-internal limiting membrane (ILM) bleed.[104] In a study by O'Hanley et al. patients with dense premacular hemorrhage who were not vitrectomized within 4 weeks of the onset of the hemorrhage, progressed to late macular traction, and poor visual outcomes.[105] Vitrectomy surgery is indicated in these eyes for visual recovery and to prevent complications.[106]

Diabetic Macular Edema

Diabetic macular edema if associated with vitreomacular traction will need surgical intervention in the form of vitrectomy.

Epiretinal membranes (ERM), macular hole, and vitreomacular traction may be seen in patients with DR. ERM in diabetic eyes have a focal attachment in comparison to a global attachment in eyes with idiopathic ERM.[107] Vitrectomy with ERM removal and concomitant ILM peeling may improve visual outcomes in patients with PDR.[108]

SURGICAL PATHOANATOMY

The growth of preretinal new vessels (PRNVs) and optic disk new vessels (ODNVs) in PDR are secondary to an aberrant angiogenic response due to inner retinal ischemia. Focal erosions of the ILM lead to development of neovascular projections into the vitreous cavity, while wider dehiscence lead to emergence of venous coils and knots.[109]

- *Formation of fibrovascular nails:* The hyaloid acts as a scaffold for the new vessels which later invade the posterior cortical vitreous by creating adhesions between ILM and posterior cortical vitreous. The RPE pump produces negative pressure in the subretinal space leading to a concave retinal configuration between tractionally elevated areas with heavy preretinal fibrosis.[110]

Role of posterior vitreous detachment (PVD): A study has reported greater incidence of complete PVD in patients with NPDR versus those with PDR, thus further stressing on the importance of the vitreous in the development and progression of DR. PVD in diabetic eyes is mostly incomplete with multiple attachments to the posterior pole and occurs due to a split in the vitreous cortex, leaving a collagen layer on the ILM. Eyes with broad areas of vitreoretinal adhesion may have higher rates of membrane reproliferation and poorer visual outcomes:[111]

- *Vitreoschisis:* Vitreoschisis is a split in the posterior vitreous cortex and is the consequence of anomalous PVD with a strong vitreomacular adhesion. When syneresis occurs, the posterior vitreous cortex splits, most of the vitreous is detached however, the outermost layer is still attached to the macula. It is particular importance to the vitreoretinal surgeon to differentiate the true cleavage point from the false cleavage point so as to enter into the right plane for dissection.[112,113]

SURGICAL TECHNIQUES

Systemic control of all parameters is essential before planning the surgery for diabetic eye disease. Co-ordination with the anesthetists and physician is crucial to have a control of blood pressure in the perioperative phase so as to reduce the risk of complication. Serial ultrasounds are important before surgery to note the exact *delineation of the traction process and to plan surgery accordingly.* Adequate visualization during surgery is extremely crucial during vitreoretinal surgery, especially for DR and so the lenticular status. With the advancements in phacoemulsification techniques, combined surgery is a choice of more now-a-days as it helps tackling cataract and better intraoperative visualization for the surgeon and opacities and stabilize the proliferative process.[114]

The Basic Steps of Vitrectomy

- *Creation of sclerotomy ports:* Preferably ports must be created at 3.5 mm from the limbus in phakic and 3 mm in aphakics with valved cannulas, if available (25 g) or nonvalved cannulas (23 g) with an angled entry. They lead to less postoperative discomfort, rapid recovery, and seldom require sutures for closure.[115]

  Relief of anteroposterior traction: Vitreous hemorrhage may be adherent to the posterior surface of the lens and careful removal is mandatory.

Careful vitrectomy to remove sequential layers of blood in the vitreous cavity is extremely crucial:

- *Posterior hyaloidotomy:* Subhyaloid blood may be diffused with free-floating blood cells and thus a small opening in the posterior hyaloid is essential to remove this retrohyaloid blood. Opening in the posterior hyaloid must be made most preferably by vitrector at the midperiphery with subsequent passive drainage of subhyaloid blood with soft-tip cannula to facilitate the visualization of the underlying membranes.[116]
- *Stoppage of intraocular bleeding:* Intraocular pressure can be increased temporarily to stop the bleeding momentarily, however, excessive rise in IOP may lead to corneal edema leading to problems in visualization. Bleeding can also be stopped using endocautery before and during proceeding to membrane dissection.[117]

   Preoperative adjuvant anti-VEGF injections also have shown to reduce proliferation and intraoperative bleeding if given 3–5 days preoperatively.[118] Bimanual surgical techniques using chandelier illumination are extremely helpful in case of significant intraoperative hemorrhage.

- *Relief of tangential traction:* After adequate vitrectomy and removal of all subhyaloid and preretinal blood, next step is to relieve the tangential traction by way of delamination and segmentation or en bloc dissection. Membranous proliferation can also be removed using a combination of all these techniques.

Removal of adherent posterior cortex from the fibrovascular plaques is important to facilitate the dissection of the fibrovascular plaques. The presence of cortical vitreous strands attached to the retina can be detected by passing a soft-tip cannula with mild suction along the retinal surface and if cortical vitreous matter is present, it will lead to bending of the cannula at the same point. It is known as the fish strike sign. Triamcinolone can also be used to identify residual vitreous matter.[119] A microvitreoretinal blade (MVR) can be used to facilitate dissection of the membrane if there is slight elevation of the taut posterior hyaloid. Along with MVR, the surgeon can make use of horizontal scissors or a pick can be used especially when there is no pre-existing separation. The site of initial dissection can be started in the midperipheral retina in area of previous laser to reduce chances of bleeding and away from the site of the FVP to reduce the chances of a retinal tear. Starting the dissection from the peripapillary site especially in cases of combined traction-rhegmatogenous detachment has been advocated. An important thing for the vitreoretinal surgeon is to correctly identify the plane of dissection especially in cases of vitreoschisis wherein the inner wall of schisis cavity can form a membrane between the fibrovascular plaque and the peripheral retina, and failure to identify the correct plane will often lead to failure of dissection.

Steps to Manage Diabetic Membranes: Segmentation and Delamination

- *Segmentation:* The tangential traction is cut or severed into smaller islands and each island of remaining tissue connected to one or two fibrovascular nails or pegs are subsequently removed.
- *Delamination:* The tangential traction is removed by severing those fibrovascular nails or pegs, one-by-one. The different types of delamination are as follows:
  - *En bloc dissection*: It entails removing the large sheet of fibrous tissue (tangential traction) in a single sheet by severing the nails using the bimanual approach.[120]
  - *Fold back delamination*: It is a technique for removing flexible, weakly fixed membranes by putting the cutter port just behind the membrane's leading edge.
  - *Conformal cutter delamination*: In cases with thickened membranes, the "conformal cutter delamination" technique can be used. This involves dissecting the thickened membranes directly by moving the cutter port forward into the leading edges of the membranes.
  - *Lift and cut*: In this technique, the cutter is applied to the edge of a rigid ERM. It is a side/oblique approach where the cutter is more used as a pic forceps and membrane is lifted. Once lifted nips are made in the membrane.
  - *Lawnmower technique*: In this technique, the cutter is used for lifting the membrane and for blunt dissection. Membrane is then shaved using the cutter.[121]

COMPLICATIONS

Intraoperative Complications

Corneal edema: Corneal edema is seen during prolonged surgical procedures or when the intraocular pressure has been elevated for a substantial period of time.

Cataract formation: Development of cataracts is a mandatory consequence of vitrectomy. It could be an iatrogenic complication and it also happens in uneventful operation.

Intraocular bleeding: Bleeding commonly occurs during peeling of fibrovascular membrane or due to sudden changes in intraocular pressure while exchanging instruments.

Iatrogenic breaks: Iatrogenic breaks can occur during dissection of fibrovascular membranes. Intraoperative break formation is much more frequent during vitrectomy for TRD and the reported rates range from 27 to 50% of eyes.

Postoperative Complications

Cataract: Cataract progresses faster after vitrectomy in diabetic eyes compared to nondiabetic eyes.

Retinal detachment: The iatrogenic retinal tears are usually seen close to the superior sclerotomies because of inadvertent peripheral vitreous traction caused by intraocular instrument manipulation. Posterior retinal breaks are the other possible cause for postoperative rhegmatogenous retinal detachment (RRD) and are usually created during fibrovascular membrane dissection over thin and atrophic retina.

Reproliferations: Inadequately treated ischemic retina during vitrectomy for DR can lead to reproliferation of diabetic fibrovascular membranes after surgery. The fibrovascular membranes may also develop along the anterior vitreous remnants creating anterior hyaloid fibrovascular membranes. The neovascular proliferations can be picked up by ultrasound bio microscopy (UBM) and can be managed by trans-scleral cryotherapy with or without vitreous lavage.

Vitreous hemorrhage: Delayed vitreous hemorrhage is seen usually 3 months after surgery and is caused by residual vascular membranes, recurrent neovascularization, and most commonly from fibrovascular ingrowths at sclerotomy entry site.[122]

Iris rubeosis and neovascular glaucoma: Diabetic retinopathy vitrectomy study (DRVS) report five reported rates of NVG from 13 to 27%. Few recent studies have reported a much-reduced rate of NVG following diabetic vitrectomies, ranging from 0.7 to 8%.[123]

Phthisis bulbi: In the DRVS study reports the rates of phthisis after diabetic vitrectomy were as high as 19%. Fortunately, recent data have shown a significantly reduced rate of phthisis, ranging from 0 to 1% following diabetic vitrectomies.

OUTCOME

Vitreous hemorrhage: Recent studies have shown a single surgery anatomical success rate between 85 and 90%. Studies show that visual improvement does occur in 80% of the operated cases of vitreous hemorrhage with no TRD, with a final visual acuity of ≥20/200 in 48–72% of the cases.

Traction RD (TRD) and combined RRD (CRD): In patients with TRD, sparing the macula, the anatomical success rate was high (82%). The rate of reattachment in patients with TRD, involving macula, was attained in 56% of the eyes. The visual outcome of patients with CRD were poorer still compared with TRD, with only 20–36% of the eyes achieving a final visual acuity of ≥20/200.[121]

Diabetic macular edema: Though, ILM peeling along with PPV has been shown to be beneficial in reducing macular edema in some studies, the visual outcome, in other studies, failed to show a significant improvement.

CONCLUSION

Early diagnosis and initiation of therapy is the key to prevent permanent visual loss due to DR. Though anti-VEGF therapy and intravitreal steroids has revolutionized management of DME yet good systemic control and adherence to therapy remains the cornerstone for successful outcome. Role of laser photocoagulation in PDR still remains gold standard. Surgical management of DR remains an enigma, even to the most experienced vitreoretinal surgeons. With the advents of newer instruments, cutters, operating microscopes, viewing systems and vitrectomy machines, PPV for DR has undergone a paradigm shift. These advances have provided a better surgical control and more precision; and simultaneously, less surgical time and less operative complications thus giving better anatomical and visual results.

REFERENCES

1. Flaxman SR, Bourne RRA, Resnikoff S, Ackland P, Braithwaite T, Cicinelli MV, et al; Vision Loss Expert Group of the Global Burden of Disease Study. Global causes of blindness and distance vision impairment 1990-2020: a systematic review and meta-analysis. Lancet Glob Health. 2017;5(12):e1221-34.
2. Abcouwer SF, Gardner TW. Diabetic retinopathy: loss of neuroretinal adaptation to the diabetic metabolic environment. Ann N Y Acad Sci. 2014;1311:174-90.
3. Schmidt-Erfurth U, Garcia-Arumi J, Bandello F, Berg K, Chakravarthy U, Gerendas BS, et al. Guidelines for the Management of Diabetic Macular Edema by the European Society of Retina Specialists (EURETINA). Ophthalmologica. 2017;237(4):185-222.
4. Zheng Y, He M, Congdon N. The worldwide epidemic of diabetic retinopathy. Indian J Ophthalmol. 2012;60(5):428-31.
5. Yau JWY, Rogers SL, Kawasaki R, Lamoureux EL, Kowalski JW, Bek T, et al; Meta-Analysis for Eye Disease (META-EYE) Study Group. Global prevalence and major risk factors of diabetic retinopathy. Diabetes Care. 2012;35(3):556-64.
6. Rema M, Premkumar S, Anitha B, Deepa R, Pradeepa R, Mohan V. Prevalence of diabetic retinopathy in urban India: The Chennai urban rural epidemiology study (CURES) eye study, I. Invest Ophthalmol Vis Sci. 2005;46(7):2328-33.
7. Raman R, Rani PK, Reddi Rachepalle S, Gnanamoorthy P, Uthra S, Kumaramanickavel G, et al. Prevalence of diabetic retinopathy in India: Sankara Nethralaya diabetic retinopathy epidemiology and molecular genetics study report 2. Ophthalmology. 2009;116(2):311-8.
8. Gadkari SS, Maskati QB, Nayak BK. Prevalence of diabetic retinopathy in India: The All India Ophthalmological Society Diabetic Retinopathy Eye Screening Study 2014. Indian J Ophthalmol. 2016;64(1):38-44.
9. International Diabetes Federation Diabetes Atlas, 9th edition. Brussels, Belgium: International Diabetes Federation; 2019.
10. Rajalakshmi R, Amutha A, Ranjani H, Ali MK, Unnikrishnan R, Anjana RM, et al. Prevalence and risk factors for diabetic retinopathy in Asian Indians with young onset type 1 and type 2 diabetes. J Diabetes Complications. 2014;28(3):291-7.

11. Klein R, Klein BE, Moss SE, Cruickshanks KJ. The Wisconsin epidemiologic study of diabetic retinopathy. XIV. Ten-year incidence and progression of diabetic retinopathy. Arch Ophthalmol. 1994;112(9):1217-28.
12. Tan GS, Gan A, Sabanayagam C, Tham YC, Neelam K, Mitchell P, et al. Ethnic differences in the prevalence and risk factors of diabetic retinopathy: the Singapore Epidemiology of Eye Diseases study. Ophthalmology. 2018;125(4):529-36.
13. Kostev K, Rathmann W. Diabetic retinopathy at diagnosis of type 2 diabetes in the UK: a database analysis. Diabetologia. 2013;56(1):109-11.
14. Lee R, Wong TY, Sabanayagam C. Epidemiology of diabetic retinopathy, diabetic macular edema and related vision loss. Eye Vis (Lond). 2015;2:17.
15. Rajalakshmi R, Prathiba V, Mohan V. Does tight control of systemic factors help in the management of diabetic retinopathy? Indian J Ophthalmol. 2016;64(1):62-8.
16. American Diabetes Association. Standards of medical care in diabetes-2013. Diabetes Care. 2013;36 (Suppl 1):S11-66.
17. Chiefari E, Ventura V, Capula C, Randazzo G, Scorcia V, Fedele M, et al. A polymorphism of HMGA1 protects against proliferative diabetic retinopathy by impairing HMGA1-induced VEGFA expression. Sci Rep. 2016;6:39429.
18. Lee CS, Lee AY, Baughman D, Sim D, Akelere T, Brand C, et al. The United Kingdom Diabetic Retinopathy Electronic Medical Record Users Group: Report 3: Baseline retinopathy and clinical features predict progression of diabetic retinopathy. Am J Ophthalmol. 2017;180:64-71.
19. Bressler SB, Beaulieu WT, Glassman AR, Gross JG, Jampol LM, Melia M, et al. Factors Associated with Worsening Proliferative Diabetic Retinopathy in Eyes Treated with Panretinal Photocoagulation or Ranibizumab. Ophthalmology. 2017;124(4):431-9.
20. Wilkinson CP, Ferris FL 3rd, Klein RE, Lee PP, Agardh CD, Davis M, et al; Global Diabetic Retinopathy Project Group. Proposed international clinical diabetic retinopathy and diabetic macular edema disease severity scales. Ophthalmology. 2003;110(9):1677-82.
21. Singh R, Ramasamy K, Abraham C, Gupta V, Gupta A. Diabetic retinopathy: An update. Indian J Ophthalmol. 2008;56(3):178-88.
22. Bressler NM, Edwards AR, Antoszyk AN, Beck RW, Browning DJ, Ciardella AP, et al; Diabetic Retinopathy Clinical Research Network. Retinal thickness on Stratus optical coherence tomography in People with diabetes and minimal or no diabetic retinopathy. Am J Ophthalmol. 2008;145(5):894-901.
23. Raman R, Bhende M. Diabetic Macular Edema. Sci J Med & Vis Res Foun. 2015;XXXIII:50-6.
24. Sun JK, Jampol LM. The Diabetic Retinopathy Clinical Research Network (DRCR.net) and Its Contributions to the Treatment of Diabetic Retinopathy. Ophthalmic Res. 2019;62(4):225-30.
25. Grading diabetic retinopathy from stereoscopic color fundus photographs-an extension of the modified Airlie House classification. ETDRS report number 10. Early Treatment Diabetic Retinopathy Study Research Group. Ophthalmology. 1991;98 (5 Suppl):786-806.
26. Vujosevic S, Benetti E, Massignan F, Pilotto E, Varano M, Cavarzeran F, et al. Screening for diabetic retinopathy: 1 and 3 nonmydriatic 45-degree digital fundus photographs vs 7 standard early treatment diabetic retinopathy study fields. Am J Ophthalmol. 2009;148(1):111-8.
27. Lim G, Bellemo V, Xie Y, Lee XQ, Yip MYT, Ting DSW. Different fundus imaging modalities and technical factors in AI screening for diabetic retinopathy: a review. Eye Vis (Lond). 2020;7:21.
28. Boucher MC, Gresset JA, Angioi K, Olivier S. Effectiveness and safety of screening for diabetic retinopathy with two nonmydriatic digital images compared with the seven standard stereoscopic photographic fields. Can J Ophthalmol. 2003;38(7):557-68.

29. Jain AB, Jaya Prakash V, Bhende M. Techniques of Fundus Imaging. Sci J Med & Vis Res Foun. 2015;XXXIII(2):100-7.
30. Williams GA, Scott IU, Haller JA, Maguire AM, Marcus D, McDonald HR. Single-field fundus photography for diabetic retinopathy screening: a report by the American Academy of Ophthalmology. Ophthalmology. 2004;111(5):1055-62.
31. Staurenghi G, Viola F, Mainster MA, Graham RD, Harrington PG. Scanning laser ophthalmoscopy and angiography with a wide-field contact lens system. Arch Ophthalmol. 2005;123(2):244-52.
32. Saurabh K, Roy R, Goel S. Correlation of multicolor images and conventional color fundus photographs with foveal autofluorescence patterns in diabetic macular edema. Indian J Ophthalmol. 2020;68(1):141-4.
33. Pece A, Isola V, Holz F, Milani P, Brancato R. Autofluorescence imaging of cystoid macular edema in diabetic retinopathy. Ophthalmologica. 2010;224(4):230-5.
34. Aiello LM, Berrocal J, David MD, Ederer F, Goldberg MF, Harris JE, et al. The diabetic retinopathy study. Arch Ophthalmol. 1973;90(5):347-8.
35. Early photocoagulation for diabetic retinopathy. ETDRS report number 9. Early Treatment Diabetic Retinopathy Study Research Group. Ophthalmology. 1991;98(5):766-85.
36. Bresnick GH: Diabetic macular edema: a review. Ophthalmology. 1986;93(7):989-97.
37. Wessel MM, Nair N, Aaker GD, Ehrlich JR, D'Amico DJ, Kiss S. Peripheral retinal ischemia, as evaluated by ultra-widefield fluorescein angiography, is associated with diabetic macular oedema. Br J Ophthalmol. 2012;96(5):694-8.
38. Nguyen QD, Brown DM, Marcus DM, Boyer DS, Patel S, Feiner L, et al. Ranibizumab for diabetic macular edema: results from 2 phase III randomized trials: RISE and RIDE. Ophthalmology. 2012;119(4):789-801.
39. Korobelnik JF, Do DV, Schmidt-Erfurth U, Boyer DS, Holz FG, Heier JS, et al. Intravitreal aflibercept for diabetic macular edema. Ophthalmology. 2014;121(11):2247-54.
40. Gerendas B, Simader C, Deak GG, Prager SG, Lammer J, Waldstein SM, et al. Morphological parameters relevant for visual and anatomic outcomes during anti-VEGF therapy of diabetic macular edema in the RESTORE trial. Invest Ophthalmol Vis Sci. 2014;55:1791.
41. Karst SG, Lammer J, Mitsch C, Schober M, Mehta J, Scholda C, et al. Detailed analysis of retinal morphology in patients with diabetic macular edema (DME) randomized to ranibizumab or triamcinolone treatment. Graefes Arch Clin Exp Ophthalmol. 2018;256(1):49-58.
42. Sun JK, Lin MM, Lammer J, Prager S, Sarangi R, Silva SS, et al: Disorganization of the retinal inner layers as a predictor of visual acuity in eyes with center-involved diabetic macular edema. JAMA Ophthalmol. 2014;132(11):1309-16.
43. Rayess N, Rahimy E, Ying G-S, Bagheri N, Ho AC, Regillo CD, et al. Baseline choroidal thickness as a predictor for response to anti-vascular endothelial growth factor therapy in diabetic macular edema. Am J Ophthalmol. 2015;159(1):85-91.
44. American Academy of Ophthalmology Preferred Practice Pattern Retina/Vitreous Committee: HYPERLINK "https://www.aao.org/preferred-practice-pattern/diabetic-retinopathy-ppp"Diabetic Retinopathy PPP 2019, October 2019. https://www.aao.org/preferred-practice-pattern/diabetic-retinopathy-ppp.
45. de Carlo TE, Chin AT, Bonini Filho MA, Adhi M, Branchini L, Salz DA, et al. Detection of microvascular changes in eyes of patients with diabetes but not clinical diabetic retinopathy using optical coherence tomography angiography. Retina. 2015;35(11):2364-70.
46. Takase N, Nozaki M, Kato A, Ozeki H, Yoshida M, Ogura Y. Enlargement of foveal avascular zone in diabetic eyes evaluated by en face optical coherence tomography angiography. Retina. 2015;35(11):2377-83.
47. Choi W, Waheed NK, Moult EM, Adhi M, Lee B, De Carlo T, et al. Ultrahigh speed swept source optical coherence tomography angiography of retinal and

choriocapillaris alterations in diabetic patients with and without retinopathy. Retina. 2017;37(1):11-21.
48. Matsunaga DR, Yi JJ, De Koo LO, Ameri H, Puliafito CA, Kashani AH, et al. Optical coherence tomography angiography of diabetic retinopathy in human subjects. Ophthalmic Surg Lasers Imaging Retina. 2015;46(8):796-805.
49. Khadamy J, Abri Aghdam K, Falavarjani KG. An Update on Optical Coherence Tomography Angiography in Diabetic Retinopathy. J Ophthalmic Vis Res. 2018;13(4):487-97.
50. The Diabetes Control and Complications Trial Research Group; Nathan DM, Genuth S, Lachin J, Cleary P, Crofford O, Davis M, et al. The effect of intensive treatment of diabetes on the development and progression of long-term complications in insulin-dependent diabetes mellitus. N Engl J Med. 1993;329(14):977-86.
51. Intensive blood-glucose control with sulphonylureas or insulin compared with conventional treatment and risk of complications in patients with type 2 diabetes (UKPDS 33). UK Prospective Diabetes Study (UKPDS) Group. Lancet. 1998;352(9131):837-53.
52. Tight blood pressure control and risk of macrovascular and microvascular complications in type 2 diabetes. UKPDS 38. UK Prospective Diabetes Study Group. BMJ. 1998;317(7160):703-13.
53. Klein R, Klein BEK, Moss SE, Davis MD, DeMets DL. The Wisconsin Epidemiology Study of Diabetic Retinopathy: V. Proteinuria and retinopathy in a population of diabetic persons diagnosed prior to 30 years of age. In: Friedman EA L'Esperance FA (Eds). Diabetic Renal-Retinal Syndrome 3. Orlando: Grune & Stratton, Orlando; 1986.
54. Sinclair SH, Grunwald JE, Riva CE, Braunstein SN, Nichols CW, Schwartz SS. Retinal vascular autoregulation in diabetes mellitus. Ophthalmology. 1982;89(7):748-50.
55. Effect of pregnancy on microvascular complications in the diabetes control and complications trial. The Diabetes Control and Complications Trial Research Group. Diabetes Care. 2000;23(8):1084-91.
56. Effects of aspirin treatment on diabetic retinopathy. ETDRS report number 8. Early Treatment Diabetic Retinopathy Study Research Group. Ophthalmology. 1991;98:757-65.
57. Davis MD, Fisher MR, Gangnon RE, Barton F, Aiello LM, Chew EY, et al. Risk factors for high-risk proliferative diabetic retinopathy and severe visual loss: Early Treatment Diabetic Retinopathy Study Report #18. Invest Ophthalmol Vis Sci. 1998;39(2):233-52.
58. Larsson LI, Alm A, Lithner F, Dahlén G, Bergström R. The association of hyperlipidemia with retinopathy in diabetic patients aged 15–50 years in the county of Umea. Acta Ophthalmol Scand. 1999;77(5):585-91.
59. Klein BE, Moss SE, Klein R, Surawicz TS. The Wisconsin Epidemiologic Study of Diabetic Retinopathy. XIII. Relationship of serum cholesterol to retinopathy and hard exudate. Ophthalmology. 1991;98(8):1261-5.
60. Action to Control Cardiovascular Risk in Diabetes Study Group; Gerstein HC, Miller ME, Byington RP, Goff DC Jr, Bigger JT, Buse JB, et al. Effects of intensive glucose lowering in type 2 diabetes. N Engl J Med. 2008;358(24):2545-59.
61. Techniques for scatter and local photocoagulation treatment of diabetic retinopathy: Early Treatment Diabetic Retinopathy Study report number 3. Early Treatment Diabetic Retinopathy Study Research Group. Int Ophthalmol Clin. 1987;27(4):254-64.
62. Diabetic Retinopathy Clinical Research Network. A randomized trial comparing intravitreal triamcinolone acetonide and focal/grid photocoagulation for diabetic macular edema. Ophthalmology. 2008;115(9):1447-9.
63. Beck RW, Edwards AR, Aiello LP, Bressler NM, Ferris F, Glassman AR, et al. Three-year follow-up of a randomized trial comparing focal/grid photocoagulation and intravitreal triamcinolone for diabetic macular edema. Arch Ophthalmol. 2009;127(3):245-51.

64. Nguyen QD, Shah SM, Khwaja AA, Channa R, Hatef E, Do DV, et al. Two-year outcomes of the ranibizumab for edema of the macula in diabetes (READ-2) study. Ophthalmology. 2010;117(11):2146-51.
65. Fong DS, Strauber SF, Aiello LP, Beck RW, Callanan DG, Danis RP, et al. Comparison of the modified Early Treatment Diabetic Retinopathy Study and mild macular grid laser photocoagulation strategies for diabetic macular edema. Arch Ophthalmol. 2007;125(4):469-80.
66. Guyer DR, D'Amico DJ, Smith CW. Subretinal fibrosis after laser photocoagulation for diabetic macular edema. Am J Ophthalmol. 1992;113(6):652-6.
67. Luttrull JK, Dorin G. Subthreshold diode micropulse laser photocoagulation (SDM) as invisible retinal phototherapy for diabetic macular edema: a review. Curr Diabetes Rev. 2012;8(4):274-84.
68. Cilley JC, Barfi K, Benson AB 3rd, Mulcahy MF. Bevacizumab in the treatment of colorectal cancer. Expert Opin Biol Ther. 2007;7(5):739-49.
69. Wells JA, Glassman AR, Ayala AR, Jampol LM, Aiello LP, Antoszyk AN, et al. Aflibercept, bevacizumab, or ranibizumab for diabetic macular edema. N Engl J Med. 2015;372(13):1193-203.
70. Mitchell P, Bandello F, Schmidt-Erfurth U, Lang GE, Massin P, Schlingemann RO, et al. The RESTORE Study: Ranibizumab Monotherapy or Combined with Laser versus Laser Monotherapy for Diabetic Macular Edema. Ophthalmology. 2011;118(4):615-25.
71. Schmidt-Erfurth U, Lang GE, Holz FG, Schlingemann RO, Lanzetta P, Massin P, et al. Three-year outcomes of individualized ranibizumab treatment in patients with diabetic macular edema: the RESTORE extension study. Ophthalmology. 2014;121(5):1045-53.
72. Elman MJ, Ayala A, Bressler NM, Browning D, Flaxel CJ, Glassman AR, et al. Intravitreal ranibizumab for diabetic macular edema with prompt versus deferred laser treatment: 5-year randomized trial results. Ophthalmology. 2015;122(2): 375-81.
73. Brown DM, Schmidt-Erfurth U, Do DV, Holz FG, Boyer DS, Midena E, et al. Intravitreal aflibercept for diabetic macular edema: 100-week results from the VISTA and VIVID studies. Ophthalmology. 2015;122(10):2044-52.
74. Lau PE, Jenkins KS, Layton CJ. Current Evidence for the Prevention of Endophthalmitis in Anti-VEGF Intravitreal Injections. J Ophthalmol. 2018;2018:8567912.
75. Das S, Lai T, Liu S, Lam D. The Rate of Endophthalmitis After Intravitreal Injections. Asia Pac J Ophthalmol (Phila). 2016;5(2):165-6.
76. Sohn HJ, Han DH, Kim IT, Oh IK, Kim KH, Lee DY, et al. Changes in aqueous concentrations of various cytokines after intravitreal triamcinolone versus bevacizumab for diabetic macular edema. Am J Ophthalmol. 2011;152(4): 686-94.
77. Ip MS, Bressler SB, Antoszyk AN, Flaxel CJ, Kim JE, Friedman SM, et al. A randomized trial comparing intravitreal triamcinolone and focal/grid photocoagulation for diabetic macular edema: baseline features. Retina. 2008;28(7):919-30.
78. Callanan DG, Gupta S, Boyer DS, Ciulla TA, Singer MA, Kuppermann BD, et al. Dexamethasone intravitreal implant in combination with laser photocoagulation for the treatment of diffuse diabetic macular edema. Ophthalmology. 2013;120(9):1843-51.
79. Boyer DS, Faber D, Gupta S, Patel SS, Tabandeh H, Li XY, et al. Dexamethasone intravitreal implant for treatment of diabetic macular edema in vitrectomized patients. Retina. 2011;31(5):915-23.
80. Campochiaro PA, Brown DM, Pearson A, Ciulla T, Boyer D, Holz FG, et al. Long-term benefit of sustained-delivery fluocinolone acetonide vitreous inserts for diabetic macular edema. Ophthalmology. 2011;118(4):626-35.

81. Cunha-Vaz J, Ashton P, Iezzi R, Campochiaro P, Dugel PU, Holz FG, et al. Sustained delivery fluocinolone acetonide vitreous implants: long-term benefit in patients with chronic diabetic macular edema. Ophthalmology. 2014;121(10):1892-903.
82. Stefansson E. The therapeutic effects of retinal laser treatment and vitrectomy. A theory based on oxygen and vascular physiology. Acta Ophthalmol Scand. 2001;79(5):435-40.
83. Photocoagulation treatment of proliferative diabetic retinopathy. Clinical application of Diabetic Retinopathy Study (DRS) findings, DRS report number 8. The Diabetic Retinopathy Study Research Group. Ophthalmology. 1981;88(7):583-600.
84. The Diabetic Retinopathy Study Research Group. Indications for photocoagulation treatment of diabetic retinopathy: Diabetic Retinopathy Study report number 14. Int Ophthalmol Clin. 1987;27(4):239-53.
85. Four risk factors for severe visual loss in diabetic retinopathy: the third report from the Diabetic Retinopathy Study. Diabetic Retinopathy Study Research Group. Arch Ophthalmol. 1979;97(4):654-5.
86. Ferris F. Early photocoagulation in patients with either type I or type II diabetes. Trans Am Ophthalmol Soc. 1996;94:505-37.
87. Wade EC, Blankenship GW. The effect of short versus long exposure times of argon laser panretinal photocoagulation on proliferative diabetic retinopathy. Graefes Arch Clin Exp Ophthalmol. 1990;228(3):226-31.
88. Patel JI, Jenkins L, Benjamin L, Webber S. Dilated pupils and loss of accommodation following diode panretinal photocoagulation with sub-tenon local anaesthetic in four cases. Eye (Lond). 2002;16(5):628-32.
89. Writing Committee for the Diabetic Retinopathy Clinical Research Network; Gross JG, Glassman AR, Jampol LM, Inusah S, Aiello LP, Antoszyk AN, et al. Panretinal photocoagulation vs intravitreous ranibizumab for proliferative diabetic retinopathy: A randomized clinical trial. JAMA. 2015;314(20):2137-46.
90. Gross JG, Glassman AR, Liu D, Sun JK, Antoszyk AN, Baker CW, et al. Five-Year Outcomes of Panretinal Photocoagulation vs Intravitreous Ranibizumab for Proliferative Diabetic Retinopathy: A Randomized Clinical Trial. JAMA Ophthalmol. 2018;136(10):1138-48.
91. Arevalo JF, Maia M, Flynn HW Jr, Saravia M, Avery RL, Wu L, et al. Tractional retinal detachment following intravitreal bevacizumab (Avastin) in patients with severe proliferative diabetic retinopathy. Br J Ophthalmol. 2008;92(2):213-6.
92. Wykoff CC, Eichenbaum DA, Roth DB, Hill L, Fung AE, Haskova Z. Ranibizumab Induces Regression of Diabetic Retinopathy in Most Patients at High Risk of Progression to Proliferative Diabetic Retinopathy. Ophthalmol Retina. 2018;2(10):997-1009.
93. Early vitrectomy for severe vitreous hemorrhage in diabetic retinopathy. Two-year results of a randomized trial. Diabetic Retinopathy Vitrectomy Study report 2. The Diabetic Retinopathy Vitrectomy Study Research Group. Arch Ophthalmol. 1985;103(11):1644-52.
94. Recchia FM, Scott IU, Brown GC, Brown MM, Ho AC, Ip MS. Small-gauge pars plana vitrectomy: a report by the American Academy of Ophthalmology. Ophthalmology. 2010;117(9):1851-7.
95. Ho T, Smiddy WE, Flynn HW Jr. Vitrectomy in the management of diabetic eye disease. Surv Ophthalmol. 1992;37(3):190-202.
96. Flynn HW Jr, Chew EY, Simons BD, Barton FB, Remaley NA, Ferris FL 3rd. Pars plana vitrectomy in the Early Treatment Diabetic Retinopathy Study. ETDRS report number 17. The Early Treatment Diabetic Retinopathy Study Research Group. Ophthalmology. 1992;99(9):1351-7.
97. Thompson JT, de Bustros S, Michels RG, Rice TA, Glaser BM. Results of vitrectomy for proliferative diabetic retinopathy. Ophthalmology. 1986;93(12):1571-4.

98. Joussen AM, Joeres S. Benefits and limitations in vitreoretinal surgery for proliferative diabetic Retinopathy and macular edema. Dev Ophthalmol. 2007;39:69-87.
99. Two-year course of visual acuity in severe proliferative diabetic retinopathy with conventional management. Diabetic Retinopathy Vitrectomy Study (DRVS) report #1. Ophthalmology.1985;92(4):492-502.
100. Yang CM, Su PY, Yeh PT, Chen MS. Combined rhegmatogenous and traction retinal detachment in proliferative diabetic retinopathy: clinical manifestations and surgical outcome. Can J Ophthalmol. 2008;43(2):192-8.
101. Douglas MJ, Scott IU, Flynn HW Jr. Pars plana lensectomy, pars plana vitrectomy, and silicone oil tamponade as initial management of cataract and combined traction/rhegmatogenous retinal detachment involving the macula associated with severe proliferative diabetic retinopathy. Ophthalmic Surg Lasers Imaging. 2003;34(4): 270-8.
102. Favard C, Guyot-Argenton C, Assouline M, Marie-Lescure C, Pouliquen YJ. Full panretinal photocoagulation and early Vitrectomy improve prognosis of florid diabetic retinopathy. Ophthalmology. 1996;103(4):561-74.
103. Ulbig MR, Hykin PG, Foss AJ, Schwartz SD, Hamilton PA. Anterior hyaloidal fibrovascular proliferation after extracapsular cataract extraction in diabetic eyes. Am J Ophthalmol.1993;115(3):321-6.
104. Ramsay RC, Knobloch WH, Cantrill HL. Timing of vitrectomy for active proliferative diabetic retinopathy. Ophthalmology. 1986;93(3):283-9.
105. O'Hanley GP, Canny CL. Diabetic dense premacular hemorrhage. A possible indication for prompt vitrectomy. Ophthalmology. 1985;92(4):507-11.
106. Davis MD, Blodi BA. Proliferative diabetic retinopathy. In: Ryan SJ (Ed). Retina. St Louis: Mosby; 2001. pp. 1309-49.
107. Mori K, Gehlbach PL, Sano A, Deguchi T, Yoneya S. Comparison of epiretinal membranes of differing pathogenesis using optical coherence tomography. Retina. 2004;24(1):57-62.
108. Bovey EH, Uffer S, Achache F. Surgery for epimacular membrane: impact of retinal internal limiting membrane removal on functional outcome. Retina. 2004;24(5):728-35.
109. Faulborn J, Bowald S. Microproliferations in proliferative diabetic retinopathy and their relationship to the vitreous: Corresponding light and electron microscopic studies. Graefes Arch Clin Exp Ophthalmol. 1985;223(3):130-8.
110. Eliott D. Vitreoretinal Attachments in Proliferative Diabetic Retinopathy: Effect on Outcome. Vail Vitrectomy Meeting Vail. 2004.
111. Sebag J. Anomalous posterior vitreous detachment: a unifying concept in vitreo-retinal disease. Graefes Arch Clin Exp Ophthalmol. 2004;242(8):690-8.
112. Chu TG, Lopez PF, Cano MR, Freeman WR, Lean JS, Liggett PE, Thomas EL, Green RL. Posterior vitreoschisis: an echographic finding in proliferative diabetic retinopathy. Ophthalmology. 1996;103(2):315-22.
113. Schwatz SD, Alexander R, Hiscott P, Gregor ZJ. Recognition of vitreoschisis in proliferative diabetic retinopathy: a useful landmark in vitrectomy for diabetic traction retinal detachment. Ophthalmology. 1996;103(2):323-8.
114. Eliott D, Lee MS, Abrams GW. Proliferative diabetic retinopathy: Principles and techniques of surgical treatment. In: Ryan SJ (Ed). Retina. Amsterdam, The Netherlands: Elsevier Inc.; 2006. pp. 2413-49.
115. Heimann H. Primary 25- and 23-gauge vitrectomy in the treatment of rhegmatogenous retinal detachment-advancement of surgical technique or erroneous trend? Klin M Augenheilkd. 2008;225(11):947-56.
116. Flynn HW Jr, Davis JL, Parel JM, Lee WG. Applications of a cannulated extrusion needle during vitreoretinal microsurgery. Retina. 1988;8(1):42-9.

117. Charles S, Chang S, McCuen BW. New techniques for hemostasis during diabetic vitrectomy. Retina. 2003;23(1):120-2.
118. Oshima Y, Shima C, Wakabayashi T, Kusaka S, Shiraga F, Ohji M, et al. Microincision vitrectomy surgery and intravitreal bevacizumab as a surgical adjunct to treat diabetic traction retinal detachment. Ophthalmology. 2009;116(5):927-38.
119. Sonoda KH, Sakamoto T, Enaida H, Miyazaki M, Noda Y, Nakamura T, et al. Residual vitreous cortex after surgical posterior vitreous separation visualized by intravitreous triamcinolone acetonide. Ophthalmology. 2004;111(2):226-30.
120. Kakehashi A. Total en bloc excision: a modified vitrectomy technique for proliferative diabetic retinopathy. Am J Ophthalmol. 2002;134(5):763-5.
121. Sharma T, Fong A, Lai TY, Lee V, Das S, Lam D. Surgical treatment for diabetic vitreoretinal diseases: a review. Clin Exp Ophthalmol. 2016;44(4):340-54.
122. el Annan J, Carvounis PE. Current management of vitreous hemorrhage due to proliferative diabetic retinopathy. Int Ophthalmol Clin. 2014;54(2):141-53.
123. Goto A, Inatani M, Inoue T, Awai-Kasaoka N, Takihara Y, Ito Y, et al. Frequency and risk factors for neovascular glaucoma after vitrectomy in eyes with proliferative diabetic retinopathy. J Glaucoma. 2013;22(7):572-6.

CHAPTER 12

Current Trends in the Management of Neovascular Age-related Macular Degeneration

Giridhar Anantharaman, Kiran Chandran, Akanksha Rai

ABSTRACT

Neovascular age-related macular degeneration (NVAMD) is an important cause of visual morbidity in persons above the age of 50 years. It is characterized by the presence of choroidal neovascularization (CNV) which results in leakage of fluid and blood that accumulates in the intraretinal, subretinal, and subretinal pigment epithelium space. Over the last 2 decades, there have been significant advances in the management of NVAMD especially with development of intravitreal antivascular endothelial growth factor (anti-VEGF) therapy. This manuscript gives a complete overview of landmark trials and the current approaches to the treatment of NVAMD.

Keywords: Neovascular age-related macular degeneration, antivascular endothelial growth factor, clinical trials, pro-re-nata (PRN), treat and extend.

INTRODUCTION

Age-related macular degeneration (AMD or ARMD) is a leading cause of visual morbidity in the elderly populations, above the age of 50 years. The incidence of ARMD increases with increasing age. By 2050, the number of individuals affected by AMD is expected to reach 17.8 million.[1] Wet AMD otherwise called "neovascular age-related macular degeneration" accounts for 20% of all cases of AMD and can lead to significant visual loss if left untreated. It is characterized by CNV which leads to bleeding, fluid accumulation and finally fibrosis in the macula. The natural course of the disease is unfavorable and leads to significant central visual loss.

TIMELINE IN THE MANAGEMENT OF WET AGE-RELATED MACULAR DEGENERATION (FLOWCHART 1)

Between the years 70s and the 90s, the only treatment for selected cases of juxtafoveal and extrafoveal neovascular AMD was thermal laser photocoagulation based on the macular photocoagulation study.[2-6] There was no effective treatment for subfoveal NVAMD and these patients progressed

Flowchart 1: Timeline in the management of wet age-related macular degeneration.

```
┌─────────────────────────────────────┐
│   Thermal Laser Photocoagulation    │
│  For extrafoveal and juxtafoveal    │
│   classic choroidal neovascular     │
│              membrane               │
│               (1982)                │
└─────────────────────────────────────┘
                  ↓
┌─────────────────────────────────────┐
│            Verteporfin              │
│   For photodynamic therapy (PDT)    │
│               (1999)                │
└─────────────────────────────────────┘
                  ↓
┌─────────────────────────────────────┐
│             Pegaptanib              │
│   First approved anti-VEGF drug,    │
│          binds VEGF-165             │
│               (2004)                │
└─────────────────────────────────────┘
                  ↓
┌─────────────────────────────────────┐
│            Bevacizumab              │
│           Used off-label            │
│               (2005)                │
└─────────────────────────────────────┘
                  ↓
┌─────────────────────────────────────┐
│            Ranibizumab              │
│ First anti-VEGF against all         │
│         isoforms of VEGF            │
│               (2006)                │
└─────────────────────────────────────┘
                  ↓
┌─────────────────────────────────────┐
│             Aflibercept             │
│  Binds to VEGF-A, VEGF-B, and PGF   │
│               (2011)                │
└─────────────────────────────────────┘
                  ↓
┌─────────────────────────────────────┐
│            Brolucizumab             │
│   Single chain antibody fragment    │
│               (2019)                │
└─────────────────────────────────────┘
```

(PGF: placental growth factor; VEGF: vascular endothelial growth factor)

to irreversible central visual loss. In 1999, vertiporfin photodynamic therapy was the first Food and Drug Administration (FDA) approved treatment for subfoveal choroidal neovascular membrane. Based on the result of the TAP (Treatment of Age-related macular degeneration with Photodynamic therapy) trial which compared "photodynamic therapy" with sham treatment, the results showed a decrease in rate of vision loss although improvement in vision was uncommon.[7] The early 2000s marked the beginning of the revolutionary treatment of NVAMD with drugs that targeted vascular endothelial growth factor (VEGF) which plays a key role in both angiogenesis and vascular permeability.[8]

In 2004, pegaptanib sodium, a pegylated anti-VEGF-aptamer, designed to target the 165 isoforms of VEGF-A was approved by the FDA based on the results of the vision-1 trial (VEGF inhibitor study in ocular neovascularization) which showed that subjects receiving intravitreal 0.3 mg pegaptanib every 6 weeks for 1 year experienced approximately half the vision loss when compared to subjects receiving sham.[9]

Ranibizumab is a monoclonal antibody that works against all isoforms of VEGF-A and this was approved in 2006 based on the results of two pivotal studies. This was administered in a dose of 0.3 mg/0.5 mg at monthly intervals in the MARINA and ANCHOR trials.[10-12]

Bevacizumab is a recombinant humanized monoclonal immunoglobulin G (IgG)-1 antibody against all isoforms of VEGF-A and is an off-label drug used extensively in the treatment of neovascular AMD at a dose of 1.25 mg in 0.05 mL. It was first used as an off-label drug in two patients with treatment naïve NVAMD in May 2005.[13]

Aflibercept is a recombinant protein created by fusing the second immunoglobulin domain of human VEGF receptor 1 with a third domain of human VEGF receptor 2 which in turn is fixed to the constant region of human IgG-1[14-17] **(Table 1)**.

Brolucizumab (formerly ESBA1008 and RTH258), a newly developed anti-VEGF molecule for NVAMD treatment, has shown longer duration of action and improvement in visual acuity (VA) and favorable anatomical outcomes in two randomized trials. Brolucizumab is a humanized single chain variable fragment antibody with a molecular mass of approximately 26 kDa. Nd preclinical studies have shown that brolucizumab due to its small size readily penetrates the retinal layers to reach the retinal pigment epithelium (RPE) and choroid with minimal systemic concentration. Single chain antibody fragments are the smallest functional unit of an antibody and allow delivery of a greater molar dose compared to larger molecule and so it has the potential for more effective tissue penetration. Preclinical trial data have demonstrated 2.2- and 1.7-folds higher exposure in the retina and RPE, respectively and therefore, it has more potential to control intraretinal fluid, subretinal fluid, and sub-RPE fluid than compared to ranibizumab.[18,19]

TABLE 1: Antivascular endothelial growth factor drugs used for treatment of neovascular age-related macular degeneration.

Drug	Dosage	Molecular weight (kDa)*	Frequency
Pegaptanib	0.3 mg	50	Monthly
Ranibizumab	0.5 mg	48	Monthly
Bevacizumab	1.25 mg	149	Monthly
Aflibercept	2 mg	115	Bimonthly
Brolicizumab	6 mg	26	Quarterly

*kDa: kilodalton

TREATMENT REGIMEN FOR NEOVASCULAR AGE-RELATED MACULAR DEGENERATION USING ANTIVASCULAR ENDOTHELIAL GROWTH FACTOR MONOTHERAPY

The treatment of NVAMD is based on the results of the various randomized trials. Based on current evidence, there are two phases in the management of a treatment naïve patient with NVAMD.

1. *Induction phase*: The induction phase involves monthly injection of anti-VEGF drug that is guided by serial spectral domain optical coherence tomography (SD-OCT) at each visit. Intravitreal injections are continued till the macula is dry on SD-OCT. This is otherwise described as the initial loading dose.
2. *Maintenance phase*: Once the macula is dry on SD-OCT, the patient enters the maintenance phase. Based on current evidence, treatment during the maintenance plan could be:
   - Fixed intervals (monthly, bimonthly, or quarterly)
   - Pro-pre-nata treatment
   - Treat and extend

It will be of great interest to dwell on each of these treatment strategies with a summary of the important landmark clinical trials. **Table 2** gives a short overview of the important randomized trials.

Anti-VEGF injection is given at regularly spaced fixed or in discontinuous treatment regimens. The aim and objective of treatment is to titrate the need for injections without sacrificing on visual outcome.

Fixed Intervals

- *Monthly and bimonthly*: Some of the landmark clinical trials that transformed the management of NVAMD are:
  - *Minimally classic/occult trial of tanibizumab in the treatment of neovascular AMD (MARINA)*: The MARINA trial was a 2-year, multicenter, prospective, double-blind trial in which 716 subjects with nAMD with non-classical CNV were randomized to receive sham injections (n = 238), 0.3 mg ranibizumab (n = 238) or 0.5 mg ranibizumab (n = 240) injections every 4 weeks for a total of 2 years. The primary endpoint analysis assessed the superiority of ranibizumab versus sham control at 12 months with respect to the proportion of subjects losing <15 early treatment of diabetic retinopathy study (ETDRS) letters of best-corrected visual acuity (BCVA). At 12 months, 95% of the 0.5 mg ranibizumab group (ultimately approved dose) lost <15 ETDRS letters, compared with 62% in the untreated control group. Most importantly, MARINA was one of the two pivotal trials that marked the beginning of vision-improving anti-VEGF therapy; at 12 months, the mean BCVA increased 7.2 ETDRS letters from baseline in the 0.5 mg ranibizumab group, whereas

TABLE 2: Summary of landmark clinical trials in neovascular age-related macular degeneration.

Study	Duration (years)	Patient details	Type of CNV/Regimen	Anti-VEGF	Conclusion
ANCHOR	2	N = 423 Age > 50 years	Predominantly classic subfoveal CNV; Q4	Ranibizumab vs. PDT	Ranibizumab provided greater clinical benefit than verteporfin PDT.
MARINA	2	N = 716 Age > 50 years	Minimally classic or occult CNV; Q4	Ranibizumab vs. Sham	Intravitreal ranibizumab for 2 years prevented vision loss and improved mean VA with low rate of serious adverse effects.
PIER	2	N = 184 Age > 50 years	Subfoveal CNV of all subtypes; Q12	Ranibizumab	Quarterly ranibizumab inferior to monthly injection.
PrONTO	2	N = 40 Age > 50 years	Subfoveal CNV; Q4 for 3 months, followed by PRN	Ranibizumab	Comparable visual outcomes from phase III clinical studies, but fewer intravitreal injections were required.
VIEW1/VIEW2	2	N = 2419 Age > 50 years	Subfoveal CNV; Q4, Q8	Aflibercept vs. Ranibizumab	VA improvements achieved at week 52 were largely maintained through week 96 with both aflibercept and ranibizumab.
HARBOR	2	N = 1098 Age > 50 years	Subfoveal CNV; Q4, PRN	Ranibizumab 0.5 mg and 2 mg	• Patients in the less than monthly dosing arm maintained good VA gains through month 12 and 24. • 2 mg dose of ranibizumab was not significantly more effective than a 0.5-mg dose.
CATT	2; with recall at 5 years	N = 1185 Age > 50 years	Subfoveal CNV; Q4, PRN	Ranibizumab Bevacizumab	• Both ranibizumab and bevacizumab had similar effects of VA over a 2-year period. • PRN resulted in less gain in VA.

(ANCHOR: ??; CATT: comparisons of Age-related Macular Degeneration Treatments Trials; CNV: choroidal neovascularization; N: number of patients enrolled; MARINA: minimally classic/occult trial of ranibizumab in the treatment of neovascular AMD; PDT: photodynamic therapy; PRN: pro-re-nata; Q4: quarterly; Q8: bimonthly; Q12: monthly; VA: visual acuity) the sham injection group lost 10.4 ETDRS letters ($P < 0.0001$). MARINA demonstrated that monthly 0.5 mg dosing was an effective strategy to improve BCVA in subjects with nAMD with nonclassical neovascularization. In addition, MARINA, which was conducted in 2003, was the last major anti-VEGF registration trial in wet AMD to employ sham control.[10]

- *ANCHOR*: The 2-year, phase III multicenter, randomized, double-masked trial designated for the treatment of predominantly classic CNV in age-related macular degeneration (ANCHOR).

  During the 1st year of the 2 years multicenter study, patients were randomly assigned in a 1:1:1 ratio to receive monthly intravitreal injections of ranibizumab (0.3 mg or 0.5 mg) plus sham verteporfin therapy or monthly sham injections plus active verteporfin therapy. The primary endpoint was the proportion of patients losing fewer than 15 letters from base time VA at 12 months. Of the 423 patients enrolled, 94.3–96.4% of patients who received ranibizumab lost fewer than 15 letters as compared to 64.3% of those in the verteporfin group. Improvement in VA by 15 letters or more was seen in 35.7–40.3% of eyes which received ranibizumab as compared to only 5.6% of the vertiporfin group. Mean VA increased by 8.5–11.3 letters in the ranibizumab group as compared with a decrease of 9.5 letters in the verteporfin group. Ranibizumab was found to be superior to verteporfin photodynamic therapy in the treatment of wet NVAMD and for the first time there was a drug that could improve VA in the treatment of NVAMD.[11,12]

- *VIEW trials:* The VIEW-1 and VIEW-2 are two landmark clinical trials. They are important for the following reasons:
  - They enrolled one of the largest numbers of patients in any randomized trial evaluating the use of anti-VEGF therapy in NVAMD.
  - They are one of the earliest trials that looked into a modified treat-and-extend regimen in the management of NVAMD. The view trials have three parts.
    - *Part 1*: During year-1, 2,419 patients with active subfoveal NVAMD were randomized to intravitreal aflibercept 0.5 mg monthly, 2 mg monthly, 2 mg every 8 weeks after initial three loading doses and ranibizumab 0.5 mg monthly. Ranibizumab also was given as an initial loading dose regimen followed by monthly treatment. The primary endpoint was noninferiority of the aflibercept regimen to ranibizumab at the end of 1 year (losing <15 letters on ETDRS chart). All the aflibercept groups were noninferior to monthly ranibizumab at 1 year.[14]
    - *Part 2*: From 52 to 96 weeks, patients received the original dosing regimen using an as-needed treatment with defined retreatment

criteria and mandatory dosing at 12 weeks. They were therefore treated on a PRN basis with a cap at 12 weeks. All the aflibercept and ranibizumab arms were equally effective in improving BCVA and preventing best corrected visual loss at 96 weeks. The 2 mg Q 8-weekly aflibercept arm had five fewer injections through 96 weeks when compared to ranibizumab arm.[15,16]

- *Part 3*: The third part of the View trial is the extension study after completing 24 months of the trial. Here, 323 patients from the VIEW-1 trial who had completed 96 weeks were enrolled in an extension study through week 212 and received an as-needed treatment with a cap at 12 weeks when they received an injection irrespective of the findings in SD-OCT. The visual results of VIEW extension trial showed that the VA results in the VIEW-1 trial were maintained in the extension study. Mean number of injections was 12.9 in the extension study.[17]

Summarizing the results of the VIEW trials:
- Aflibercept was found to be noninferior to ranibizumab in the management of NVAMD.
- Aflibercept was noninferior to ranibizumab in a modified treat-and-extend regimen requiring less numbers of injections across 56 weeks to 212 weeks.

- *Quarterly:*
  - *PIER 1*: Phase III-b, multicenter, randomized, double-masked, sham injection-controlled trial to evaluate the efficacy and safety of ranibizumab administered monthly for 3 months and then quarterly in patients with subfoveal CNV secondary to AMD.
  Patients were randomized 1:1:1 to 0.3 mg ranibizumab, 0.5 mg ranibizumab, or sham treatment groups. The primary efficacy endpoint was mean change from baseline VA at month 12.
  Mean changes from baseline VA at 12 months were –16.3, –1.6, and –0.2 letters for the sham, 0.3 mg, and 0.5 mg groups, respectively. However, the treatment effect declined in the ranibizumab groups during quarterly dosing (e.g., at 3 months the mean changes from baseline VA had been gains of 2.9 and 4.3 letters for the 0.3 mg and 0.5 mg doses, respectively). Results of subgroups analyses of mean change from baseline VA at 12 months by baseline age, VA, and lesion characteristics were consistent with the overall results. Conclusion was the visual outcome of ranibizumab administered quarterly is far inferior when compared to monthly injection in the pivotal MARINA and ANCHOR trials.[20]
  - *EXCITE*: A 12-month, multicenter, randomized, double-masked, active-controlled, phase III-b study to demonstrate noninferiority of a quarterly treatment regimen to a monthly regimen of ranibizumab in patients with subfoveal CNV secondary to AMD. Participants

were patients with primary or recurrent subfoveal CNV secondary to AMD, with predominantly classic, minimally classic, or occult (no classic component) lesions. Patients were randomized (1:1:1) to 0.3 mg quarterly, 0.5 mg quarterly, or 0.3 mg monthly doses of ranibizumab. Treatment comprised of a loading phase (3 consecutive monthly injections) followed by a 9-month maintenance phase (either monthly or quarterly injection). Main outcome measures were mean change in BCVA and central retinal thickness (CRT) from baseline to month 12 and the incidence of adverse events (AEs). At month 12, BCVA gain in the monthly regimen was higher than that of the quarterly regimens. The noninferiority of a quarterly regimen was not achieved with reference to 5.0 letters.[21]

Summary
The fixed dosing regimen could be monthly, bimonthly, or quarterly. Quarterly injection results in poorer visual outcome when compared to monthly or bimonthly treatment. The reason why the quarterly regimen was attempted is to see whether the same results as described in the pivotal studies could be achieved with lesser number of injection and less burden on patients.

Recent trials using quarterly dosing: The most recent trial looking into quarterly dosing is the Hawk and Harrier trial. The two 96 weeks multicenter phase 3 clinical trials compare the efficacy of brolucizumab 6 mg (Hawk and Harrier) and brolucizumab 3 mg (Hawk) versus 2 mg aflibercept in 1817 subjects with treatment of naïve NVAMD. In both these studies, there was a 3-month loading phase followed by dosing every 12 weeks for the brolucizumab group and 8 weekly for the aflibercept group. It is a known inferiority trial and at 2 years brolucizumab was noninferior to aflibercept. There was an improvement of 6.6 and 6.1 ETDRS letters in brolucizumab group when compared to 6.8 letters in the aflibercept group with reduced number of injections in the brolucizumab group. Therefore, brolucizumab at a dosage of 6 mg is the recently approved anti-VEGF drug with a prolonged duration of action of up to 12 weeks.[18,19]

Pro-re-nata Treatment

Pro-re-nata is a Latin phrase commonly used in medicine to mean "as needed" or "as the situation arises". Therefore, by PRN treatment what we mean is after the initial induction phase we follow-up the patient on a monthly interval and treat as needed based on VA and SD-OCT. **Figures 1 and 2** describe a representative case managed on a PRN-based treatment.

Some of the important studies that looked into PRN treatment are:

PrONTO: Prospective optical coherence tomography (OCT) imaging of patients with NVAMD treated with intraocular ranibizumab (PrONTO) study

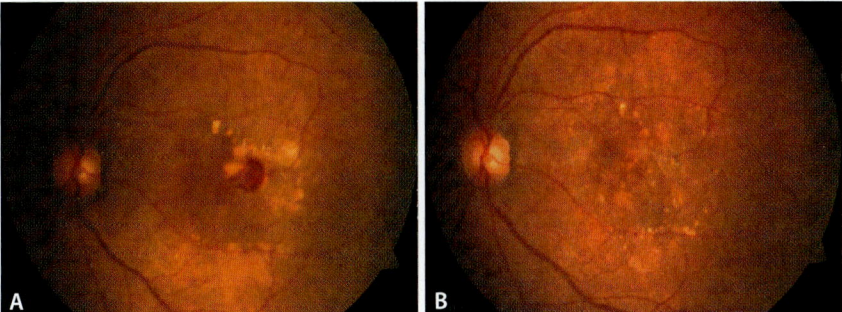

Figs. 1A and B: Color fundus photograph of the outer segment showing choroidal neovascular membrane with subretinal heme (A), prior to starting antivascular endothelial growth factor (anti-VEGF) treatment. Fundus photograph showing complete resolution of subretinal heme after four anti-VEGF injection's during the pro-re-nata treatment (B).

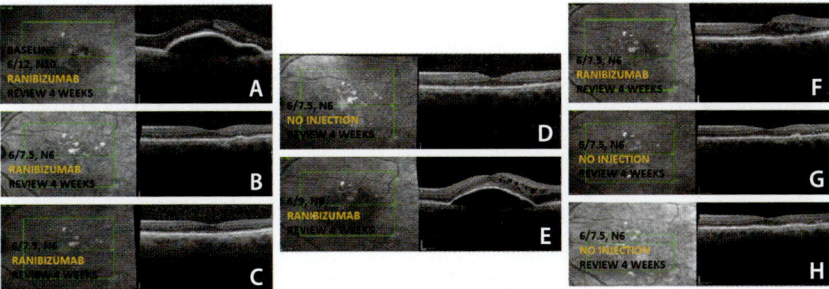

Figs. 2A to H: This illustration demonstrates a pro-re-nata injection protocol in which the patient was given an initial 3-month loading dose of intravitreal antivascular endothelial growth factor (anti-VEGF) injection and subsequent treatment was given only in case of instability (intra- or subretinal fluid) on the basis of 4-weekly assessment on spectral domain optical coherence tomography (SD-OCT). The baseline OCT (A) shows a notched fibrovascular pigment epithelial detachment (PED) with intraretinal fluid (IRF), confirming the diagnosis of neovascular age-related macular degeneration. Three loading doses of anti-VEGF injection were given monthly (A to C). At the end of 3 months, the macula sections were dry. Hence, no intravitreal injection was given (D) and the patient was asked to follow-up 1 month later. SD-OCT done next visit showed a PED with pockets of IRF (E) due to which another dose of anti-VEGF was administered. In the subsequent follow-up (F), the PED had collapsed, but there was persisting IRF and, hence, anti-VEGF injection was given. In the final two follow-ups (G and H), no injection was administered as there was no fluid on OCT sections.

assessed the long-term efficacy of a variable dosing regimen of ranibizumab. It was a 2-year prospective, single center, uncontrolled, variable-dosing regimen with intravitreal ranibizumab based on OCT findings. Treatment-naïve wet AMD patients with neovascularization involving the central fovea and CRT of at least 300 μm measured by OCT were enrolled to receive three consecutive monthly intravitreal injections of ranibizumab (0.5 mg). During the 1st year, retreatment with ranibizumab was performed at each monthly visit if any criterion was fulfilled.[22]

Criteria for reinjection after three loading doses in PrONTO study (1st year):
- Decrease of 5 letters of VA (ETDRS) and fluid on OCT
- Increase of 100 μ in CRT on OCT
- Macular hemorrhage
- Classic CNV in emerging FA
- Persistent fluid on OCT 1 month after the last injection

During the 2nd year, the retreatment criterion was any qualitative increase in the amount of fluid detected using OCT. Forty patients were enrolled and 37 completed the 2-year study. At month 24, the mean VA improved by 11.1 letters ($P < 0.001$) and the OCT-CRT decreased by 212 μm ($P < 0.001$). VA improved by 15 letters or more in 43% of patients. These VA and OCT outcomes were achieved with an average of 9.9 injections over 24 months. The PrONTO study using an OCT-guided variable-dosing regimen with intravitreal ranibizumab resulted in VA outcomes comparable with the outcomes from the phase III clinical studies, but with fewer intravitreal injections.

These BCVA results obtained compare favorably with ANCHOR and MARINA, in which more injections were administered, but PrONTO was a small, single-center, uncontrolled, open-label study, and consequently the efficacy results must be interpreted in this context. Nevertheless, PrONTO is important because it supported the role for OCT-guided anti-VEGF treatment in wet AMD.

HARBOR: It was a 24-month, multicenter, randomized, double-masked, active treatment-controlled phase 3 trial to evaluate the 24-month efficacy and safety of intravitreal ranibizumab 0.5 mg and 2.0 mg administered monthly or as needed (PRN) in patients with NVAMD (wet AMD). Study population was >50 years of age with treatment-naïve subfoveal wet AMD, they were randomized to receive intravitreal injections of ranibizumab 0.5 mg or 2.0 mg monthly or PRN after 3 monthly loading doses. It was one of the first trials using SD-OCT to evaluate patients.

At month 24, results were the mean change from baseline in BCVA was (letters) +9.1 (0.5 mg monthly), +7.9 (0.5 mg PRN), +8.0 (2.0 mg monthly), and +7.6 (2.0 mg PRN). The change in mean BCVA from month 12 to 24 was (letters) −1.0, −0.3, −1.2, and −1.0, respectively. The proportion of patients who gained 15 letters from baseline in BCVA at month 24 was 34.5%, 33.1%, 37.6%, and 34.8%, respectively. The mean number of ranibizumab injections through month 24 was 21.4, 13.3, 21.6, and 11.2, respectively; 5.6 and 4.3 mean injections were required in year 2 in the 0.5 mg and 2.0 mg PRN groups, respectively. The average treatment interval in the 0.5 mg PRN group was 9.9 weeks after 3 monthly loading doses, and 93% of these patients did not require monthly dosing. Ocular and systemic safety profiles over 2 years were similar among all four treatment groups and were consistent with previous ranibizumab trials in AMD. Conclusion was at month 24, mean BCVA improvements were clinically meaningful and similar among all four ranibizumab treatment groups. The 0.5-mg PRN group achieved a mean gain of 7.9 letters at month 24 with an average of 13.3 injections (5.6 injections in year 2).[23]

Comparison of Age-related Macular Degeneration Treatments Trials (CATT): CATT trial in its 1st year was designed as a multi-center single blind noninferiority trial where 1,208 patients with NVAMD were randomly assigned to receive intravitreal injection of ranibizumab or bevacizumab on either a monthly or as "as-needed" schedule with monthly evaluation. The primary outcome was the mean change in VA at 1 year with a noninferiority limit of five letters on the ETDRS chart. In the second year (n = 1,107), patients initially enrolled to monthly treatment were reassigned randomly to monthly or as needed regimen without changing the drug. Patient exited the trial at 2 years and was recalled at 5 years.

Results

At 1 year, both bevacizumab and ranibizumab had equivalent effect on VA when administered both as a monthly treatment and also as "as-needed" treatment. The 5-year outcome of the CATT trial is important because it throws light on the long-term results of anti-VEGF therapy in wet AMD. At 5 years, the VA was obtained for 647 of 914 (71%) living patients with an average follow-up of 5.5 years. The mean number of examinations for AMD care after the clinical trial ended at 2 years was 25.3 and the mean number of the treatment was 15.4. At 5 years, 50% of the eyes had a VA of 20/40 or better. Geographic atrophy was present in 213 of 515 (41%) gradable eyes and was subfoveal in 85 eyes. On SD-OCT, 83% had fluid and therefore active disease.[24,25]

Conclusion

Based on the 1-year, 2-year, and 5-year data of the CATT trial, the bevacizumab was not found to be inferior to ranibizumab in terms of efficacy in the treatment of NVAMD. 50% of eyes with over 5-year follow-up retained a VA of 20/40 or better. Geographic atrophy is a long-term complication of NVAMD and can be seen in over 50% of the eyes over a period of 5 years. NVAMD is a chronic disease and requires long-term regular follow-up and appropriate regular treatment.

Summary

Various studies have evaluated and compared the PRN form of treatment with the fixed dosing monthly regimen. The results show that PRN treatment if followed meticulously can result in similar visual outcomes as compared to fixed dose monthly regimen with a reduced burden of injections. However, one of the drawbacks of the PRN treatment is that patients require regular monthly monitoring and monthly clinic visits.

Treat and Extend (Figs. 3 and 4)

What is treat-and-extend (TREX)? The TREX is another variable dosing regimen where the patient receives a loading dose regimen initially to dry the macula. Subsequently, the intervals are increased by 2–4 weeks depending

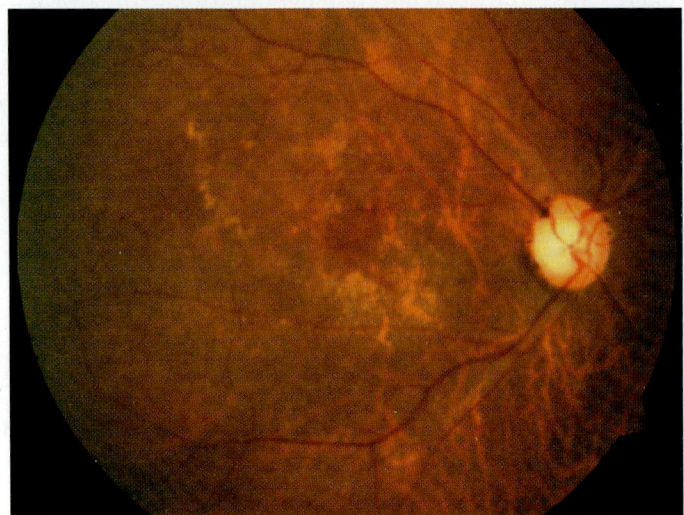

Fig. 3: Color fundus photograph of the right eye (OD) showing a small subretinal hemorrhage at the macula. Multiple drusen scattered in the macula along with a grayish-yellow membrane in the fovea are also seen.

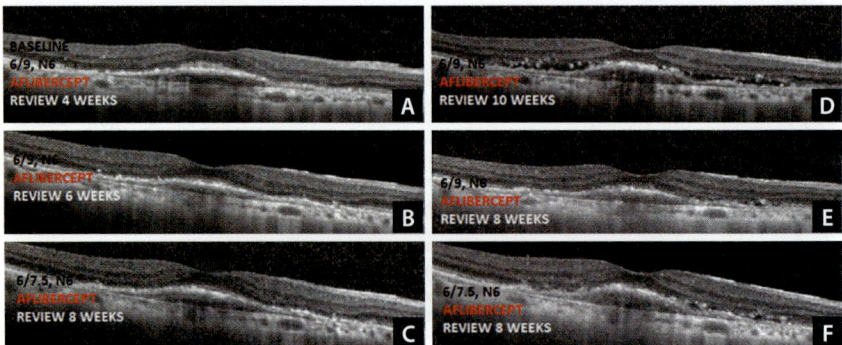

Figs. 4A to F: A representative case to describe the treat-and-extend protocol. (A) Shows a dry macula after the initial loading dose of aflibercept at 4-week intervals. (B and C) The next follow-up is extended to 6 weeks and the spectral domain-optical coherence tomography (SD-OCT) shows a dry macula. Therefore, the subsequent follow-up is extended by another 2 weeks and again the OCT and visual acuity is repeated and it shows that the visual acuity has improved and OCT is dry. Subsequently, the follow-up is extended to 10 weeks (D) when OCT shows reappearance of subretinal fluid. Therefore, the subsequent visit is shortened by 2–8 weeks and the visual acuity has improved and OCT shows a dry macula. The subsequent visit is kept at 8 weeks intervals (E and F).

on the discretion of the physician. As an example, the patient after the loading dose has his next examination 6 weeks after the previous examination and receives an injection irrespective of the findings in SD-OCT.

If the macula was dry in OCT, the next follow-up is increased by a further 2 weeks, i.e., 8 weeks from the time of the previous injection. At this visit, the patient receives an injection and if the macula is dry the next check-up is increased by a further 2 weeks. However, if the macula is found to have fluid, then he receives the injection and the next check-up is shortened by 2 weeks. In all the TREX trials, there is a cap on the maximum extension of follow-up and injection to 12 weeks. There are various trials which have evaluated the TREX regimen.

What are the advantages of the TREX regimen?
- It reduces the number of visits for patients to the clinic and this improves patient compliance. This is important considering that most patients are very old and find it difficult to visit clinics.
- It can help in sustaining the initial visual improvement as we are not waiting for the disease to manifest which results in decrease in VA.

What are the possible drawbacks of TREX regimen?
- There is a school of thought that this regimen may result in unnecessary over treatment of patients. Therefore, it is important for physicians to identify ideal patients for the TREX regimen. Patients who need intravitreal injections very frequently during the course of treatment in the first 12–18 months to maintain a dry macula are probably the ideal patients to be switched to TREX regimen.
- There are some reports that long-term use of anti-VEGF injection on a regular basis can result in geographical atrophy although we do not have enough evidence to conclude whether the geographical atrophy is secondary to the disease or the intervention. Long-term studies on anti-VEGF treatment for wet AMD have shown that nearly 50% of the eyes with 5–7 years of follow-up have some element of geographical atrophy.

A short summary of the various trials with TREX regimen is given here:
- *LUCAS*: Compared the efficacy and safety of bevacizumab versus ranibizumab when administered according to a TREX protocol for the treatment of NVAMD. It was a multicenter, randomized, noninferiority trial with a noninferiority limit of five letters. Participants were patients aged ≥50 years with previously untreated NVAMD in one eye and BCVA between 20/25 and 20/320. Patients were randomly assigned to receive ranibizumab 0.5 mg or bevacizumab 1.25 mg intravitreal injections. Monthly injections were given until inactive disease was achieved. The patients were then followed with a gradual extension of treatment interval by 2 weeks at a time up to a maximum of 12 weeks. If signs of recurrent disease appeared, the treatment interval was shortened by 2 weeks at a time.[26]

Main outcome measures change in VA at 1 year: Between March 2009 and July 2012, 441 patients were randomized at 10 ophthalmological centers in Norway. The 1-year visit was completed by 371 patients. In the per protocol analysis at 1 year, bevacizumab was equivalent to ranibizumab, with 7.9 and 8.2 mean letters gained, respectively [95% confidence interval (CI) of mean difference, –of mean diff$P = 0.845$]. The intention-to-treat analysis was concordant.

Conclusion

Bevacizumab and ranibizumab had equivalent effects on VA at 1 year when administered according to a TREX protocol. The VA results at 1 year were comparable to those of other clinical trials with monthly treatment.

- *TREX-AMD*: Prospectively assessed a TREX management strategy with monthly dosing of intravitreal ranibizumab in treatment-naïve NVAMD patients. It was a multicenter, randomized, controlled clinical trial.

    Sixty treatment-naïve NVAMD patients were randomized to 1:2 to monthly or TREX management. Patients with BCVA from 20/32 to 20/500 (Snellen equivalent) were randomized to receive intravitreal 0.5 mg ranibizumab monthly or according to a TREX protocol. The TREX patients were treated monthly for at least three doses, until resolution of clinical and SD-OCT evidence of exudative disease activity; the interval between visits then was individualized according to a strict prospective protocol. The main outcome measure was mean BCVA change from baseline. At baseline, mean BCVA was 20/60 (Snellen equivalent), and mean CRT was 511 μm. Fifty-seven eyes (95%) completed the study, at which point mean BCVA improved by 9.2 and 10.5 letters in the monthly and TREX cohorts, respectively ($P = 0.60$). The mean number of injections administered through month 12 was 13.0 and 10.1 (range, 7–13) in the monthly and TREX cohorts, respectively ($P < 0.0001$). Among TREX patients, 7 (18%) were maximally extended, 4 (10%) demonstrated fluid at every visit, and at month 12, 18 (45%) had achieved an extension interval of 8 weeks or more; the mean maximum extension interval between injections after the first 3 monthly doses was 8.4 weeks (range, 4–12 weeks). Most TREX patients who demonstrated recurrent exudative disease activity [17/24 (71%)] were unable to extend beyond their initial maximum extension interval. The TREX neovascular AMD management strategy used in this prospective, randomized, controlled trial resulted in visual and anatomic gains comparable with those obtained with monthly dosing. However, only 45% of the patient could achieve an extension of 8 weeks or more.[27,28]

- *TREND*: TReat and extEND (TREND) study evaluated the efficacy and safety of ranibizumab 0.5 mg in treat-and-extend (T&E) versus monthly regimens in patients with NVAMD). It is a 12-month VA assessor-masked, multicenter, randomized, interventional study. 650 treatment-naïve nAMD patients were randomized 1:1 to receive ranibizumab 0.5 mg either T&E or monthly regimen.

The primary objective was to show noninferiority of ranibizumab 0.5 mg T&E versus monthly regimen, as assessed by the change in best-corrected BCVA from baseline to the end of the study. Secondary objectives included change in retinal central subfield thickness (CSFT) from baseline to the end of study, treatment exposure, and safety. The T&E regimen was noninferior ($P < 0.001$) to the monthly regimen. In both treatment groups, most BCVA improvements occurred during the first 6 months and were maintained until the end of the study. This study found ranibizumab 0.5 mg administered according to a T&E regimen was statistically noninferior and clinically comparable with a monthly regimen in improving VA from baseline to the end of study.[29,30]

SUMMARY

Intravitreal anti-VEGF therapy has revolutionized the management of NVAMD. Currently, the diagnosis and management of NVAMD is based on clinical examination and SD-OCT. Fundus fluorescein angiography and indocyanine green angiography can be done once at the time of diagnosis to complete the work-up and identify the subtype of the NVAMD. Once a patient is diagnosed with neovascular AMD, following the loading dose of intravitreal anti-VEGF injection, the patient is examined ideally on monthly intervals with VA and SD-OCT. Further intravitreal injection is based on activity in SD-OCT and VA assessment. This is called the "pro-re-nata" form of treatment. TREX is a useful option to be considered in eyes that requires frequent injections in the 1st year of treatment. NVAMD is a chronic disease which requires long-term regular follow-up and appropriate treatment. With a compliant, patient and optimum treatment at least 50% of eyes maintain a VA of 20/40 or better after 5–7 years of treatment. Patient education should go hand in hand with clinical expertise. Low visual aid is a usual adjuvant to therapy especially in eyes with poor near visual function.

ACKNOWLEDGMENT

I would like to acknowledge the help and assistance of Mr Murukan Velayudhan, Administrative Officer and my Secretary in preparing this manuscript.

REFERENCES

1. Klein BEK, Klein R. Forecasting age-related macular degeneration through 2050. JAMA. 2009;301(20):2152-3.
2. Fine SL. Macular photocoagulation study. Arch Ophthalmol. 1980;98(5):832.
3. Laser photocoagulation for juxtafoveal choroidal neovascularization. Five-year results from randomized clinical trials. Macular Photocoagulation Study Group. Arch Ophthalmol. 1994;112(4):500-9.

4. Macular Photocoagulation Study Group. Argon laser photocoagulation for neovascular maculopathy after 5 years: results from randomized clinical trials. Arch Ophthalmol. 1991;109:1109-14.
5. Macular Photocoagulation Study Group. Argon laser photocoagulation for senile macular degeneration: results of a randomized clinical trial. Arch Ophthalmol. 1982;100:912-8.
6. Macular Photocoagulation Study Group. Laser photocoagulation of subfoveal neovascular lesions of age-related macular degeneration: updated findings from two clinical trials. Arch Ophthalmol. 1993;111:1200-9.
7. Treatment of Age-related Macular Degeneration with Photodynamic Therapy (TAP) Study Group. Photodynamic therapy of subfoveal choroidal neovascularization in age-related macular degeneration with verteporfin: one year results of 2 randomized clinical trials—TAP report No. 1. Arch Ophthalmol. 1999;117:1329-45.
8. Miller JW, Le Couter J, Strauss EC, Ferrara N. Vascular endothelial growth factor A in intraocular vascular disease. Ophthalmology. 2013;120:106-14.
9. Gragoudas ES, Adamis AP, Cunningham ET, Feinsod M, Guyer DR; VEGF Inhibition Study in Ocular Neovascularization Clinical Trial Group. Pegatanib for neovascular age-related macular degeneration. N Engl J Med. 2004;351:2805-16.
10. Rosenfeld PJ, Brown DM, Heier JS, Boyer DS, Kaiser PK, Chung CY, et al. Ranibizumab for neovascular age-related macular degeneration. N Engl J Med. 2006;355:1419-31.
11. Brown DM, Michels M, Kaiser PK, Heier JS, Sy JP, Ianchulev T, et al. Ranibizumab versus verteporfin photodynamic therapy for neovascular age-related macular degeneration: two-year results of the anchor study. Ophthalmology. 2009;116:57-65.
12. Kaiser PK, Brown DM, Zhang K, Hudson HL, Holz FG, Shapiro H, et al. Ranibizumab for predominantly classic neovascular age-related macular degeneration: subgroup analysis of first-year anchor results. Am J Ophthalmol. 2007;144:850-7.
13. Rosenfeld PJ. Lessons learned from Avastin and OCT-The Great, the Good, the Bad, and the Ugly: The LXXV Edward Jackson Memorial Lecture. Am J Ophthalmol. 2019;204:26-45.
14. Schmidt-Erfurth U, Chong V, Kirchof B, Korobelnik JF, Papp A, Anderesi M, et al. Primary results of an international phase III study using intravitreal VEGF trap-eye compared to ranibizumab in patients with wet AMD (VIEW 2). Invest Ophthalmol Vis Sci. 2011;52:1650.
15. Schmidt-Erfurth U, Kaiser PK, Korobelnik JF, Brown DM, Chong V, Nguyen QD, et al. Intravitreal aflibercept injection for neovascular age-related macular degeneration: ninety-six–week results of the VIEW studies. Ophthalmology. 2014;121:193-201.
16. Heier JS, Brown DM, Chong V, Korobelnik JF, Kaiser PK, Nguyen QD, et al. Intravitreal aflibercept (VEGF trap-eye) in wet age-related macular degeneration. Ophthalmology. 2012;119(12):2537-48.
17. Kaiser PK, Singer S, Tolentino M, Vitti R, Erickson K, Saroj N, et al. Long-term safety and visual outcome of intravitreal aflibercept in neovascular age-related macular degeneration. VIEW 1 Extension Study. Ophthalmol Retina. 2017;1:304-13.
18. Dugel PU, Koh A, Ogura Y, Jaffe GJ, Schmidt-Erfurth U, Brown DM, et al. HAWK and HARRIER: Phase 3, multicenter, randomized, double-masked trials of brolucizumab for neovascular age-related macular degeneration. Ophthalmology. 2020;127:72-84.
19. Dugel PU, Singh RP, Koh A, Ogura Y, Weissgerber G, Gedif K, et al. HAWK and HARRIER 96-week outcomes from the phase 3 trials of brolucizumab for neovascular age-related macular degeneration. Ophthalmology. 2021;128(1):89-99.
20. Regillo CD, Brown DM, Abraham P, Yue H, Ianchulev T, Schneider S, et al. Randomized, double-masked, sham-controlled trial of ranibizumab for neovascular age-related macular degeneration. PIER study year 1. Am J Ophthalmol. 2008;145:239-48.
21. Schmidt-Erfurth U, Eldem B, Guymer R, Korobelnik JF, Schlingemann RO, Axer-Siegel R, et al. Efficacy and safety of monthly versus quarterly ranibizumab treatment

in neovascular age-related macular degeneration: the excite study. Ophthalmology. 2011;118:831-9.
22. Lalwani GA, Rosenfeld PJ, Fung AE, Dubovy SR, Michels S, Feuer W, et al. A variable-dosing regimen with intravitreal ranibizumab for neovascular age-related macular degeneration: year 2 of the PrONTO study. Am J Ophthalmol. 2009;148:43-58.e1.
23. Ho AC, Busbee BG, Regillo CD, Wieland MR, Van Everen SA, Li Z, et al. Twenty-four-month efficacy and safety of 0.5 mg or 2.0 mg ranibizumab in patients with subfoveal neovascular age-related macular degeneration. Ophthalmology. 2014;121:2181-92.
24. Comparison of Age-related Macular Degeneration Treatments Trials (CATT) Research Group, Martin DF, Maguire MG, Fine SL, Ying GS, Jaffe GJ, et al. Ranibizumab and Bevacizumab for Treatment of Neovascular age-related Macular Degeneration. N Engl J Med. 2011;364(20):1897-908.
25. Comparison of Age-related Macular Degeneration Treatments Trials (CATT) Research Group, Maguire MG, Martin DF, Ying GS, Jaffe GJ, Daniel E, et.al. Five-Year Outcomes with Anti–Vascular Endothelial Growth Factor Treatment of Neovascular Age-related Macular Degeneration: The Comparison of Age-related Macular Degeneration Treatments Trials (CATT) Research Group. Ophthalmology. 2016;123:1751-61.
26. Berg K, Pedersen TR, Sandvik L, Bragadóttir R. Comparison of ranibizumab and bevacizumab for neovascular age-related macular degeneration according to LUCAS treat-and-extend protocol. Ophthalmology. 2014;122:146-52.
27. Wykoff CC, Croft DE, Brown DM, Wang R, Payne JF, Clark L, et al. Prospective trial of treat-and-extend versus monthly dosing for neovascular age-related macular degeneration TREX-AMD 1 year results. Ophthalmology. 2015;122:2514-22.
28. Wykoff CC, Ou WC, Brown DM, Croft DE, Wang R, Payne JF, et al. Randomized trial of treat-and-extend versus monthly dosing for neovascular age-related macular degeneration. Ophthalmology Retina. 2017;1:314-2.
29. Silva R, Berta A, Larsen M, Macfadden W, Feller C, Monés J, et al. Treat-and-extend versus monthly regimen in neovascular age-related macular degeneration: results with ranibizumab from the TREND study. Ophthalmology. 2018;125(1):57-65.
30. Khanna S, Komati R, Eichenbaum DA, Hariprasad I, Ciulla TA, Hariprasad SM. Current and upcoming anti-VEGF therapies and dosing strategies for the treatment of neovascular AMD: a comparative view. BMJ Open Ophthalmology. 2019;4:e000398.

CHAPTER 13

Newer Approaches to Management of Retinal Degenerative Disorders: Gene Therapy and Cell Replacement Therapy

Lingam Gopal, Su Xinyi, Mayuri Bhargava, Zeng Ping liu, Swathi Lingam

ABSTRACT

There has been tremendous progress in the management of retinal disorders in the last few decades. The advent of antivascular endothelial growth factor (VEGF) drugs has helped to manage many vascular chorioretinal disorders including age-related macular degeneration (AMD), diabetic retinopathy, etc. However, not much was available as treatment option for retinal degenerative disorders such as retinitis pigmentosa (RP) or end-stage age-related macular degeneration where in the retina and retinal pigment epithelium are atrophic. Two approaches have offered hope to manage these conditions—"gene therapy" and "cell replacement therapy". This article is a concise review of the present status of gene therapy and cell replacement therapy. The article is aimed at clinician ophthalmologists and, hence, includes some introductory paragraphs that some may consider as redundant. At the present time, these approaches are mostly in developmental phase. It is hoped that the future will see them becoming available to the clinicians so as to bring the much-needed succor to the patients suffering from inherited degenerative disorders of the retina.

Keywords: Retinitis pigmentosa, age-related macular degeneration, gene therapy, retinal pigment epithelium, retinal progenitor cell

INTRODUCTION

Over the last 4 decades, there has been tremendous progress in the management of retinal disorders. The progress has been mainly in the areas of vitreoretinal surgery and intravitreal injections for proliferative disorders of the retina including diabetic retinopathy and age-related macular degeneration (AMD). However, one large segment of retinal disorders has remained outside the scope of interventional treatment including hereditary retinal degenerations, geographic atrophy (GA) of macula secondary to AMD, etc.

Progress on two fronts has given hope to provide active treatment for these disorders: (1) gene therapy and (2) cell replacement therapy. Advances in genetics have enabled the identification of causative gene mutations in many monogenic inherited retinal degenerative conditions. Molecular and cellular biology has also enabled the functional understanding of why these genes are important during normal physiology, and after a mutation has occurred. Advance in molecular biology has also enabled strategies for gene replacement therapy and is thus already available in clinical practice. However, its success is dependent on the presence of sufficient functional retinal tissue to enable effective gene replacement. In the case of long-standing disease, whereby the retina is already atrophic, cell replacement therapy might be a more appropriate strategy.

This chapter summarizes the concepts and present status of these therapies related to retinal degenerative disorders and aimed at the clinician ophthalmologist.

GENE THERAPY

INTRODUCTION[1]

In order to understand the concepts of gene therapy, a modicum of understanding is needed of normal genetics and how defects in genes affect normal function.

Humans have 22 pairs of autosomes and one of sex chromosomes (XX or XY). The deoxyribonucleic acid (DNA) in the chromosomes acts as a reservoir of information. Genes are segments of the DNA that are responsible for generation of polypeptides (specific proteins)—a process termed also as "gene expression". The coding regions are located in the exons. Interspersed in-between exons are the noncoding sequences called introns. Transcription is the first stage whereby information is transferred from DNA to messenger ribonucleic acid (mRNA). "Promoter" is the region that initiates the process of transcription. "Enhancers" regulate the gene expression. mRNA is constructed as a complement of the gene sequence from one of the strands of the DNA. "Splicing" describes the process of removal of the intron sequences from the mRNA that do not code for the protein. "Translation" is the process where the information carried by the mRNA is used to construct the protein (a process that occurs in the cytoplasm with help of ribosomes). "Codon" is a sequence of three DNA or RNA nucleotides. They code for individual amino acids as well as act as initiators (initiation codon) or terminators (stop codon) of the process of translation. Further protein processing includes proper folding of the protein and other post-translational modifications.

POLYMORPHISMS AND MUTATIONS[2]

Polymorphism refers to the variants found in general population (>1%). Polymorphisms are common and probably not connected with disease causation. The variation can involve difference in one nucleotide, single nucleotide polymorphism (SNP), and deletions or insertions. The polymorphisms mostly involve noncoding regions and thus do not usually affect function.

Mutations, on the other hand, are rarer variations (<1%) and can be associated with significant effect on the protein expression, and thereby cause many genetic disorders. A mutation can cause disease due to the following reasons: absence of the protein; reduced levels of the protein; and altered structure of the protein (mutant protein). Or, it may have no effect (silent mutation). Mutations can involve change in one nucleotide (point mutation), insertion or deletions of one or more nucleotides.

"Nonsense mutations" refer to premature termination of the sequence due to a stop codon forming earlier than needed. "Missense mutations" refer to change in the sequence resulting in incorporation of a different amino acid. However, not all mutations lead to change in protein expression (silent mutations).

Deletions and insertions can affect the protein expression variably. "Frame shift mutation" refers to change in the reading frame caused by the insertion or deletion of nucleotides leading to effect downstream on the amino-acid sequence thus resulting in a mutant protein. Deletion of large segments of DNA leads to loss of several genes that are normally close to each other. Deletion can also bring together genes that are normally far apart. Other modifications include translocations (interchange of regions), amplifications (more than one copy of the genes leads to increased levels of proteins), and inversions (reversal of a segment of DNA).

"Synonymous mutations" refer to a mutation that does not change the final protein. This is possible since more than one code can produce the same amino acid. "Nonsynonymous mutations" change the protein sequence.

The terms 'dominant and recessive' in clinical terminology refers to the phenotype. A heterozygote with one normal allele and one abnormal allele is expected to be having a normal phenotype if the defective gene is recessive. It produces an abnormal phenotype if the defective gene is dominant.

Dominance in genetics describes the relationship of one allele with respect to the other. A dominant allele will suppress or mask the effect of its counterpart. Homozygous is a term used when the DNA sequence in a gene is identical in both alleles (could be normal or abnormal) versus heterozygous when the DNA sequence is different.

A homozygous functional (wild type) gene produces normal protein product. A homozygous abnormal (nonfunctional) gene would result in absence of production of normal protein product. A heterozygous gene with one functional and one nonfunctional allele can have varied phenotype depending on whether the functional allele is dominant or recessive and on the amount of normal protein that is produced by one normal allele.

- *Haplosufficiency*: The amount of protein produced is enough for normal functioning although it is 50% of normal. Sometimes the normal allele can actually produce >50% (upregulation) and effectively compensate for lack of protein from defective gene.

- *Haploinsufficiency*: The amount of protein made by the single functional allele is insufficient and the phenotype resembles a homozygote with both alleles being dysfunctional.
- *In-between*: Wherein the phenotype is not normal but not as severe as a homozygote with dysfunctional protein.

"Loss of function" and "gain of function" are yet another way of describing the outcome of a mutation in terms of what the gene is normally expected to produce. "Loss of function" is when the normal protein is not made at all or made in insufficient quantities. This happens when the mutant gene does not produce any protein (null mutation) or produces insufficient amounts (leaky loss of function). "Gain of function" is when the mutant gene produces a different protein, and this can produce a different phenotype. In most cases these mutant genes are "dominant" (to the normal allele) and, hence, express themselves. If both alleles are mutant, the cells may or may not be viable.

Dominant-negative mutations describe the condition where the mutant protein disrupts the activity of the normal protein. For example, dominant-negative mutation in the tumor suppressor gene can permit continued proliferation of the cells despite DNA damage (suppressed apoptosis) leading to tumor formation. **Flowchart 1** summarizes the important genetic variations.

Flowchart 1: Genetic variations.

```
Change in sequence can involve single nucleotide (single nucleotide
polymorphism/point mutations); insertion or deletion of number of nucleotides (indel)
```

Polymorphisms
- Common; seen in >1% of population; usually involve noncoding regions; usually no effect on function

Mutations
- Uncommon; seen in <1% of population; can involve coding regions; and can affect function

Missense mutations
- Change in nucleotide sequence can result in different protein expression/or could be silent mutation
- Tend to have dominant effect

Nonsense mutations
- Premature codon results in premature termination of sequence; however, a truncated protein is usually prevented from forming by NMD (point nonsense mediated mRNA decay); usual effect is of haploinsufficiency (lack of enough protein)
- Mostly recessive when normal allele supplies normal protein
- Can be dominant, if NMD fails resulting in abnormal protein that masks effect of normal protein (dominant-negative)

GENE THERAPY APPROACHES[3,4]
Direct Approaches Targeting the Disease Gene

Gene supplementation/augmentation: Where there is haploinsufficiency and gene product is less or absent (as in most recessive disorders), supplementation is a useful strategy.

Gene surgery/editing: In most autosomal dominant conditions, the abnormal gene would need to be silenced/inactivated. The gene editing tools include meganucleases, zinc-finger nucleases (ZFNs), transcription activator-like effector nucleases (TALEN) and clustered regularly interspaced short palindromic repeats (CRISPR). CRISPR is the latest technology that permits precision cleaving of the DNA relatively easily compared to the older techniques. CRISPR-Cas9 system was first identified in bacteria. These bacteria when invaded by virus, cleave the viral genome, and incorporate short segments of the viral genome between the CRISPR sequences. If exposed to the same virus again, the bacterium is able to cleave the virus using Cas endonucleases guided by CRISPR RNA and transactivating CRISPR RNA. The bacterium uses the protospacer adjacent motif (PAM) in the virus to discriminate between the virus sequences and the sequence present between CRISPR sequences in its own genome (the segment of the virus genome that was originally incorporated into its genome). Similar approach can be used to cleave the human genome at the site of defective gene as long as the site of cleavage is close to a proper PAM sequence.

A DNA double-strand break (DSB) is thus induced at the loci of choice. This break gets repaired by providing a DNA template using either homology directed repair (HDR) or nonhomologous end joining (NHEJ).

Indirect Approaches not Based on Diseased Gene

Here, the disease genes are not the target of the therapy. Instead, the therapeutic gene is used to support the survival of the affected cells. These include trials with adeno-associated virus (AAV)8 CRISPR-mediated disruption of neural retinal leucine (Nrl) zipper. This process may convert rods into cone-like cells that may make them less susceptible to the retinitis pigmentosa (RP) gene mutations. Inhibiting cell death pathways is another approach to preserve the retinal cells. Use of necrostatin-1s (RIP1 inhibitor) and N-acetyl cysteine (NLRP3 inhibitor) has been shown to preserve rod function and survival. Similar approach has been used to have a neuroprotective effect by knocking out prodegenerative genes in ganglion cells. The approach of targeting genes not connected directly with the disease causation was also used to disrupt genes for vascular endothelial growth factor A (VEGF-A) and VEGF receptor 2 in a mice model of laser induced neovascularisation (an approach that may have application in treatment of AMD).

Mutation independent gene replacement: Tsai et al.[5] reported use of ablate and replace strategy wherein the *Rhodopsin (RHO)* genes (both wild type and mutated alleles) were ablated with CRISPR and gene replacement helps to restore normal RHO function. This approach can potentially work irrespective of the type of mutation in the *RHO* gene.

Delivery of Gene/CRISPR Components to the Target Tissue[6]

This involves: (1) depositing the material as close to the tissue as possible, and (2) guiding the entry of the gene/CRISPR components into the cell.

The first step is carried out by intraocular injections. **Table 1** gives the modes of intraocular injection that have been tried with their advantages and disadvantages.

The next step is to guide the entry of the gene/CRISPR components into the cell. This step requires a vector. **Tables 2 and 3** describe the various viral and nonviral vectors that have been used in the delivery of genes/CRISPR components.

TABLE 1: Approaches for intraocular injection of gene/CRISPR components.

Mode of delivery	Advantages	Disadvantages
Intravitreal injection	• Simple outpatient technique • Access to relatively large retinal surface	• Internal limiting membrane barrier • Better access to inner retina • Humoral immune response to AAV capsids can occur
Subretinal injection	• Direct access to outer retinal layers (photoreceptor layer) • Humoral immune response to AAV capsids less likely	• Needs complex vitreoretinal surgery • Area of deposition of material is limited mostly to the bleb created by injection • Risk of retinal thinning, macular holes, etc.
Suprachoroidal injection	Relatively simpler technique using microneedles or surgical cannulation	Mostly reaches the choroid and RPE, but not efficient for retina
Transchoroidal subretinal injection	• Uses microneedles similar to one above without needing vitrectomy • Has been shown to be incorporated in retinal layers at site of injection—more efficiently than intravitreal or suprachoroidal injections	Potential to target macula would be limited by reduced access to sclera in posterior pole
Intravitreal injection after ILM peel	• Needs vitrectomy first with ILM peel followed by intravitreal injection or layering of the denuded area with vector • Avoids need to induce retinal detachment	• Would still need vitrectomy first • Humoral response to AAV capsids can occur

(AAV: adeno-associated virus; CRISPR: clustered regularly interspaced short palindromic repeats; ILM: internal limiting membrane)

TABLE 2: Viral vectors for delivery of gene/CRISPR components.

Viral Vectors		
Adeno-associated virus (AAV)	• Single-stranded DNA of 4.7 Knt • Nonpathogenic, nonreplicating, and nonintegrating • Vector DNA remains as episomes (no risk of insertional mutagenesis) • 13 serotypes and several variants available • Stable in postmitotic cells providing sustained transgene expression	• Can package only up to ~4.5 kb of transgene DNA • For larger packages dual AAV approach (two vectors carrying two separate packages) needs to be used • Not replicated in dividing cells
Adenovirus	• Double-stranded DNA • Can transduce dividing and non-dividing cells • Can package up to 37 kb • Remains as episome (no risk of insertional mutagenesis) • About 50 serotypes with different tropisms (affinity to specific tissues) exist	• Higher chances of antiviral immune response that can limit transgene expression • Sustained expression only in nondividing cells
Lenti virus	• Single-stranded RNA genome • Can infect dividing and nondividing cells • Sustained expression in dividing and nondividing cells since the viral DNA integrates with chromosome of cells • Can package up to 9–10 kb	• Insertional mutagenesis is a possibility • Can elicit antiviral immune response

(CRISPR: clustered regularly interspaced short palindromic repeats; DNA: deoxyribonucleic acid; RNA: ribonucleic acid)

Optogenetic Therapy[12]

Optogenetic therapy refers to a technology wherein artificial photoreceptors are generated in the retina using the surviving retinal cells. These genetically encoded light sensors sit on the membranes of the retinal cells. Two microbial molecules are currently being used to produce light sensitivity in various retinal cells **(Table 4)**.

These sensors can be genetically targeted toward specific retinal cells (bipolar cells/amacrine cells/ganglion cells) to try and simulate the natural retinal circuit. Researchers are trying different strategies using these molecules.

Gene Therapy for Retinal Disorders

The eye is suited for gene therapy approaches due to several reasons.
- The eye is immune-privileged due to presence of blood ocular barrier. Thus, immune reaction toward the viral vector and consequent suppression of the exogenous gene expression may be relatively less.

TABLE 3: Nonviral vectors for delivery of gene/CRISPR components.

Nonviral Vectors		
• Gene is packaged into a plasmid DNA and directly injected to site of interest • Easy to package large genes • Vector production is easy • No risk of mutagenicity • Rate of transfection is less than with viral vectors • Lower transgene expression	Nanoparticles	*Delivery facilitation* Lipid nanoparticles have been used to facilitate transfection of the plasmid DNA into the cells, e.g., lipofectamine 3000[7]
	Electroporation	• Use of electric impulses transiently increases membrane permeability and permits entry of the plasmid DNA into the cell • Mainly used in vitro but has been used in vivo in mouse experiments[8]
	Optoporation	• Optical transfection of cells using femtosecond near infrared laser • Proof of concept demonstrated in vitro[9]
Extracellular exosomes:[10] • Vesicles formed from outpouching of cell membrane. An ectosome is formed from plasma membrane and exosome is formed from endosome • 40–160 nm in size vesicles containing distinct intracellular contents including membrane proteins, nuclear proteins, extracellular matrix proteins, metabolites, mRNA, fragments of DNA • Complex and partly understood biological role—considered as way of intercellular communication • Contain host cell elements and hence can be used for disease diagnosis and monitoring by sampling body fluids		• By engineering the contents of the exosomes and utilizing their competence to enter cells easily, these vesicles can be used as vehicles to deliver cargo of interest to specific target cells.[11] Tissue targeting is made possible by engineering the surface ligands • In the management of degenerative disorders of retina, the role of exosomes is being explored

(CRISPR: clustered regularly interspaced short palindromic repeats; DNA: deoxyribonucleic acid; mRNA: messenger ribonucleic acid)

TABLE 4: Optogenetic therapy.

	Molecule	*Derived from*	*Action*	*On light activation*
ChR2	Channel rhodopsin-2	*Chlamydomonas reinhardtii*	Light-gated cation channel	Depolarizes
NpHR	Halorhodopsin	*Natronomonas pharaonis*	Light-activated chloride pump	Hyperpolarizes

- *Allows localized gene delivery*: Subretinal injection allows localized gene delivery within a specified area. This allows efficient delivery of a high concentration of vector, achieved with a small injectable volume. In addition, the small volume of the eye limits the spread and scatter of the injected components.
- *Ease of live in-vivo imaging for follow-up*: The retina can be visualized with simple tools such as fundus photography, fluorescein angiography, autofluorescence, and optical coherence tomography. Its function can be evaluated by noninvasive techniques such as electroretinography. Often the fellow eye can serve as untreated control since hereditary retinal degenerations tend to be bilateral and often symmetrical.

TABLE 5: Summary of clinical trials of gene therapy in retinal disorders.

Disorder	Targeted gene	Vector used	Status of trials	Remarks
Leber's congenital amaurosis[13,14]	RPE65	AAV	FDA approved (LUXTURNA)	Multiluminance mobility test shows 1.6 light levels better score for treated patients. No serious adverse events
Achromatopsia	CNGB3; CNGA3	AAV	Phase 1/2	Anecdotal improvement. No consistent positive result
Choroideremia[15]	REP1	AAV	Phase 1/2; Phase 3	VA improved in 14 treated eyes versus controls; maximum sensitivity on dark adapted microperimetry improved
Retinitis pigmentosa[16]	MERTK	AAV	Phase 1	3/6 had short-term improvement
Retinitis pigmentosa	PDE6B	AAV	Phase 1/2	Ongoing
Retinitis pigmentosa	RLBP1	AAV	Phase 1/2	Ongoing
Retinoschisis[17]	RS1	AAV	Phase 1/2	Well-tolerated
Stargardt's disease	ABCA4	Lentivirus	Phase 1/2	Proposed
Usher syndrome 1B	MYO7A	Lentivirus	Phase 1/2	Study terminated
X-linked retinitis pigmentosa[18]	RPGR	AAV	Phase 1/2	5/6 patients showed improved mobility at lux levels 1, 4, and 16 (1 lux is equal to deep twilight and 256 lux is like office setting)

(AAV: adeno-associated virus; FDA: Food and Drug Administration; VA: visual acuity)

Several retinal disorders are under consideration for gene therapy. The torch bearer of this progress has been the treatment of RPE65 mutation related Leber's congenital amaurosis (LCA). The landmark experiments in the Briard dogs have paved the way for clinical trials in humans. Luxturna (Voretigene neparvovec, AAV2-hRPE65v2) has now been approved for human use by the Food and Drug Administration (FDA). Gene therapy for other diseases is either in preclinical phase or in early clinical trials. **Table 5** summarizes the present status of gene therapy for retinal disorders.

Issues with Gene Therapy for Retinal Disorders

It is obvious that we need to make much more progress before gene therapy can become a standard-of-care in the management of hereditary and other retinal disorders.

Major issues include:
- Vector integration wherein the vectors ("Adeno" virus and "Lenti" virus) can integrate with the host genome at site of the DSB induced by the CRISPR Cas system.

- "Off target" effects refer to the potential of CRISPR application to produce off target cleavage. This issue is being addressed by development of high-fidelity Cas nucleases and use of CRISPR/Cas inhibitors.
- The prolonged existence of Cas nuclease can also be a source of problem by inducing inflammatory reaction. A sort of self-destructing system that is delivered with the vector reduces the period of activity of the Cas nuclease as well as reduce the "off target" effects.
- *Immune reaction*:[19] AAV has been reported to be associated with significant local and systemic immune response despite administration of steroids. This immune response causes significant inflammation leading deterioration of vision. It can also result in loss of efficacy after initial improvement.

CELL THERAPY FOR RETINAL DISORDERS

INTRODUCTION

Cell therapy for retinal disorders refers to use of stem cells to rescue or replace degenerating or degenerated cells in retinal layers in various disorders. Since it attempts to replace dead cells, potentially, stem-cell therapy can be useful even for end stages of disease.

STEM CELLS AND REGENERATION

Stem cells are cells that have regenerative potential to differentiate into specialized cells. "Pluripotent" describes the ability of cells to generate any cell in the body. Pluripotent stem cells can be derived from embryos (embryonal stem cells/ESC). "Induced pluripotent stem cells (iPSC)", on the other hand, refers to human adult cells that have been programed to return to an embryonic stem cell like state.

In contrast, "adult stem cells" that are found in a particular organ or tissue are often multipotent, i.e., they are restricted to becoming a more limited population of cells (e.g., cell types specific to that organ). Adult stem cells which exist in almost all individual organs (except the heart) serve as a reservoir for internal repair system. In the eye, stem like cells have been identified in the ciliary margin zone of mammals.[20,21]

"Pluripotent" cells have the ability to generate all the cell types that make up the body. Typical example are the ESCs. "Multipotent" describes cells that can develop into more than one cell type but not as diverse as pluripotent.

THE EYE AS A TARGET FOR CELL-BASED THERAPY

Similar to the advantages quoted in gene therapy, the eye seems to offer some unique features that can be beneficial while administering cell therapy for retinal disorders. These include:

- Access retina, subretinal space, etc. which is well established by advanced vitreoretinal surgical techniques.
- The retina can be well evaluated post-therapy, both structurally and functionally by relatively noninvasive techniques including photography, optical coherence tomography, electrophysiological studies, fluorescein and indocyanine green angiography, autofluorescence, microperimetry, etc.
- Subretinal space is relatively immune-privileged.
- The number of cells needed to be injected is relatively small due to the relatively small size of the structures of the eye. This can result in reduced risk of immune rejection by virtue of reduced antigen load.
- Retinal pigment epithelium (RPE) cells are at end-stage of fully differentiated cells from stem cell, therefore the risk of tumorigenicity is minimum in comparison to other stem-cell-derived cell products.
- Retinal progenitor cells (RPC) have low immunogenicity. The risk of immune rejection is even lower than RPE cells.

Retinal diseases that can be potentially targeted for cell therapy: Age-related macular degeneration and inherited retinal dystrophies such as RP and Stargardt's disease are currently the diseases being explored for this innovative approach.

Age-related Macular Degeneration

Dry AMD starts as damage of RPE first followed by degeneration of the overlying photoreceptor layer, clinically seen as areas of GA. Lack of specific treatment leads to increase in these areas over time and when it involves the fovea, visual acuity is severely affected. In the presence of a relatively intact photoreceptor layer, replacement of RPE can potentially improve the function of the overlying retina. In neovascular AMD, late stages are characterized by loss/severe damage to RPE. In such cases, removal of the choroidal neovascular membrane and replacement of RPE can potentially recover vision.

Retinitis Pigmentosa

Although a disease primarily of the photoreceptor layer, the RPE can secondarily be affected, especially in the late stages. Potentially photoreceptor replacement alone may suffice if the RPE underlying is not irreparably damaged.

Stargardt's Disease

This is primarily a macular dystrophy that affects visual acuity quite early in life. The primary tissue of damage is RPE with secondary photoreceptor atrophy.

CELLS PROPOSED TO BE REPLACED

Retinal degenerative disorders affect primarily the RPE or the photoreceptors. However, there are several disorders where both these layers are damaged severely in the late stages of the disease. Thus, replacing either the RPE and/or photoreceptors can be a treatment strategy in these diseases.

Potential Source of Stem Cells

- *Embryonic stem cells (ESCs):* These are derived from the inner cell mass of the human embryo at the blastocyst stage. ESCs are pluripotent and can form any type of tissue—ectodermal, mesodermal, and endodermal. In the eye, ESC derived RPE has been used. However, the use of embryonal stem cells is mired in ethical concerns. In addition, immune rejection is a possibility. The donor can also harbor genes causing disease. Tumorigenicity is a possibility with accumulation of oncogenic mutations over several replications.
- *Induced pluripotent stem cells (iPSC):* Somatic cells such as skin fibroblasts are reprogramed to become stem cells. The cells are pluripotent. There are issues of the cells harboring disease causing genes of the donor and may also retain the epigenetic features of the cell of origin (e.g., fibroblast). Rejection chances are said to be less with iPSCs. Tumorigenicity is a possibility. Use of viral vectors for the cell line generation as well as use of *MYC* transduction in the generation of iPSC can potentially trigger tumorigenicity. iPSC derived RPE as well as progenitor retinal cells have been used.
- *Autologous-induced pluripotent cells:* The concept of using patients own tissue to generate pluripotent cells and then to differentiate them into RPE for implantation is very appealing since it seems to eliminate the risk of immunogenicity and need for use of immunosuppressants. Skin fibroblasts and more recently $CD34^+$ cells from blood have been used as a source.
- *Adult stem cells:* These are multipotent stem cells. Most commonly used are the bone marrow derived hematopoietic stem cells (HSCs), bone marrow derived mesenchymal stem cells, and neural progenitor cells (derived from neural stem cells).[22] Adult Muller cells can also be a source of RPCs. Proto-oncogenic activation and tumorigenicity are possible. Culture of RPE cells from cadaver eyes has shown presence of RPE stem cells which could be guided to differentiate back into RPE cells.[23,24]
- *Cord blood and cord lining cells:*[25] Cells found in cord blood are mainly HSCs. The cord lining membrane is a source of mesenchymal stem cells and epithelial stem cells. The source is considered as a medical waste and so inexpensive. Stemness is retained even after several replication cycles. Cells from umbilical cord proliferate but do not produce tumors. Stem cells from umbilical cord express some embryonic stem cell

markers, hence they are somewhere between adult stem cells and ESCs. While there are reports of umbilical cord derived stem cells being used for wound healing, diabetes, liver degeneration, limbal cell deficiency, etc., applications for retinal regeneration have still not been tried/or in its infancy. Mesenchymal stem cells may have to be dedifferentiated to iPSC before being differentiated into RPE or photoreceptors.

RATIONALE FOR CELL-BASED THERAPY

- *Cell replacement:* Surgeons have dissected and translocated patches of choroid/RPE under the fovea in eyes with end stages of AMD and have shown some success in terms of integration of the grafted tissue and functional improvement in vision.[26] Similar results are expected if one can integrate the injected RPE cells with the host tissue and effectively replace the nonfunctional RPE. In the retina, RPE and the photoreceptor layers are the main tissues targeted for replacement.
- *Neurotrophic effect:* The cells may serve as a source of factors that can potentially rescue retinal cells/RPE that are under stress as well as protect them. RPE cells have been shown to express a variety of trophic factors which have been shown to rescue photoreceptors that are located some distance away from site of the injection, clearly indicating the effect to be due to trophic factors.[27]

Different Approaches for Retinal Pigment Epithelium Transplantation

Injection of Loose Cells

One approach to transplant RPE cells is to inject suspension of cultured RPE cells through a fine needle directly into the subretinal space.[28]

Advantages: The main advantage of this procedure is the ease of administration. Following vitrectomy and induction of posterior vitreous detachment, a 38-gauge needle is used to penetrate the retina and the cell suspension is injected.

Disadvantages: The cells can clump and get multilayered. Postoperative supine position of the patient can influence the pattern of RPE cell spread. There is no surety as to the polarity of the deposited RPE cells. Risk exists of some RPE cells refluxing into the vitreous cavity and layering on the retinal surface with risk of induced proliferative vitreoretinopathy.[29]

Other issues: In the center of GA, usually the retina is atrophic as well as firmly adherent to the bare choroid. It would be difficult to induce retinal detachment in this area and even if injectable the benefit to the overlying retina is likely to be minimal in the stage of total atrophy. In the border areas, there is likely to be RPE loss/dysfunction but with relatively intact retinal architecture. The benefit of RPE transplant is likely to be highest in these areas.[30] Graft survival and functionality would also depend on the status of Bruch's membrane (aging/thickening/rigidity/atrophy); inflammation that can coexist in AMD due to imbalance in complement related activity; choroidal ischemia; and subretinal scarring. Compared to cell suspensions, implanted monolayers have been found to have better long-term survival.[31]

Clinical trials: Human embryonic stem-cell-derived RPE cells have been used in eyes with dry AMD and Stargardt's disease.[30] The authors concluded that the procedure is safe with no serious adverse events. More than half of the 18 treated patients have experienced improved vision. No case of tumorigenicity or immunogenic inflammation was observed.

Subretinal Transplantation of Monolayer of Retinal Pigment Epithelium Cells

Although there is a report of RPE cell sheet being implanted without any substrate,[32] most reports have used some substrate (biocompatible) on which the RPE cells are grown and the RPE cell sheet with the substrate is implanted. The substrate is expected to be semipermeable to enable the choriocapillaris to support the RPE cells layer and the outer retina overlying the implant. The scaffold materials tested include nonabsorbable synthetic substances such as polyethylene terephthalate (PET), polyester, parylene C membrane; absorbable (biodegradable) synthetic membranes such as polylactic-co-glycolic acid (PLGA), biological tissue such as amniotic membrane.

The surgery involves vitrectomy; induction of posterior vitreous detachment; creation of a retinal detachment posteriorly at the site of intended implantation; making a retinotomy roughly the size of the width of the implant; introduction of the implant with RPE cells under the retina using specialised injectors;[33,34] and fluid air exchange to dry the subretinal space.

While most studies were on human embryonal cell-derived RPE cells, adult RPE stem-cell-derived RPE cells were also tried in nonhuman primates.[35] The authors used PET sheet as scaffold material on which RPE cells were cultured and implanted.

Advantages: It makes intuitive sense to introduce RPE cells as a monolayer thus mimicking its natural distribution and perhaps giving the best opportunity to integrate with host tissues. The polarity of the cells and tight junctions between cells is also assured. The substrate with RPE cells can be deliberately placed at the site of choice.

Disadvantages/Challenges: The surgery is far more complicated than for injection of suspension of RPE cells. As alluded to above, specialized tools are needed to load and inject the implant subretinally. The size of the implant is limited by the size of sclerotomy and size of the retinotomy. Larger sclerotomy and larger retinotomy have more risk of intraoperative and postoperative complications. Hence, one has to strike a compromise. The introduction of the implant under the retina should be also done carefully to avoid the cells being lost by inadvertent contact with retinotomy edge. Failure to dry the retina adequately can result in the implant shifting substantially postoperatively away from the intended site. The induction of a bleb of retinal detachment can be challenging. Potentially the process can result in damage to RPE as well as producing macular hole. Techniques have been evolved to reduce this risk of damage to RPE and macula.[36]

Clinical trials: Koss et al. tested submicron parylene C membrane as a substrate on which human embryonic stem-cell-derived RPE was grown and implanted in minipigs.[37] The group followed it up with phase 1 human trials of five subjects.[38] The OCT pictures showed integration of the RPE monolayer with photoreceptors. One eye improved while others maintained the preoperative vision. da Cruz et al. have also reported a phase 1 trial of use of polyester membrane coated with human vitreonectin on which confluent RPE cells were seeded. In two patients that were included in this study, visual improvement was noted in both after 1 year of follow-up.[34] Adverse events in this study included exposure of suture that is used to anchor fluocinolone acetonide implant (used for local immune suppression) and retinal detachment, both unrelated to the RPE patch.

Issues with Stem-cell-derived Retinal Pigment Epithellium Cell Transplants

- *Need for current good manufacturing practice (cGMP) conditions*: Use of cultured RPE cells demands presence of cGMP facilities to ensure quality product free of contamination.
- *Time taken to produce the final product*: This can vary depending on the process adopted. Use of spontaneous differentiation process requires longer manufacturing time compared to directed differentiation protocols. Longer the time taken, greater the risk of contamination.
- *Contamination*: The final cell product must be free of infective organisms and also pluripotent stem cells. Contamination with pluripotent cells increases risk of teratoma formation. However, studies have shown that the conditions needed for RPE cell maturing are detrimental for the survival of iPSC.
- *Accumulation of chromosomal abnormalities and mutations on serial passages*: Upregulation of oncogenes and downregulation of tumor suppressor genes can result in increased risk of tumorigenicity.
- *Characterizing the cultured RPE cells*: It is important to ensure that the final product being implanted is close to natural RPE. Otherwise, its ability to function and support the photoreceptor layer will be hampered even if anatomically the implant is in the right place. To this end, researchers have adopted several techniques to validate the cells

for use. da Cruz et al.[34] have used immunocytochemistry, electron microscopy, pigment epithelial-derived factor secretion profile [enzyme-linked immunosorbent assay (ELISA)] and functional phagocytosis to characterize the cells as RPE. Miyagishima et al. have evolved a set of investigations that evaluate the adenosine triphosphate (ATP)-driven signaling pathways that are critical for the RPE function including transepithelial potential (TEP), total transepithelial resistance, ratio of apical to basolateral membrane resistance, intracellular calcium imaging, and mRNA and miRNA expression profiling.[39]

- *Immunogenicity*: Barring autologous RPE cell transplantation, all other sources of RPE cells can trigger immunological reaction in the form of graft rejection. Hence, immunosuppression is needed in most cases of allogenic RPE cell transplantation. Autologous cell therapy, however, has a fairly long manufacturing process. The source of cells is nonocular in origin such as skin fibroblasts.[32] CD34+ cells from blood have been recently used as a source of autologous tissue to generate iPSC.[40,41] The authors note that unlike with skin fibroblasts, iPSC derived from CD34+ cells have remained free of any induced chromosomal changes and so reduced risk of tumorigenicity. **Table 6** summarizes the clinical trials that have used RPE cells as suspension while **Table 7** summarizes the clinical trials that have used RPE cells as a monolayer with or without scaffold.

Photoreceptor Transplantation

For most retinal degenerative conditions, the final common pathway for visual loss is the loss of the photoreceptors. Ability to replace the diseased photoreceptors will be a quantum jump in the concept of regenerative medicine with respect to retinal degenerative disorders.

Retinal Pigment Epithelium versus Photoreceptor Transplantation

The eye as a target organ holds some advantages for cell therapy which have been elucidated above. These advantages hold good for photoreceptor transplant as well. Recovery of visual acuity essentially requires a functioning macular area which is a relatively small area. Fewer than 250,000 photoreceptors can provide therapeutic benefit thus effectively reducing the antigenic load.[45] In contrast, recovering peripheral field of vision is lot more challenging. The area that needs to be covered and correspondingly the number of cells to be transplanted is much more. It has been estimated that about 150,000 functioning rods can generate a recordable scotopic electroretinogram (ERG) signal.[46] However, in terms of visual field gain, the challenge is more in terms of the area that needs to be covered than the absolute number of cells that needs to be replaced.

Transplanted RPE needs to maintain contact with the outer segments of photoreceptors to be functional. For photoreceptor transplant to be

TABLE 6: Summary of clinical trials using RPE suspension.

Clinical trial	Cell type	Trial details	Outcome
Phase 1: Safety and tolerability of subretinal Transplantation of hESC derived RPE (MA09-hRPE) cells in patients with advanced dry age-related macular degeneration (dry AMD) NCT01344999[30,42]	Human embryonic stem cell derived RPE cell suspension (50,000–150,000 cells)	• Nine patients each of AMD and Stargardt's disease • Vitrectomy with subretinal injection of about 150 mL • Immunosuppression with tacrolimus and mycophenolate • 1 year follow-up	• Poor tolerance to immunosuppressive • 1 case of endophthalmitis • *VA in AMD:* Three eyes with >14 letter improvement in VA • *VA in Stargardt's disease:* Three improved by 15 letters and one lost 10 letters • No adverse reaction due to the cells
A Phase I/IIa, Open-label, single-center, prospective study to determine the safety and tolerability of subretinal transplantation of human embryonic stem cell derived retinal pigmented epithelial (MA09-hRPE) cells in patients with advanced dry age-related macular degeneration (AMD) NCT01674829[43]	Human embryonic stem-cell-derived RPE cell suspension	• Two each of Asian patients with AMD and Stargardt's disease • Vitrectomy with subretinal injection of about 150 mL • Immunosuppression with tacrolimus and mycophenolate • 1 year follow-up	• Mild reaction to immunosuppression • *VA in AMD:* 1 to 9 letter improvement • *VA in Stargardt's disease:* 12–19 letters improvement • No immune rejection/tumorigenicity • Epiretinal membrane noted in AMD patients
An open-label, non-randomized, multi-center study to assess the safety and effects of autologous adipose-derived stromal cells injected intravitreal in dry macular degeneration NCT02024269	Autologous adipose-derived stromal cells—intravitreal		• Study withdrawn after severe reaction and loss of vision noted
Phase 1/2a, multicenter, randomized, dose escalation, fellow-eye controlled, study evaluating the safety and clinical response of a single, subretinal administration of human umbilical tissue-derived cells (CNTO 2476) in subjects with visual acuity impairment associated with geographic atrophy secondary to age-related macular degeneration NCT01226628[44]	Human umbilical tissue-derived RPE cell suspension	• 33 patients with dry AMD • Cells delivered by transchoroidal injection after scleral cut down using iTrack 275 microcatheter to induce a bleb of retinal detachment • 50 mL of solution injected • 1 year follow-up • No immune suppression	• Retinal detachment in six eyes and retinal perforation in 13 eyes • No immune rejection or tumorigenicity

(RPE: retinal pigment epithelium; VA: visual acuity)

TABLE 7: Summary of clinical trials using RPE monolayer.

Clinical trial	Cell type	Trial details	Outcome
Safety and feasibility of the transplantation of autologous induced pluripotent stem cell (iPSC)-derived retinal pigment epithelium (RPE) cell sheets in patients with exudative (wet-type) age-related macular degeneration[32]	Autologous iPSC-RPE from skin fibroblasts	• One patient of AMD • Removal of CNVM and implantation of RPE sheet after vitrectomy and retinotomy • No scaffold • No immunosuppression • 1 year follow-up	• Grafted sheet survived • No change in VA • No graft rejection or tumorigenicity • CME present • Second patient not implanted because of concerns about genetic change In the iPSC-derived RPE cells
Phase 1 clinical study of an embryonic stem-cell-derived retinal pigment epithelium patch in age-related macular degeneration (AMD), NCT01691261[34]	Human embryonal cell-derived RPE cell monolayer	• RPE monolayer on a polyester Membrane scaffold—inserted after vitrectomy and retinotomy • Local immune suppression with fluocinolone implant • 1 year follow-up	• Exposure of suture of implant, retinal detachment reported as adverse events • No immune rejection or tumorigenicity • VA improved by 21–29 letters
A bioengineered retinal pigment epithelial monolayer for advanced, dry AMD NCT02590692[38]	Human embryonal cell-derived RPE cell monolayer	• Four patients with dry AMD • RPE attached to a small subretinal parylene membrane (diffusion properties similar to Bruch's membrane) inserted after vitrectomy and retinotomy • Immunosuppression with tacrolimus • 1 year follow-up	• VA: 17 letter improvement in one eye • No immune rejection or tumorigenicity

(CME: cystoid macular edema; CNVM: choroidal neovascular membrane; RPE: retinal pigment epithelium; VA: visual acuity) functional, the cells have to establish synaptic connections with bipolar cells on one hand and maintain functional contact with the underlying RPE on the other. The health of other layers of retina is important for the functionality of the transplanted cells to be evident.

REPLACEMENT VERSUS REJUVENATION

Several animal studies have shown that cell therapy for neurosensory retina seems to function by three mechanisms: (1) Transplanted cells maturing into photoreceptors and actually integrating with host retina;[47] (2) Transplanted cells acting as a source for transfer of materials to the defective host cells;[48] and (3) Transplanted cells acting as a source of paracrine factors such as brain-derived neurotrophic factor (BDNF), hepatocyte growth factor (HGF), and glial cell-derived neurotrophic factor (GDNF) that perform the task of neuroprotection and help the defective cells rejuvenate.[49,50]

Theoretically, for acting as a source of neuroprotective paracrine factors, these cells can potentially be deposited remotely from the site where they are needed (e.g., intravitreal injections) and, hence, can potentially have a wider area of impact. In contrast, for cells to integrate with the circuitry or for direct transfer of materials to defective cells they need to be deposited in the subretinal space and correspondingly the area of therapeutic benefit is restricted.

Source of Cells

Fetal-derived retinal progenitor cells: These are obtained from human fetuses of 14–20 weeks of gestation.[51,52]

Similar to RPE, embryonal stem cells (ESC), induced pleuripotent stem cells (iPSC), human umbilical cord derived stem cells (hUTC), and bone marrow derived cells (mononuclear cells, CD34+ stem cells, and mesenchymal stem cells) can be used as source to generate RPCs.

Researchers have been able to induce these stem cells to differentiate into the major retinal cell types including photoreceptors. Three-dimensional self-organizing retinal tissue could also be generated from iPSC and ESC which have shown high degree of maturation and formation of outer segments that respond to light.

Retinal progenitor cells: Refer to immature cells found in developing neural retinal tissue that are multipotent (not pluripotent) and can potentially differentiate into any of the retinal neuronal cells or glial cells. They can be cultured in vitro.[53] They are less tumor prone compared to pluripotent cells such as iPSC or ESC. Fetal-derived RPCs have been used in human phase 1 studies and shown to be safe.[54]

Embryonal stem cells and iPSC stem cells have been used to generate retinal sheets that have been transplanted in animal models with some evidence of integration but lacking organized histoarchitecture.[55,56]

Human umbilical cord tissue-derived stem cells: Cells derived from umbilical cord were used as source of neuroprotection when injected subretinally.[57]

Bone marrow derived CD34+ stem cells: Cells from bone marrow contain a small quantity (<0.2%) of CD34+ stem cells which have potential to integrate with retina. The cells have to be harvested from bone marrow but cannot be expanded (grown) in culture, hence limiting the number of cells available for injection.[58] The advantage of this source of cells is they can be autologous and hence devoid of immune rejection issues, and do not have abnormal proliferative tendencies (teratogenic).

Bone marrow derived mesenchymal stem cells:[58] They constitute <0.1% of the bone marrow derived cells but can expand (be grown) in culture. However, their ability to differentiate into retinal neural cells is limited and perhaps is better used for their neuroprotective effect from secretion of paracrine factors. Use of mesenchymal stem cells has also been found to be associated with higher risk of inflammation. The cells also appear to be heterogeneous depending on the culture conditions.

What is transplanted?
- *Cell suspension*: In most studies suspension of the cells was injected subretinally.
- *Sheets of self-organized retinal tissue*: Following the development of 3D culture techniques to develop self-organized retinal tissue, attempts have been made to implant the sheets of retinal tissue.[55] In principle, mouse studies have shown integration of graft cells to the host although the outcome depended on the state of retinal damage in the host retina, and the age of the grafts (young versus old grafts).[55] 3D culture methods were also used to develop embryoid bodies that formed optic cups from which the developing cells were harvested and used for injection.[59] This facilitated collection of large number of progenitor cells.
- *Implantation of fetal retina with RPE*: Radtke et al. cut-out pieces of fetal retina with RPE from donor eyes of fetuses at gestational age of 11–16 weeks and directly implanted the pieces in the subretinal space of human patients with AMD and RP.[60]

Factors that Seem to Influence Engraftment

There is piecemeal evidence from various studies that identify few factors that seem to influence the successful engraftment of the implanted cells into the host tissue.
- Photoreceptor precursors of a particular stage (Rod precursors expressing *Nrl*) are required in large numbers.[61]
- A disrupted external limiting membrane improves integration of transplanted cells.[62]

TABLE 8: Summary of clinical trials on neural retinal transplant.

	Study type	Patients	Type of implant	Outcome
Kaplan et al.[64]	Safety study	2 RP patients with no PL vision	Sheet of human photoreceptors from cadaver eyes implanted subretinally	No vision improvement; no rejection
Humayun et al.[65]	Pilot study	8 RP patients	Human fetal retinal microaggregate suspension	Mild increase in light sensitivity in 3/8 patients that disappeared in 3 months; tolerated well
NCT02320812 jCyte, Inc	I/IIa	28 RP patients	500,000–3,000,000 cells single dose	No data
NCT03073733 jCyte, Inc	IIb	82 RP patients	3,000,000–6,000,000 cells in single dose	No data
NCT02464436 ReNeuron ltd.	I/II	21 RP patients	?	No data
ChiCTR-TNAC-08000193	I	8 RP patients	1,000,000	No data

(PL: perception of light; RP: retinitis pigmentosa)

- Using 3D culture techniques and implanting the self-organized retinal tissue, Assawachananont et al. have shown in a mouse model that younger grafts (Day 11–17) have better integration compared to older than 18-day grafts.
- Chondroitinase ABC treatment has been shown to improve synaptogenesis between transplanted cells and host neurons in a retinal degeneration model.[63]

IMMUNOGENICITY OF RETINAL PROGENITOR CELLS TRANSPLANTATION

In contrast to allogenic RPE cell transplantation which seems to suffer from high chances of graft rejection without immunosuppression, allogenic RPC transplants seem to be better tolerated. In experimental animals, the evidence is strong. In mice, it was found that cultured neural progenitor cells do not express major histocompatibility complex (MHC) class I or II antigens and allografts were well tolerated. Early human trials have also indicated the tolerance of allografts without immunosuppression.[54] **Table 8** summarizes the clinical trials for neural retinal transplant.

REFERENCES

1. Kassem HSh, Girolami F, Sanoudou D. Molecular genetics made simple. Glob Cardiol Sci Pract. 2012;2012(1):6.
2. Karki R, Pandya D, Elston RC, Ferlini C. Defining "mutation" and "polymorphism" in the era of personal genomics. BMC Med Genomics. 2015;8:37.

3. Takahashi VKL, Takiuti JT, Jauregui R, Tsang SH. Gene therapy in inherited retinal degenerative diseases: a review. Ophthalmic Genet. 2018;39(5):560-8.
4. DiCarlo JE, Mahajan VB, Tsang SH. Gene therapy and genome surgery in the retina. J Clin Invest. 2018;128(6):2177-88.
5. Tsai YT, Wu WH, Lee TT, Wu WP, Xu CL, Park KS, et al. Clustered regularly interspaced short palindromic repeats-based genome surgery for the treatment of autosomal dominant retinitis pigmentosa. Ophthalmology. 2018;125(9):1421-30.
6. Yu W, Wu Z. Ocular delivery of CRISPR/Cas genome editing components for treatment of eye diseases. Adv Drug Deliv Rev. 2021;168:181-95.
7. Sunshine JC, Sunshine SB, Bhutto I, Handa JT, Green JJ. Poly-(β-amino ester)-nanoparticle mediated transfection of retinal pigment epithelial cells in vitro and in vivo. PLoS One. 2012;7(5):e37543.
8. Matsuda T, Cepko CL. Electroporation and RNA interference in the rodent retina in vivo and in vitro. Proc Natl Acad Sci USA. 2004;101(1):16-22.
9. Batabyal S, Kim S, Wright W, Mohanty S. Laser-assisted targeted gene delivery to degenerated retina improves retinal function. J Biophotonics. 2021;14(1):e202000234.
10. Kalluri R, LeBleu VS. The biology, function, and biomedical applications of exosomes. Science. 2020;367(6478):eaau6977.
11. Jiang XC, Gao JQ. Exosomes as novel bio-carriers for gene and drug delivery. Int J Pharm. 2017;521(1-2):167-75.
12. Simunovic MP, Shen W, Lin JY, Protti DA, Lisowski L, Gillies MC. Optogenetic approaches to vision restoration. Experiment Eye Res. 2019;178:15-26.
13. Russell S, Bennett J, Wellman JA, Chung DC, Yu ZF, Tillman A, et al. Efficacy and safety of voretigene neparvovec (AAV2-hRPE65v2) in patients with RPE65-mediated inherited retinal dystrophy: a randomised, controlled, open-label, phase 3 trial. Lancet. 2017;390(10097):849-60.
14. Jacobson SG, Cideciyan AV, Ratnakaram R, Heon E, Schwartz SB, Roman AJ, et al. Gene therapy for Leber congenital amaurosis caused by RPE65 mutations: safety and efficacy in 15 children and adults followed up to 3 years. Arch Ophthalmol. 2012;130(1):9-24.
15. MacLaren RE, Groppe M, Barnard AR, Cottriall CL, Tolmachova T, Seymour L, et al. Retinal gene therapy in patients with choroideremia: initial findings from a phase 1/2 clinical trial. Lancet. 2014;383(9923):1129-37.
16. Ghazi NG, Abboud EB, Nowilaty SR, Alkuraya H, Alhommadi A, Cai H, et al. Treatment of retinitis pigmentosa due to MERTK mutations by ocular subretinal injection of adeno-associated virus gene vector: results of a phase I trial. Hum Gene. 2016;135:327-43.
17. Cukras C, Wiley HE, Jeffrey BG, Sen HN, Turriff A, Zeng Y, et al. Retinal AAV8-RS1 gene therapy for X-linked retinoschisis: initial findings from a Phase I/IIa trial by intravitreal delivery. Mol Ther. 2018;26(9):2282-94.
18. Cehajic-Kapetanovic J, Xue K, Martinez-Fernandez de la Camara C, Nanda A, Davies A, Wood LJ, et al. Initial results from a first-in-human gene therapy trial on X-linked retinitis pigmentosa caused by mutations in RPGR. Nat Med. 2020;26:354-9.
19. Bucher K, Rodríguez-Bocanegra E, Dauletbekov D, Fischer MD. Immune responses to retinal gene therapy using adeno-associated viral vectors: implications for treatment success and safety. Prog Retin Eye Res. 2020:100915.
20. Ahmad I, Das AV, James J, Bhattacharya S, Zhao X. Neural stem cells in the mammalian eye: types and regulation. Semin Cell Dev Biol. 2004;15(1):53-62.
21. Tropepe V, Coles BL, Chiasson BJ, Horsford DJ, Elia AJ, McInnes RR, et al. Retinal stem cells in the adult mammalian eye. Science. 2000;287(5460):2032-6.
22. Smith LE. Bone marrow-derived stem cells preserve cone vision in retinitis pigmentosa. J Clin Invest. 2004;114(6):755-7.

23. Blenkinsop TA, Saini JS, Maminishkis A, Bharti K, Wan Q, Banzon T, et al. Human adult retinal pigment epithelial stem cell-derived RPE monolayers exhibit key physiological characteristics of native tissue. Invest Ophthalmol Vis Sci. 2015;56:7085-99.
24. Blenkinsop TA, Salero E, Stern JH, Temple S. The culture and maintenance of functional retinal pigment epithelial monolayers from adult human eye. Methods Mol Biol. 2013;945:45-65.
25. Saleh R, Reza HM. Short review on human umbilical cord lining epithelial cells and their potential clinical applications. Stem Cell Res Ther. 2017;8(1):222.
26. Karasu B, Erdoğan G. Autologous translocation of the choroid and retinal pigment epitelial cells (RPE) in age-related macular degeneration: monitoring the viability of choroid and RPE patch with indocyanine green angiography (ICGA) and fundus autofluorescence (FAF). Photodiagnosis Photodyn Ther. 2019;28:318-23.
27. Lund RD, Adamson P, Sauvé Y, Keegan DJ, Girman SV, Wang S, et al. Subretinal transplantation of genetically modified human cell lines attenuates loss of visual function in dystrophic rats. Proc Natl Acad Sci USA. 2001;98:9942-7.
28. Alexander P, Thomson HA, Luff AJ, Lotery AJ. Retinal pigment epithelium transplantation: concepts, challenges, and future prospects. Eye (Lond). 2015;29(8):992-1002.
29. Del Priore LV, Kaplan HJ, Hornbeck R, Jones Z, Swinn M. Retinal pigment epithelial debridement as a model for the pathogenesis and treatment of macular degeneration. Am J Ophthalmol. 1996;122(5):629-43.
30. Schwartz SD, Tan G, Hosseini H, Nagiel A. Subretinal transplantation of embryonic stem cell-derived retinal pigment epithelium for the treatment of macular degeneration: an assessment at 4 years. Invest Ophthalmol Vis Sci. 2016;57:ORSFc1. doi: 10.1167/iovs.15-18681. PMID: 27116660.
31. Diniz B, Thomas P, Thomas B, Ribeiro R, Hu Y, Brant R, et al. Subretinal implantation of retinal pigment epithelial cells derived from human embryonic stem cells: improved survival when implanted as a monolayer. Invest Ophthalmol Vis Sci. 2013;54(7):5087-96.
32. Mandai M, Watanabe A, Kurimoto Y, Hirami Y, Morinaga C, Daimon T, et al. Autologous induced stem-cell-derived retinal cells for macular degeneration. N Engl J Med. 2017;376(11):1038-46.
33. Stanzel BV, Liu Z, Brinken R, Braun N, Holz FG, Eter N. Subretinal delivery of ultrathin rigid-elastic cell carriers using a metallic shooter instrument and biodegradable hydrogel encapsulation. Invest Ophthalmol Vis Sci. 2012;53(1):490-500.
34. da Cruz L, Fynes K, Georgiadis O, Kerby J, Luo YH, Ahmado A, et al. Phase 1 clinical study of an embryonic stem cell-derived retinal pigment epithelium patch in age-related macular degeneration. Nat Biotechnol. 2018;36(4):328-37.
35. Liu Z, Parikh BH, Tan QSW, Wong DSL, Ong KH, Yu W, et al. Surgical Transplantation of Human RPE Stem Cell-Derived RPE Monolayers into Non-Human Primates with Immunosuppression. Stem Cell Reports. 2021;16(2):237-51.
36. Tan GSW, Liu Z, Ilmarinen T, Barathi VA, Chee CK, Lingam G, et al. Hints for gentle submacular injection in non-human primates based on intraoperative OCT guidance. Transl Vis Sci Technol. 2021;10(1):10.
37. Koss MJ, Falabella P, Stefanini FR, Pfister M, Thomas BB, Kashani AH, et al. Subretinal implantation of a monolayer of human embryonic stem cell-derived retinal pigment epithelium: a feasibility and safety study in Yucatán minipigs. Graefes Arch Clin Exp Ophthalmol. 2016;254(8):1553-65.
38. Kashani AH, Lebkowski JS, Rahhal FM, Avery RL, Salehi-Had H, Dang W, et al. A bioengineered retinal pigment epithelial monolayer for advanced, dry age-related macular degeneration. Sci Transl Med. 2018;10(435):eaao4097.
39. Miyagishima KJ, Wan Q, Corneo B, Sharma R, Lotfi MR, Boles NC, et al. In pursuit of authenticity: induced pluripotent stem cell-derived retinal pigment epithelium for clinical applications. Stem Cells Transl Med. 2016;5(11):1562-74.

40. Mack AA, Kroboth S, Rajesh D, Wang WB. Generation of induced pluripotent stem cells from CD34⁺ cells across blood drawn from multiple donors with non-integrating episomal vectors. PLoS One. 2011;6(11):e27956.
41. Sharma R, Khristov V, Rising A, Jha BS, Dejene R, Hotaling N, et al. Clinical-grade stem cell-derived retinal pigment epithelium patch rescues retinal degeneration in rodents and pigs. Sci Transl Med. 2019;11(475):eaat5580.
42. Schwartz SD, Hubschman JP, Heilwell G, Franco-Cardenas V, Pan CK, Ostrick RM, et al. Embryonic stem cell trials for macular degeneration: a preliminary report. Lancet. 2012;379(9817):713-20.
43. Song WK, Park KM, Kim HJ, Lee JH, Choi J, Chong SY, et al. Treatment of macular degeneration using embryonic stem cell-derived retinal pigment epithelium: preliminary results in Asian patients. Stem Cell Reports. 2015;4(5):860-72.
44. Ho AC, Chang TS, Samuel M, Williamson P, Willenbucher RF, Malone T. Experience With a Subretinal Cell-based Therapy in Patients With Geographic Atrophy Secondary to Age-related Macular Degeneration. Am J Ophthalmol. 2017;179:67-80.
45. Zarbin M. Cell-Based Therapy for Degenerative Retinal Disease. Trends Mol Med. 2016;22(2):115-34.
46. Pearson RA, Barber AC, Rizzi M, Hippert C, Xue T, West EL, et al. Restoration of vision after transplantation of photoreceptors. Nature. 2012;485(7396):99-103.
47. Klassen HJ, Ng TF, Kurimoto Y, Kirov I, Shatos M, Coffey P, et al. Multipotent retinal progenitors express developmental markers, differentiate into retinal neurons, and preserve light-mediated behavior. Invest Ophthalmol Vis Sci. 2004;45(11):4167-73.
48. Ortin-Martinez A, Tsai EL, Nickerson PE, Bergeret M, Lu Y, Smiley S, et al. A reinterpretation of cell transplantation: GFP transfer from donor to host photoreceptors. Stem Cells. 2017;35(4):932-9.
49. Cao J, Murat C, An W, Yao X, Lee J, Santulli-Marotto S, et al. Human umbilical tissue-derived cells rescue retinal pigment epithelium dysfunction in retinal degeneration. Stem Cells. 2016;34(2):367-79.
50. Singh MS, Park SS, Albini TA, Canto-Soler MV, Klassen H, MacLaren RE, et al. Retinal stem cell transplantation: balancing safety and potential. Prog Retin Eye Res. 2020;75:100779.
51. Hendrickson A, Bumsted-O'Brien K, Natoli R, Ramamurthy V, Possin D, Provis J. Rod photoreceptor differentiation in fetal and infant human retina. Exp Eye Res. 2008;87(5):415-26.
52. del Cerro M, Notter MF, del Cerro C, Wiegand SJ, Grover DA, Lazar E. Intraretinal transplantation for rod-cell replacement in light-damaged retinas. J Neural Transplant. 1989;1(1):1-10.
53. Klassen HJ, Ng TF, Kurimoto Y, Kirov I, Shatos M, Coffey P, et al. Multipotent retinal progenitors express developmental markers, differentiate into retinal neurons, and preserve light-mediated behavior. Invest Ophthalmol Vis Sci. 2004;45(11):4167-73.
54. Liu Y, Chen SJ, Li SY, Qu LH, Meng XH, Wang Y, et al. Long-term safety of human retinal progenitor cell transplantation in retinitis pigmentosa patients. Stem Cell Res Ther. 2017;8(1):209. doi: 10.1186/s13287-017-0661-8. PMID: 28962643; PMCID: PMC5622579.
55. Assawachananont J, Mandai M, Okamoto S, Yamada C, Eiraku M, Yonemura S, et al. Transplantation of embryonic and induced pluripotent stem cell-derived 3D retinal sheets into retinal degenerative mice. Stem Cell Reports. 2014;2(5):662-74.
56. Mandai M, Fujii M, Hashiguchi T, Sunagawa GA, Ito SI, Sun J, et al. iPSC-Derived Retina Transplants Improve Vision in rd1 End-Stage Retinal-Degeneration Mice. Stem Cell Reports. 2017;8(1):69-83. doi: 10.1016/j.stemcr.2016.12.008. Erratum in: Stem Cell Reports. 2017;8(2):489. Erratum in: Stem Cell Reports. 2017;8(4):1112-3.
57. Lund RD, Wang S, Lu B, Girman S, Holmes T, Sauvé Y, et al. Cells isolated from umbilical cord tissue rescue photoreceptors and visual functions in a rodent model of retinal disease. Stem Cells. 2007;25(3):602-11.

58. Park SS, Moisseiev E, Bauer G, Anderson JD, Grant MB, Zam A, et al. Advances in bone marrow stem cell therapy for retinal dysfunction. Prog Retin Eye Res. 2017;56:148-65.
59. Eiraku M, Takata N, Ishibashi H, Kawada M, Sakakura E, Okuda S, et al. Self-organizing optic-cup morphogenesis in three-dimensional culture. Nature. 2011;472(7341):51-6.
60. Radtke ND, Aramant RB, Petry HM, Green PT, Pidwell DJ, Seiler MJ. Vision improvement in retinal degeneration patients by implantation of retina together with retinal pigment epithelium. Am J Ophthalmol. 2008;146(2):172-82.
61. MacLaren RE, Pearson RA, MacNeil A, Douglas RH, Salt TE, Akimoto M, et al. Retinal repair by transplantation of photoreceptor precursors. Nature. 2006;444(7116):203-7.
62. West EL, Pearson RA, Tschernutter M, Sowden JC, MacLaren RE, Ali RR. Pharmacological disruption of the outer limiting membrane leads to increased retinal integration of transplanted photoreceptor precursors. Exp Eye Res. 2008;86(4):601-11.
63. Suzuki T, Akimoto M, Imai H, Ueda Y, Mandai M, Yoshimura N, et al. Chondroitinase ABC treatment enhances synaptogenesis between transplant and host neurons in model of retinal degeneration. Cell Transplant. 2007;16(5):493-503.
64. Kaplan HJ, Tezel TH, Berger AS, Wolf ML, Del Priore LV. Human photoreceptor transplantation in retinitis pigmentosa: a safety study. Arch Ophthalmol. 1997;115(9):1168-72.
65. Humayun MS, de Juan E Jr, del Cerro M, Dagnelie G, Radner W, Sadda SR, et al. Human neural retinal transplantation. Invest Ophthalmol Vis Sci. 2000;41(10):3100-6.

Ocular Myasthenia Gravis

CHAPTER 14

Asmita Mahajan, Pradeep Sharma

ABSTRACT

Myasthenia gravis is an autoimmune disease affecting neuromuscular transmission and presenting with easy fatiguablity of muscles. The extra ocular muscles are particularly predisposed due to their high firing frequencies and singly innervated fibers. Clinical manifestations include ocular features such as ptosis, diplopia and ophthalmoplegia and generalized features such as slurred speech, difficulty in chewing and respiratory muscle weakness. Myasthenia gravis can be diagnosed clinically using ice-pack test or sleep test or using acetyl cholinesterase inhibitors such as edrophonium and neostigmine. Immunological testing may be done for anti-AChR-Ab and anti-MuSK-Ab. Electrophysiological testing in the form of repetitive nerve stimulation and single-fiber electromyography has high sensitivity but is not pathognomonic for myasthenia as it indicates a disturbed neuromuscular transmission. Treatment is mainly aimed at alleviating the symptoms of diplopia and ophthalmoplegia. Medical treatment in the form of acetylcholinesterase inhibitors which increase the duration of action of neurotransmitters can be given orally every three to four hours and lead to marked improvement in some patients. However, they do not influence the natural course of the disease. Corticosteroids or immunosuppressant therapy is helpful for patients with MG who have not met treatment goals with ACh inhibitors. Acute exacerbations and myasthenic crisis are treated using plasmapheresis or intravenous immunoglobulins. Myasthenia is frequently associated with thymic hyperplasia or thymoma and these patients may respond to thymectomy as well.

Keywords: Ocular myasthenia, ptosis, neurotransmitters, ophthalmoplegia, electromyography, immunosuppressant, thymectomy.

INTRODUCTION

Myasthenia gravis (MG) is an autoimmune disease which affects the neuromuscular junction (NMJ) and causes fatigability of muscles. About 85% of patients may present to an ophthalmologist. This presentation is termed as "ocular myasthenia gravis (OMG)".[1] Up to 23.3–80% of patients of OMG may transform to generalized myasthenia gravis (GMG) during their lifetime.[2,3] MG has a non-uniform age distribution with a bimodal distribution in several studies. The first peak is seen in the second and third decades and shows a female preponderance and the second peak in the sixth to eighth decades with male preponderance. Though the incidence of MG is higher in females worldwide, in India, it has been more commonly reportedly in males.[4]

Presentation of the disease in <10 years of age or after 70 years of age is rarely seen.

The major histocompatibility complex (MHC) plays an important genetic susceptibility locus for MG. The early-onset of MG is associated with MHC haplotype human leukocyte antigen (HLA)-B8, DR3-DQ2, and hyperplastic thymus. HLA-B7 and DR2 have been described for patients with late onset of MG and is associated with an atrophic thymic histology.[5]

PATHOPHYSIOLOGY

The NMJ is the site of neuromuscular transmission where acetylcholine (ACh) molecules are released and traverse across the synapse to bind to receptors on the postsynaptic membrane of the muscle. This leads to its depolarization and subsequent muscular contraction. Antiacetylcholine receptor antibodies (AChR-Abs) which block these receptors have been seen in up to 80–90% of patients with GMG and about 50% patients of pure ocular myasthenia.[6] They produce deficient neuromuscular transmission by three different mechanisms: (1) they directly bind to the ACh receptors (AChRs) leading to alteration of their function; (2) they promote cross-linking of receptors and their endocytosis; and (3) antibodies also activate complement system leading to destruction of the postsynaptic surface.[7]

This ultimately results in defective transmission at the NMJ and weakness of the muscle which increases with sustained muscle activation. Patients, therefore, present with increased fatigability of muscles with prolonged use, and improvement of symptoms with rest.

Myasthenia has variable affliction for muscle groups and several factors specific to the extraocular muscles (EOMs) place them at a higher risk for involvement: (1) The ocular motor neuron firing frequencies are extremely high, which exacerbate any transmission defect; (2) EOMs have singly innervated fibers with less prominent synaptic folds. The AChRs and sodium channels on the postsynaptic membrane are fewer in number which reduces the safety factor and predisposes to neuromuscular transmission failure.[8]

CLINICAL FEATURES

Patients characteristically present with a fluctuating weakness of muscles which improves on resting and is exacerbated by prolonged activity. Thus, a diurnal variation of symptoms is seen where the patients are asymptomatic in the morning or have minimal symptoms and present with ptosis or diplopia in the evening. Generalized myasthenia involves the limbs and the respiratory muscles whereas exclusive ocular myasthenia presents with involvement of the EOMs, levator palpebrae superioris (LPS), and orbicularis oculi.[6]

Ptosis due to the involvement of the LPS complex is one of the most common manifestations of ocular myasthenia. It may be unilateral or bilateral and in bilateral cases, it is mostly asymmetrical. Ptosis may increase after prolonged upgaze. This is referred to as "lid fatigability". The **Cogan "twitch response"** or irritable lid phenomenon is another sign described by David Cogan in OMG. It is demonstrated by having a patient change his gaze from infraversion (for 10-15 seconds) to the primary position. Cogan explained this sign on the basis of rapid recoverability of fatigued muscles after a period of relaxation of the lid while the patient has been looking down. The lid shows an elevation when the gaze is raised to the primary position but this elevation is maintained only for a fraction of a second and, therefore, appears as a twitch. When associated with several blinks, it may appear as a flutter or "irritable lid".[9] Cogan's lid twitch is, however, not specific to myasthenia.[10] When the ptotic eyelid is lifted manually, enhancement of ptosis of the contralateral eye may be noted, explained by Hering's law of equal innervation to yoke muscles. Tone of orbicularis should also be assessed in these patients by trying to open the eyes against forced closure of eyelids. The eyelids tend to drift apart easily and even when not opened forcefully, the underlying sclera may be seen. This is called the **"peek sign"**.

Myasthenia is a great imitator, especially of peripheral nerve lesions or supranuclear gaze palsy and, hence, in every patient of diplopia or ophthalmoplegia which does not fit into a typical pattern of peripheral nerve lesion, it should be considered in the differential diagnosis. The muscle most frequently affected in myasthenia is probably the medial rectus.[11] Orbicularis weakness is also seen frequently.[12]

Over 15% of OMG patients will also show bulbar weakness leading to slurred speech, or difficulty in chewing or swallowing. Neck and extremity weaknesses may also be seen in about 5% of patients.[13]

Myasthenia gravis usually spares the pupil and this serves as a useful sign to distinguish these patients from cases of pupil involving third nerve palsy. However, clinically evident pupillary abnormalities have been reported by Yamazaki A et al., like anisocoria, a sluggish pupillary response to light and fatigue of accommodation.[14,15] These patients may also exhibit intrasaccadic fatigue, i.e., a decline in the saccadic velocity during a long saccade.[16]

DIAGNOSIS

Ice Pack Test

The ocular motility deficits and ptosis are measured and an ice pack is placed over the patient's closed eyelids for a period of 2-5 minutes. The ptosis and motility defects are measured again. This test is considered positive if the

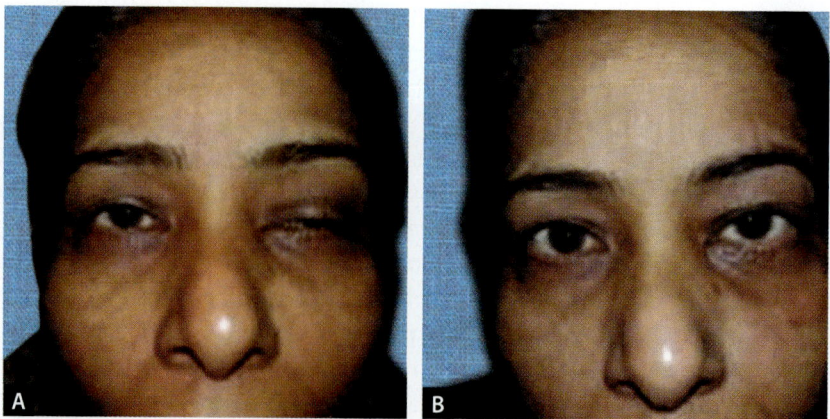

Figs. 1A and B: Patient before and after ice pack application. Note improvement in ptosis of left eye.

upper eyelid elevates by at least 2 mm following ice application (**Figs. 1A and B**). This occurs because activity of acetylcholinesterase is reduced on cooling and this leads to increased levels of ACh transmitter at NMJ.[17]

Sleep Test

This test is mainly of historical importance. It involves measurement of improvement in manifestations of OMG, i.e., resolution of ptosis or ophthalmoplegia after a period of rest of about 30 minutes. Reappearance of the myasthenic signs over the next 5 minutes adds further confirmation.[18]

Edrophonium Test

Edrophonium is a reversible acetylcholinesterase inhibitor which results in an increase of ACh in the NMJ. Historically, it has served as a diagnostic tool for MG. In 2018, the Food and Drug Administration (FDA) discontinued edrophonium in the United States due to its high rate of false-positive results.[19]

Neostigmine Test

Neostigmine test is a longer-acting AChE being increasingly used as an alternative to edrophonium for diagnostic testing. 1 cc of a 1/2,000 solution (0.5 mg) is injected intravenously over 1 minute. Improvement is often seen instantly and is maximal over the next 5 minutes. Therefore, measurement of ptosis and diplopia recorded should be repeated after 5 minutes of injection. Occasionally, in very mild cases, the response to an intravenous dose of 0.5 mg of neostigmine is unequivocal. In such cases, the test should be repeated on another day with 1 mg neostigmine. Atropine sulfate (0.6 mg) should always be kept at hand to be injected subcutaneously if side effects of neostigmine become manifest but should never to be injected with the neostigmine.[20]

Immunologic Testing

As discussed previously, increase in anti-AChR-Ab titer is observed in 80-90% of cases of MG and about 50% of OMG cases. In OMG cases, high titers signify increased risk of systemic MG in future.[21] Of anti-AChR-Ab negative patients, 30% will have autoantibodies against muscle-specific kinase (anti-MuSKAb) expressed on skeletal muscle. Patients who are negative for both AChR and MuSKAbs are classified as "seronegative MG".

ELECTROPHYSIOLOGIC TESTING

Repetitive Nerve Stimulation Studies

The nerve to be studied is electrically stimulated with a supramaximal stimulus 6-10 times at 2 or 3 Hz (slow rate) and the compound muscle action potential (CMAP) recorded with surface electrodes. In MG, the number of individual muscle fiber action potentials is reduced, hence, the CMAP is decreased in amplitude. A characteristic decrement (>10%) by the fourth or fifth response is typically seen. More than 70% patients show abnormal response when proximal muscles are tested in generalized MG (Oh et al., 1992). But in patients with mild generalized MG and ocular MG, this percentage is much lower.[22,23] A decremental response to repetitive nerve stimulation (RNS) is not specific and may be seen in other myasthenic syndromes like Lambert-Eaton and also in myopathies.

Single-fiber Electromyography

Single-fiber electromyography (SFEMG) is the most sensitive diagnostic test for detecting abnormal neuromuscular transmission. When a motor axon is depolarized, the action potentials travel distally and excite the muscle fibers of a single motor unit more or less at the same time. The variation in the time interval between the action potentials of muscle fibers in a motor unit is called as "jitter". SFEMG measures their variation (jitter) with an especially contracted single-fiber EMG needle electrode or facial concentric needle electrode with a small recording surface. Increased jitter values are sensitive but not pathognomonic for myasthenia as they indicate a disturbed neuromuscular transmission. Overall, SFEMG has a sensitivity of 85-100% for OMG when used on the frontalis or orbicularis oculi muscle.[24]

IMAGING STUDIES

As many as 70% of patients with myasthenia may have thymic hyperplasia or a thymoma.[25] Baseline computed tomography (CT) of the chest is, therefore, advisable in patients diagnosed with myasthenia.

TREATMENT

Treatment is chiefly medical and aims at symptomatic relief by improving muscle weakness and alleviating symptoms of diplopia and ptosis.

Acetylcholinesterase Inhibitors

Acetylcholinesterase inhibitors can help in by alleviating muscle weakness by increasing the duration of action of neurotransmitters. Pyridostigmine has a rapid onset of action (15–30 minutes) with peak action at approximately 2 hours, and is effective for 3–4 hours after which it has to be repeated. It leads to marked improvement in some patients and little to none in others. In particular, patients with muscle-specific tyrosine kinase-positive disease have a poor response to anticholinesterase agents. Adverse effects of pyridostigmine occur due to the cholinergic properties of the drug and oral glycopyrrolate 1 mg can be added with each pyridostigmine dose to block those bothersome symptoms. Excessive pyridostigmine use may even cause cholinergic crisis.[26]

Neostigmine is an alternative drug of the same class but with a less favorable side effect profile. In general, limb and bulbar symptoms (dysphagia, fatigable chewing, and dysarthria) respond better to anticholinesterase drugs than the ocular manifestations. Among ocular symptoms, ptosis responds better than diplopia. Acetylcholinesterase inhibitors, however, do not influence the natural course of the disease and about 36% of patients with OMG, who were treated with pyridostigmine and not steroids developed GMG within 2 years in a study.[27]

Corticosteroids

Corticosteroids or immunosuppressant therapy should be used in all patients with MG who have not met treatment goals after an adequate trial of pyridostigmine.[25] There are multiple regimens for corticosteroid use in MG and we usually start with 20 mg/day that is increased weekly to a maximum of 1 mg/kg/day based on the patient's response. There is a risk of myasthenia exacerbation within 7–10 days with initial high-dose oral prednisone therapy, which may even require intubation or assisted ventilation. Once remission is achieved, the dose is slowly tapered (as rapid reductions may precipitate myasthenic crisis) at a rate of 20% or less at 4–8-weekly intervals with conversion into an alternate day dosing schedule. Oral corticosteroids produce significant improvement in 66–85% of OMG patients. A permanent remission is seen in only a minority of patients (<10%).[28]

Immunosuppressive Therapy

Azathioprine (AZA) interferes with T-cell and B-cell proliferation by blocking nucleotide synthesis and is used both as monotherapy (e.g., in steroid-resistant patients) and with conjunction with oral corticosteroids.

It is started at 50 mg daily or 1 mg/kg and is increased weekly by 50 mg/day to a target dose of 2–3 mg/kg daily, divided into two or three doses. When used as monotherapy, the clinical response may be delayed by >6 months associated with a progressive fall in AChR-Ab titers. AZA-related side effects are leukopenia, thrombocytopenia, nausea, vomiting, and hepatotoxicity. Thus, complete blood count and liver function tests should be performed for monitoring.[28]

Cyclosporine A, an inhibitor of calcineurin, decreases the antigen-stimulated interleukin-2 production in T-cells. It is a third-line drug and is of use in patients who are dependent or intolerant of steroids and/or azathioprine. Mycophenolate mofetil (MMF), a selective inhibitor of T- and B-lymphocyte proliferation by blocking purine synthesis, is a relatively new drug in the treatment of MG. It is used both as a steroid-sparing agent as well as monotherapy although it did not show much apparent steroid-sparing effect in recent randomized controlled trials (RCTs).

Plasmapheresis

Plasma exchange or plasmapheresis separates the patient's plasma from whole blood and replaces it with saline, albumin, or plasma-protein fraction thus removing the circulating antibodies in the patient of MG. Patients are treated in about five sessions over a span of 1–2 weeks. The role of plasmapheresis has been limited to management of myasthenic exacerbations or crisis.

Intravenous Immunoglobulin

Intravenous immunoglobulin (IVIG) is a fractionated blood product derived from up to 10,000 human plasma donors and consists primarily of IgG. It accelerates the catabolism of antibodies and suppresses its production in addition to inhibiting complement activation. The usual IVIG dose is 0.4–1 g/kg body weight given over 3–5 days. There are conflicting reports on the efficacy of IVIG in ocular myasthenia and its use may be restricted to myasthenic crisis only.

Thymectomy

Thymectomy has for long been known to have a benefit in patients with MG. However, it may not be effective in pure OMG and is usually recommended only in patients with documented thymic enlargement. Response to thymectomy may be delayed for several years.[29]

CONCLUSION

Ocular myasthenia gravis leads to easy fatiguablity of extra-ocular muscles and a clinical presentation of ptosis, diplopia and ophthalmoparesis. About 15% patients may have bulbar signs as well. Ice-pack test, neostigmine test and immunological testing can be done in clinical settings to confirm the diagnosis. Treatment is chiefly medical using oral acetyl cholinesterase inhibitors.

REFERENCES

1. Grob D, Brunner N, Namba T, Pagala M. Lifetime course of myasthenia gravis. Muscle Nerve. 2008;37(2):141-9.
2. Hong YH, Kwon SB, Kim BJ, Kim BJ, Kim SH, Kim JK, et al; Korean Research Group for Neuromuscular Diseases. Prognosis of ocular myasthenia in Korea: a retrospective multicenter analysis of 202 patients. J Neurol Sci. 2008;273(1-2):10-4.
3. Bever CT Jr, Aquino AV, Penn AS, Lovelace RE, Rowland LP. Prognosis of ocular myasthenia. Ann Neurol. 1983;14(5):516-9.
4. Singhal BS, Bhatia NS, Umesh T, Menon S. Myasthenia gravis: A study from India. Neurol India. 2008;56:352-5.
5. Levinson AI. Chapter 65: Myasthenia gravis. In: Rich RR, Fleisher TA, Shearer WT, Schroeder HW, Jr., Frew AJ, Weyand CM (Eds). Clinical Immunology: Principles and Practice, 5th Edition. Amsterdam, Netherlands: Elsevier; 2019. pp. 879-90.
6. Lindstrom JM, Seybold ME, Lennon VA, Whittingham S, Duane DD. Antibody to acetylcholine receptor in myasthenia gravis: prevalence, clinical correlates, and diagnostic value. Neurology. 1976;26:1054-9.
7. Hughes B, De Casillas M, Kaminski H. Pathophysiology of myasthenia gravis. Semin Neurol. 2004;24(01):21-30.
8. Porter JD. Extraocular muscle: cellular adaptations for a diverse functional repertoire. Ann N Y Acad Sci. 2002;956:7-16.
9. Cogan DG. Myasthenia Gravis: A review of the disease and a description of lid twitch as a characteristic sign. Arch Ophthalmol. 1965;74(2):217-21.
10. Keane JR. Vertical diplopia. Semin Neurol. 1986;6:147-54.
11. Trouth AJ, Dabi A, Solieman N, Kurukumbi M, Kalyanam J. Myasthenia gravis: a review. Autoimmune Disease. 2012;2012:874680.
12. Nair AG, Patil-Chhablani P, Venkatramani DV, Gandhi RA. Ocular myasthenia gravis: a review. Indian J Ophthalmol. 2014;62(10):985-91.
13. Myasthenia Gravis Foundation of America. (2008) Myasthenia Gravis: A Manual for the Health Care Provider. [online] Available from https://books.google.co.in/books/about/Myasthenia_Gravis.html?id=U_jvPgAACAAJ&redir_esc=y [Last accessed April, 2021].
14. Yamazaki A, Ishikawa S. Abnormal pupillary responses in myasthenia gravis: a pupillographic study. Br J Ophthalmol. 1976;60(8):575-80.
15. Cooper J, Pollak GJ, Ciuffreda KJ, Kruger P, Feldman J. Accommodative and Vergence Findings in Ocular Myasthenia. J Neuro-Ophthalmol. 2000;20(1):5-11.
16. Yee RD, Cogan DG, Zee DS, Baloh RW, Honrubia V. Rapid eye movements in myasthenia gravis. II. Electro-oculographic analysis. Arch Ophthalmol. 1976;94:1465-72.
17. Sethi KD, Rivner MH, Swift TR. Ice pack test for myasthenia gravis. Neurology. 1987;37(8):1383.
18. Odel JG, Winterkorn JMS, Behrens MM. The sleep test for myasthenia gravis: a safe alternative to Tensilon. J Clin Neuroophthalmol. 1991;11:288-92.
19. Naji A, Owens ML. Edrophonium. Treasure Island (FL): StatPearls Publishing; 2021. [online] Available from https://www.ncbi.nlm.nih.gov/books/NBK430685/?term=%22Edrophonium%22 [Last accessed April, 2021].
20. Tether JE. Intravenous neostigmine in diagnosis of myasthenia gravis. Ann Intern Med. 1948;29:1132-8.

21. Benatar M. A systematic review of diagnostic studies in myasthenia gravis. Neuromuscul Disord. 2006;16:459-67.
22. Engel AG. Myasthenia gravis and myasthenic syndromes. Ann Neurol. 1984;16:519-34.
23. Stalberg E, Sanders DB. Electrophysiological tests of neuromuscular transmission. In: Stalberg E, Young RR (Eds). Clinical neurophysiology. London: Butterworths; 1981. pp. 88-116.
24. Arul SV. Single-fiber EMG: A review. Ann Indian Acad Neurol. 2011;14:64-7.
25. Osserman KE, Tsairis P, Weiner LB. Myasthenia gravis and thyroid disease: clinical and immunologic correlation. J Mt Sinai Hosp NY. 1967;34:469-83.
26. Sanders DB, Wolfe GI, Benatar M, Evoli A, Gilhus NE, Illa I, et al. International Consensus Guidance for Management of Myasthenia Gravis: Executive summary. Neurology. 2016;87:419-25.
27. Kupersmith MJ, Moster M, Bhuiyan S, Warren F, Weinberg H. Beneficial effects of corticosteroids on ocular myasthenia gravis. Arch Neurol. 1996;53:802-4.
28. Antonio-Santos AA, Eggenberger ER. Medical treatment options for ocular myasthenia gravis. Curr Opin Ophthalmol. 2008;19:468-78.
29. Evoli A, Batocchi AP, Provenzano C, Ricci E, Tonali P. Thymectomy in the treatment of myasthenia gravis: report of 247 patients. J Neurol. 1988;235:272-6.

Index

Page numbers followed by *b* refer to box, *f* refer to figure, *fc* refer to flowchart, and *t* refer to table.

A

Acetylcholine 230
Acetylcholinesterase 232
    inhibitors 229, 234
Achromatopsia 212
Active retinal vasculitis, diagnosis of 81
Active Sentry handpiece 138
Acute posterior multifocal placoid pigment epitheliopathy 81, 88, 89, 96, 116
Adeno-associated virus 208-210, 212
Adenosine triphosphate 219
Adenovirus 210
Adnexal surgery 41
Adult stem cells 213, 215
Aflibercept 167, 189
Age-related eye disease study 27
Age-related macular degeneration 16, 26, 29, 61, 65, 121, 187, 192, 204, 214
    treatment of 188, 191, 197
Alcon Verion system 147
American Diabetic Association 154
Amniotic membrane transplant 38
Ampiginous choroiditis 91, 116
Anemia 154
Angiography, traditional 82
Angio-optical coherence tomography, interpretation of 79
Angiotensin-converting enzyme 2 3, 6
Angle-closure glaucoma 11
Anterior corneal stroma 54
Anterior segment-optical coherence tomography 68, 69
Anteroposterior traction, relief of 175
Antiacetylcholine receptor antibodies 230
Antibiotics 52
Anti-inflammatory treatment 110
Antimetabolites 115
Antivascular endothelial growth factor 83, 152, 166, 189t, 190, 204
    drugs 27
    treatment 28, 195f
Antiviral therapy 13
Apoptosing retinal cells, detection of 69
Artificial intelligence 16-18, 30, 61, 62, 62f, 65, 70, 72, 73
    concept of 61
    hierarchy 19f
    model 18f
    risk of 30
    system 23
Artificial neural network 61, 63, 64f
Aspirin 165
Atropine sulfate 232
Autoimmune disease 229
Azathioprine 114, 234

B

Bacteria 105
Balanced salt solution 144f
Benzalkonium chloride 53
Best corrected visual acuity 163
Bevacizumab 167, 169, 189, 197
Birdshot chorioretinopathy 81, 90, 96
Birdshot lesions 90
Black box artificial intelligence 71
Blindness 152
Blood
    pressure 62
    retinal barrier 80
Body mass index 62
Bone marrow derived cells 222, 223
Bowman's and endothelial layers 48
Brain 2
    derived neurotrophic factor 222
Branch retinal vein occlusion 4, 10
Brolicizumab 189
Bruch's membrane 126

B-scans 79
Bullous keratopathy 48, 50, 129
Bunsen-Roscoe's law 52

C

Cannula vacuum 143-146
    continuous curvilinear capsulorhexis 143, 144
Capillary flow deficit 81
Capsular tear using bent 26G needle 144*f*
Capsulorhexis
    advances in 143
    overlay for 148*f*
Capsulotomy 145
Cardiovascular disease 165
Catalys 141
Cataract 16, 30, 64, 138, 152, 178
    formation 177
    removal 129
    surgery 129, 147, 150
        complicated 136
        image-guided 147
Cell
    based therapy, rationale for 216
    replacement therapy 204, 216
    source of 222
    suspension 223
    therapy 213
Central artery occlusion 4, 10
Central corneal thickness 50
    measurement of 66
Central foveal thickness 158
Central retinal
    artery occlusion 1
    thickness 90, 162, 194
    vein occlusion 10
Central vision 113
Centurion vision system, active fluidics of 138
Cerebrospinal fluid 12
Chest, computed tomography of 233
Choriocapillaris 79, 116, 120
    flow, impairment of 164
    hypoperfusion 109
    nonperfusion 110
    segmentation 95*f*
Choriocapillaritis, inflammatory 81
Chorioretinal inflammatory lesions 94
Chorioretinopathy, central serous 120, 123, 124
Choroid 111, 112

Choroidal capillaries 125
Choroidal hyperpermeability 123, 124*f*, 125*f*
Choroidal hyper-reflectivity 111
Choroidal hypofluorescence, cause of 92
Choroidal morphology 127
Choroidal neovascular membrane 86*f*, 103, 195*f*, 221
Choroidal neovascularization 27, 79, 82, 84, 86, 94-96, 112, 123, 191
Choroidal stroma, inflammatory lesions in 81
Choroidal thickness 121
Choroidal vascular polyps 125
Choroidal veins 121
Choroidal vessels, large 109
Choroideremia 212
Choroiditis 103, 107*f*, 110, 111
    active 111
    control of 115
    exacerbations of 113
Choroid-sclera junction 121
Circle scan technology 141
Clinically significant macular edema 158
Cogan's lid twitch 231
Collagen 48
    crosslinking
        accelerated protocol for 52*b*
        pathways 47, 48, 49*fc*
    fibrils 49
Confocal microscopy 54
Confocal scanning laser ophthalmoscopy 160
Conjunctival swab 4
Conjunctivitis 1
Continuous curvilinear capsulorhexis 143
Continuous thermal capsulotomy system 146
Conventional laser photocoagulation 166
Convolutional neural network 19, 20*f*, 21, 22, 63
Cord
    blood 215
    lining cells 215
Cornea 29, 54, 55, 64, 132
    exposure of 11
Corneal collagen 48, 50

Corneal crosslinking 47
　advances in 47
　indications for 48b
Corneal decompensation 136
Corneal ectasias 47, 49, 65
Corneal ectatic disorders 48
Corneal edema 177
Corneal stability, evidence of 53
Corneal stroma 53
Corneal surface 55
Corneal thickness 56
Coronavirus disease 1, 6, 10, 12
Corrected visual acuity 50
Corticosteroid 103, 113, 169, 229, 234
　administration of 115
　drug delivery of 115
　side effects 114
　therapy 107
Cotton-wool spots 4
COVID-19 1, 5t, 7t, 11, 12t
　infection 3, 4, 13
　treatment of 11, 13
Cranial mononeuropathies 152
Cranial nerve palsy 1
Cushing syndrome 123
Cyclosporine 114, 235
Cystoid macular edema 92, 93t, 129, 221

D

Deep capillary plexus 79, 86, 96
　disruption of 95f
Deep neural networks 18, 19
Deeper choroidal vessels, imaging of 97
Dengue fever 11
Dense scotomas 112
Deoxyribonucleic acid 50, 205, 210, 211
Descemet's stripping 135
Dextran T-500 54
Diabetes Control and Complications Trial 164
Diabetes mellitus 159
　gestational 159
Diabetes, eye examination in 159t
Diabetic macular edema 25, 153, 157, 157f, 162f, 163, 164f, 166, 168-170, 174, 179
　classification of 157t
　management of 166
Diabetic membranes 177
Diabetic retinopathy 16, 17, 18, 24, 61, 65, 152, 153, 155, 163, 166, 204

　classification 22f
　clinical research network 155
　disease severity scale 155t
　management of 152, 166t
　nonsight threatening 158f
　screening 159
　　artificial intelligence in 159
　　telemedicine for 159
　sight-threatening 158, 158f
　study, early treatment of 158, 190
　vitrectomy study 173, 178
　Wisconsin Epidemiologic Study of 154
Digital fundus photography 160
Digital retinal photography 159
Diplopia 229, 235
Disk, neovascularization of 156, 163, 166
Dresden protocol 47, 51
Dry eye 152
Dysarthria 234
Dyslipidemia 154

E

Edema 153
　macular 61
Edrophonium test 232
Electromyography 229
Electrophysiologic testing 233
Electroretinogram 219
Embryonal stem cells 213, 215, 222
En bloc dissection 177
Endophthalmitis 115
Endoscopic surgery 36
　traditional 41
Endothelial loss leading 129
Enzyme-linked immunosorbent assay 10, 219
Epiretinal membrane 27, 36, 40, 174
Erythrocytes 79
Ethylenediaminetetraacetic acid 53
European Society of Retina Specialists 161
Extraocular muscle 230
　palsy 152
Eye 1, 64, 133f
　care professional 64
　disease
　　diagnosis of 30
　　treatment of 30
　early detection 17
　large 132

F

Femtosecond assisted arcuate keratotomy 141f
Femtosecond laser 141
  assisted cataract surgery 140
  platforms 140
Fetal derived retinal progenitor cells 222
Fetal retina, implantation of 223
Fibrovascular nails, formation of 175
Fibrovascular proliferation 172, 174
Fluocinolone 170
  acetonide 170
Fluorescein angiography 81, 161
Focal choroidal excavation 120, 127
Food and Drug Administration 25, 188, 212, 232
Fourier-domain optical coherence tomography 141
Fovea 112
Foveal avascular zone 93, 96
Fuchs endothelial dystrophy 50
Fundus autoflourescence 103, 107, 108, 108f, 109f, 161
  imaging 123
Fundus fluorescein angiography 78, 80-84, 89, 93, 95, 96, 107, 109, 110f, 111f, 124, 126, 153, 161, 163t, 201
Fungi 105

G

Ganglion cell layer 10
Gene
  delivery of 209
  expression 205
  intraocular injection of 209t
  supplementation 208
  surgery 208
  therapy 204, 205, 210, 212
    approaches 208
    clinical trials of 212t
Ghost cell glaucoma 173
Glaucoma 16, 29, 61, 64, 66, 152
  applications in 67t
  artificial intelligence in 66
  diagnosis of 61, 66, 71
  neovascular 153, 178
  subsequent 129
  visual defects in 70
Glaucomatous optic neuropathy 68
Glial cell-derived neurotrophic factor 222
Glued intrascleral haptic fixation 129, 132, 134, 135
Glycosylation 48
Goldmann applanation tonometry 71

H

Haller's layer 123
Handshake technique 131, 133f
Haptic tuck 136
Hazy cornea 42
Hematopoietic stem cells 215
Hemorrhage
  dense premacular 173, 174
  macular 196
  massive subretinal 126f
  premacular 155, 174
  preretinal 161f
  small subretinal 198f
  subretinal 97
  vitreous 153, 155, 156, 173, 175, 178
Hepatocyte growth factor 222
Herpes simplex virus 105
Herpetic keratouveitis, development of 56
Human immunodeficiency virus 12
Human leukocyte antigen 90, 105
Human umbilical cord derived stem cells 222, 223
Hyaloid, posterior 156
Hyaloidotomy, posterior 176
Hydroxychloroquine therapy 13
Hyperautofluorescent foci 123
Hyperautofluorescent lesions 108
Hyperglycemia 154
Hyperplasia 109, 229
Hypertension 154, 165
  systemic 123
Hypoosmolar dextran-free riboflavin 54

I

Iatrogenic breaks 177
Ice pack
  application 232f
  test 231, 235
Immune reaction 213
Immunogenicity 219
Immunoglobulin, intravenous 235
Immunomodulatory agent 113-115

Immunosuppressant therapy 103, 113, 229, 234
Indocyanine green angiography 78, 81, 82, 82*t*, 84, 87, 89, 95, 107, 110, 124, 126
Induced pluripotent stem cells 213, 215, 222
Infection 13
Inflammation, chronic 90
Inflammatory choroidal neovascularization 94
Inflammatory cystoid macular edema 92
Inner plexiform layer 10, 11, 79
Inner retinal layers 116
Internal limiting membrane 79, 162, 174, 209
International Biomedical Devices 146
International Classification of Diabetic Retinopathy 155
Intraepithelial junctions 53
Intraocular bleeding 177
    stoppage of 176
Intraocular inflammation 78, 103
    idiopathic 105
Intraocular lens 129, 143, 147
Intraocular pressure 12, 66, 138, 169
    estimation, automation of 71
    measurement, artificial intelligence in 70
Intraocular ranibizumab 194
Intrastromal corneal rings, use of 48
Intravascular blood flow 112
Intravenous pulse methylprednisolone 113
Intravitreal antivascular endothelial growth factor 152, 167, 172, 187, 195*f*
Intravitreal implants 115
Intravitreal injection 166, 168, 209, 222
Intravitreal triamcinolone acetonide 134
Iridodialysis, large 135
Iris rubeosis 178
Irritable lid phenomenon 231
Irvine-Gass syndrome 94
Ischemia 113
Ischemic optic neuropathy 12, 152

K

Kawasaki disease 12
Keratectasias 48, 56
Keratitis
    corneal crosslinking 47
    infective 47, 52, 53, 56
    microbial 48, 50
Keratoconus 16, 29, 47, 65
    management of 56
    screening 30
    treatment of 30, 47
Keratocyte apoptosis 54
Keratoglobus 47
Keratometry 54, 56
Keratoplasty 135
Kidney 2
    disease, diabetic 154

L

Laser
    assisted in situ keratomileusis 48, 55
    correction surgery 47
    photocoagulation 166, 170
        complications of 171
Lawnmower technique 177
Leber's congenital amaurosis 212
Lens fragmentation 141
Lensar laser system 147
LenSx laser 141
Lenti virus 210
Levator palpebrae superioris 231
Lid fatigability 231
Liver 2
Loose cortex using 25G cannula, aspiration of 145*f*
Lucky seven sign 131
Lung 2

M

Machine learning 18, 23, 61, 62
Macula 107*f*, 199
Major adverse cardiovascular events 62
Major histocompatibility complex 224, 230
Master-slave systems 37
Medrobotics flex robotic systems 41
Meganucleases 208
Mesenchymal stem cells 216, 222, 223
Messenger ribonucleic acid 211
Microbial deoxyribonucleic acid 105
Micropulse diode laser 167
Microscopes, advances in 141
Microvitreoretinal blade 176

miLoop® 146, 147f
Missense mutations 206
Mononuclear cells 222
Multifocal choroidal lesions 108
Multifocal choroiditis 81, 83, 84t, 107, 107f
Multimodal imaging techniques 84t
Multiple diseases, detection of 71
Multiple evanescent white dot syndrome 92, 96
Multisystem autoimmune inflammatory disorder 85
Mutant protein 206
Mutations 205
    independent gene replacement 209
Myasthenia gravis 229-231
    generalized 229, 231
    ocular 229, 231, 235
Myasthenic crisis 229
Mycobacterium tuberculosis 91, 105, 115
Mydriatic fundus imaging 160
Myopia 47, 121

N

Neostigmine 234
    test 232, 235
Neovascular age-related macular degeneration 94, 191t
    management of 187
    treatment of 189t, 190
Neovascularization elsewhere 156, 163, 166
Neural retinal transplant 224t
Neural stem cells 215
Neuromuscular junction 229
Neuromuscular transmission 230
Neurons, artificial 63
Neurosurgical stereotactic biopsies 36
Neurotransmitters 229
New intelliAxis refractive capsulorhexis 147
Ngenuity three-dimensional system 142f
Nonproliferative diabetic retinopathy 155, 156f, 158, 159, 166
    mild 153, 155
    moderate 153, 155
    severe 153, 155
Nonsense mutations 206

Nonsteroidal anti-inflammatory drugs 136
Nucleic acids 50
Nucleotide 205
Nucleus management, advances in 146

O

Ocular diseases, artificial intelligence in 24
Ocular inflammation 83
Ocular surface
    disorder 152
    neoplasia, development of 56
Oncology 64
Ophthalmic surgery 36
Ophthalmology 16, 17, 23, 36, 65t
    artificial intelligence in 16, 64
    current applications in 38
Ophthalmoparesis 235
Ophthalmoplegia 229
Optic disk 66, 104f
    images 66
    new vessels 174
Optic nerve head 68, 69
Optic neuritis 12
Optical coherence tomography 10, 16, 27, 42, 61, 64, 68, 69, 78, 85, 87, 88, 107, 111, 124, 126, 149, 153, 157, 162, 163t, 194
    angiography 78-82, 84-87, 89-95, 97, 112, 163, 164f
    applications of 83
    limitations of 97
Optiwave refractive analysis
    screen of 150f
    system 149, 150f
Optogenetic therapy 210, 211t
Oral acetyl cholinesterase inhibitors 236
Oral glycopyrrolate 234
Oral prednisolone 113
Orbicularis oculi 231
Orbital operations 41
Orbital surgery 36, 41
Orbitofacial surgery 36
Outer retina 112f
Outer retinal destruction, severe 112
Oxidative pathways 48

P

Pachychoroid 120, 127
    neovasculopathy 120, 123, 125f

phenotype 121, 125
pigment epitheliopathy 120, 122
spectrum 127
Pan uveitis 12
Panretinal photocoagulation 153, 161, 166, 170
Paracentral acute middle maculopathy 4, 10
Paracentral scotomas 116
Pars plana 129
    infusion 130
    vitrectomy 169
Pegaptanib 189
Pellucid marginal degeneration 47
    diagnosis of 50
Peripapillary pachychoroid syndrome 120, 126
Peripheral ulcerative keratitis 56
Persistent epithelial defect 56
Phacoemulsification 138, 146, 147, 150
    advances in 138
Phacomachines, advances in 138
Phenocaine-assisted cataract surgery 143
Photoactivated riboflavin 50
Photodynamic therapy 188
Photoreceptor transplantation 219
Photorefractive keratectomy 48
Phthisis bulbi 178
Piezoelectric micromotor 42
Pigment disturbance, severe 116
Pigment epithelial detachment 27, 65, 126
Pivot joint 39
Placental growth factor 188
Placoid chorioretinits 116
Plasma exchange 235
Plasmapheresis 235
Platelet-derived growth factor-AA 169
Pluripotent cells, autologous-induced 215
Polyethylene terephthalate 217
Polymerase chain reaction 3, 6, 10, 12, 91
Polymethylmethacrylate 130
Polymorphisms 205
Polypoidal choroidal vasculopathy 120, 125, 126f
Porcine corneas 48
Porcine eyes 38
Posterior capsular rupture 133f

Posterior multifocal placoid pigment epitheliopathy 116
Posterior segment surgery 36, 40
Posterior vitreous detachment, role of 175
Posterior yttrium aluminum garnet 134
Postlaser-assisted in situ keratomileusis 48
Postoperative rhegmatogenous retinal detachment 178
Preceyes surgical system 39f
Prednisolone 114
Pregnancy 154
Preretinal new vessels, growth of 174
Primary open-angle glaucoma 70
Progression, estimation of 70
Proliferative diabetic retinopathy 155, 156, 156f, 161, 166, 170
management of 170
Pro-re-nata treatment 194
Proteinuria 165
Pterygium excision 38
Ptosis 229, 231, 232f, 235
Punctate inner choroidopathy 84, 85, 85f, 86
Pupil block 129
Pyridostigmine 234

R

Ranibizumab 167, 189, 197, 201
Recombinant tissue plasminogen activator 41
Refraction spherical equivalent 55
Refractive analysis system 149
Refractive error, detection of 65
Refractive surgery 48
Remedio's fundus 65
Repetitive nerve stimulation studies 233
Respiratory viruses 3
Retina 16, 56, 136
    inherited degenerative disorders of 204
    subspecialties of 64
Retinal atrophy 90
Retinal central subfield thickness 201
Retinal degenerations, hereditary 204
Retinal degenerative disorders 215
    management of 204
Retinal detachment 65, 178
Retinal diseases 214

Retinal disorders 212, 212t, 213
   gene therapy for 210
   management of 204
Retinal hemorrhages 4, 153
Retinal images, datasets of 18
Retinal ischemic mechanisms 94
Retinal nerve fiber layer 65, 68
Retinal pigment epithelium 79, 84, 103, 112f, 162, 167, 189, 204, 214, 219-221
   cells, monolayer of 217
   transplantation 216
Retinal progenitor cell 204, 214, 222
   transplantation, immunogenicity of 224
Retinal thickness 23
Retinal vascular disorders 152
Retinal vasculitis 80, 90, 113
Retinal vein occlusion 1, 94
Retinitis pigmentosa 204, 212, 214, 224
Retinopathy 165
   central serous 27
   of prematurity 16, 29, 61, 65
Retinoschisis 212
Rhegmatogenous retinal detachment 173
Rhino-orbital mucormycosis 13
Riboflavin 49, 50, 53
   concentration 53
Ribonucleic acid 1, 50, 210
Ritonavir 13
Robot-assisted orbital surgery 41
Robotic intraocular vitreoretinal surgery 39f
Robotic pterygium, steps of 39f
Robotic surgery 36, 37, 44, 45
   systems 42
Robotic system 37
   use of 41

S

Scheimpflug imaging technology 141
Schlagel lines 83
Scleral flaps 129
Sclerotomy 134, 135
   anterior 132
   ports, creation of 175
Scotomas, central 116
Self-organized retinal tissue, sheets of 223
Semi-active Robotic systems 36
Serous macular detachment 123
Serous retinal detachment 87f
Serpiginous choroiditis 81, 91, 103, 104, 104f, 106, 108f, 116, 117f
   active 110f
   lesions of 114f
Severe acute respiratory syndrome coronavirus 2 1
Sex chromosomes 205
Singapore Eye Disease Study 154
Single nucleotide polymorphism 205
Single-fiber electromyography 233
Sleep test 232
Small incision
   cataract surgery 134
   lenticule extraction 55
Snellen visual acuity 90
Sørensen-dice similarity coefficient 23
Spectral domain optical coherence tomography 68, 83, 84, 141
Stargardt's disease 212, 214
Stem cell 213, 222
   derived retinal pigment epithellium cell transplants 218
   potential source of 215
Sterile infiltrates, development of 52
Steroids 13, 52
   intravitreal 169
Strabismus
   eye 41
   surgery 41
Stroma, anterior 54
Stromal haze 53, 56
Subfoveal choroid thickness 121
Subretinal fibrosis 109
Subretinal fluid
   accumulation 126
   volume 23
Subretinal injection 209
Superficial capillary plexus 79, 86, 90, 95f
Suprachoroidal injection 209
Suture materials 44
Systemic autoimmune disease 105
Systemic corticosteroids 113
   dose of 115
Systemic lupus erythematosus 123

T

T-cell inhibitor 115
Telerobotic surgery 42, 43
   field of 43

Tetracaine 53
Three-dimensional digital visualization 141
Thymectomy 229, 235
Thymoma 229
Thyroid eye disease 41
Toric alignment, advances in 147
Toric intraocular lens 150*f*
    alignment of 148*f*
    intraoperative 149*f*
    popularity of 147
Tractional retinal detachment 153, 173, 178
Transchoroidal subretinal injection 209
Transcription activator-like effector nucleases 208
Transepithelial potential 219
Transform glaucoma management 73
Transmembrane serine protease 2
Transoral robotic surgery 41
Transplanted cells
    acting 222
    maturing 222
Triamcinolone 169
Trometamol 53
Tuberculosis 103, 115

U

Ultrasound biomicroscopy 178
United Kingdom Prospective Diabetes Study 164
Usher syndrome 212
Uveitic macular edema 96
Uveitis 78, 80-82
    idiopathic posterior 90
    posterior 78, 103

V

Vacuum rhexis using 25G cannula 145*f*
Varicella-zoster virus 105
Vascular chorioretinal disorders 204
Vascular endothelial growth factor 10, 86, 153, 188, 208
Vasculitis, inflammatory 96
Verion 147
    planning module of 148*f*

Vessels, radial network of 79
Victus 141
Viruses 105
Visual acuity 17, 23, 27, 52, 54, 106, 189, 212, 220, 221
    stability of 49
    uncorrected 55
Visual axis 129
Visual defects, progression of 70
Visual field 70
    analysis 70
Visual impairment 138
Vitamin 51
Vitesse hypersonic vitrectomy system 139
Vitrectomy 136, 152, 172
    basic steps of 175
    incomplete 136
    indications for 172
Vitreomacular traction 27
Vitreoretinal surgery 40, 172
Vitreoretinopathy, proliferative 216
Vitreoschisis 175
Vogt-Koyanagi-Harada disease 82, 85, 87, 87*f*, 96, 121

W

Weck-Cel sponge 132
Wet age-related macular degeneration, management of 187, 188*fc*
White blood cell count 6
Whitestar signature system 140
Wilkinson's classification 158
Wound healing, epithelial 56

X

X-linked retinitis pigmentosa 212

Y

Yellowish-white retinal lesion 110

Z

Zeiss Artevo 800 142, 142*f*
Zeiss cataract suite 148, 149*f*
Zinc-finger nucleases 208
Zonulopathy 129, 130